Discarded

Brooks - Cork Library
Shelton State

SSCC

Nurses as Consultants

Essential Concepts and Processes

Susan L. Norwood, EdD, ARNP
Gonzaga University
Spokane, Washington

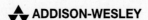

▲▲ **ADDISON-WESLEY**

An imprint of Addison Wesley Longman, Inc.

Menlo Park, California • Reading, Massachusetts • New York • Harlow, England
Don Mills, Ontario • Sydney • Mexico City • Madrid • Amsterdam

Executive editor: *Patricia L. Cleary*
Developmental editor: *Mark F. Wales*
Editorial assistant: *Marla Nowick*
Managing editor: *Wendy Earl*
Production supervisor: *Sharon Montooth*
Cover designer: *Yvo Reizebos*
Text designer and compositor: *Brad Greene*
Illustrator: *Wendy Davis*
Manufacturing supervisor: *Merry Free Osborn*

Copyright © 1998 by Addison Wesley Longman, Inc.

All rights reserved. No part of this publication may be reproduced, stored in a retrieval system, or transmitted, in any form or by any means, electronic, mechanical, photocopying, recording, or any other media or embodiments now known or hereafter to become known, without the prior written permission of the publisher. Manufactured in the United States of America. Published simultaneously in Canada.

Library of Congress Cataloging-in-Publication Data

Norwood, Susan.
    Nurses as consultants : essential concepts and processes /
Susan Norwood.
       p.   cm.
    ISBN 0-8053-5427-1
    1. Nursing Consultants--Vocational guidance. I. Title.
    [DNLM: 1. Nurses. 2. Consultants. WY 90 N895n 1998]
  RT86.4.N67 1998
  610.73'06'9--dc21
  DNLM/DLC
  for Library of Congress   97-22981
                                                CIP

ISBN 0-8053-5427-1
1 2 3 4 5 6 7 8 9 10-MA-01 00 99 98 97

Addison Wesley Longman, Inc.
2725 Sand Hill Road
Menlo Park, California 94025

Brooks - Cork Library

Shelton State

Community College

Reviewers ∼

Carolyn B. Adams, RN, EdD, CNAA
Intercollegiate Center for Nursing
Washington State University
Spokane, Washington

Theresa Capriotti, RN, MSN, DO
Villanova University College of Nursing
Villanova, Pennsylvania

Richard W. Redman, RN, PhD
University of Michigan School of Nursing
Ann Arbor, Michigan

Denise Robinson, RN, PhD, FNP
Northern Kentucky University
Highland Heights, Kentucky

Carolyn W. Schultz, RN, EdD
Pacific Lutheran University
Tacoma, Washington

~ Preface

C onsultation—working with others to help them resolve problems—is not a new role for nurses. However, in today's increasingly complex and rapidly changing health care environment, there is a growing need and increasing opportunities for nurses to provide formal consultation services. Proficiency in consultation is, in fact, generally acknowledged to be a core competency for nurses assuming advanced nursing roles as clinicians, educators, and managers/administrators.

Despite the expectation that nurses in advanced roles provide consultation, little attention has been given to addressing the essential concepts and skills needed to be an effective nurse consultant. Instead, nurses providing consultation have tended to equate clinical expertise with the ability to provide consultation and to acquire specific consultation skills through trial and error. If we have sought a theoretical basis for our consultation practice, we have had to rely on resources developed for professionals in other disciplines. *Nursing* consultation, however, deals with problems that occur in an environment that is different from that which characterizes consultation as it is practiced by other professionals. Borrowing consultation theory and strategies from other disciplines risks overlooking the nuances of *nursing* consultation, and relying on trial and error for skill development is time-consuming and can be dangerous. As nurses, we need our own consultation theory and strategies—and this text has been developed to meet that need.

About the Book

Nurses as Consultants presents nursing consultation as a five phase process (gaining entry, problem identification, action planning, evaluation, and disengagement) of working with individuals or groups to help them resolve actual or potential problems related to the health status of clients or to health care delivery. The coverage is specifically developed for nurses who are pursuing graduate degrees and preparing themselves to assume advanced nursing roles as clinicians (clinical nurse specialists or nurse practitioners), educators, or managers/administrators. This book is also appropriate for senior-level leadership courses in baccalaureate nursing programs, especially RN completion programs. Finally, this book will benefit any nurse who is already practicing consultation, but doing so without the benefit of any formal preparation or theoretical grounding.

The Teaching Approach

Nurses as Consultants is organized in five sections. Section 1 describes the nature of nursing consultation relationships, presents an overview of the five-phase nursing consultation process, differentiates interaction patterns in nursing consultation, and discusses consultative roles and skills. The second section discusses contextual issues that shape nursing consultation relationships: characteristics of organizations, group dynamics, and the dynamics of change. Section 3 provides an in-depth discussion of each phase of the nursing consultation process and emphasizes strategies for successfully completing each phase. In Section 4, business, legal, and ethical issues in

Brooks - Cork Library
Shelton State
Community College
SSCC

Discarded

nursing consultation are considered. The final section of the book explores contemporary intrapreneurial and entrepreneurial opportunities for nurse consultants and offers strategies for envisioning one's own future as a nurse consultant.

The book incorporates three teaching approaches:

- Theory-based approach: The *nursing consultation process model* that is used as the book's framework draws on the best and most relevant practices of consultation theory developed in the human service and organization development literature.

- Applied approach: Every chapter emphasizes how to translate theoretical concepts into actual consultation practices.

- Case examples are used liberally throughout to illustrate how nurses actually practice consultation to address a variety of problems in diverse practice settings.

Special features incorporated throughout the text enhance its professional relevance and readability:

- a chapter overview and list of guiding questions

- boxed features of assessment questions, consultation strategies, and consultation scenarios

- documentation guidelines

- examples of consultation contracts

- end-of-chapter learning activities (which provide a suitable foundation for course assignments)

- an annotated listing of additional readings

Nurses as Consultants: Essential Concepts and Processes provides nurses with both the theoretical background and the practical strategies that nurses need to successfully respond to the exciting and challenging demands for nursing consultation in today's health care environment.

∿ Acknowledgments

Writing one's first book is quite a journey! It is at once exhilarating, challenging, and humbling. Sometimes it is also frustrating, painful, and tiring. Certainly, it is not a journey that can be successfully completed alone, and I would be remiss not to recognize those who have contributed to the journey in various ways.

First, I would like to acknowledge the unwavering support of my parents, William and Irene Norwood. They have instilled in me a value for lifelong learning, the desire to strive for excellence, and the responsibility to serve others. For this, as well as for just being there, I thank them. To the rest of my family, who helped me celebrate the project's major milestones, and to David, who entered the journey at its midpoint and brought perspective and some fun to its second half: I thank you, too.

I also want to gratefully acknowledge the support I received from my colleagues in the Department of Nursing at Gonzaga University. First, Dale Abendroth gave me the opportunity to team-teach a course on nursing consultation with her. This opportunity piqued my interest and commitment to this nursing role and uncovered the need for this text. Dale was also generous with ideas, resources, and enthusiasm throughout this project. My chairperson, Dr. Gail Ray, facilitated the completion of this book by protecting my workload. My other colleagues were also steadfast in their interest and support. My dean and mentor, Dr. Richard Wolfe, has continually provided sage advice and expressed confidence in my abilities. It is also important to acknowledge the influence of Father Patrick Ford, my initial advisor in the Doctoral Studies Program at Gonzaga University, who instilled in me a quest for excellence in writing and a belief in the power of the well-written word. Finally, a thank you to the students at Gonzaga University who have helped me clarify the ideas presented in this book and whose experiences have provided the basis for many of the book's scenarios.

I was first put into contact with Addison-Wesley Nursing by Dr. Patricia Ladewig, and I cannot imagine having a better team to work with. Patti Cleary, Executive Editor, recognized the need for this book; her commitment to the project never wavered. Mark Wales, Senior Developmental Editor, literally transformed a fledging writer into a confident and competent one. He taught me how to write to teach rather than to report—his guidance and support were invaluable. Marla Nowick, Editorial Assistant, graciously fielded my questions throughout the project. Sharon Montooth, Production Editor, and Siobhan Scarry, Copy Editor, with their eyes for detail, gave the manuscript its final polishing. Finally, reviewers are the anonymous voice in any book project. They too have my gratitude: their perceptive comments and generous suggestions were essential to making this book meaningful, relevant, and user-friendly. To all of you, thank you.

Susan Norwood

Contents ∿

1

The Nature of Nursing Consultation

Few nurses regarded themselves, or were regarded by others,
as experts in the field with credentials worthy of consultation
until after the 1950s. (Robinson 1982)

Key terms: consultation, consultee, client, client system

Introduction

The word "consultant" often brings to mind the picture of an expensive outside expert who has been brought in to fix an organization-wide problem. Many nurses have been on the "receiving end" of consultation, often in connection with work redesign and downsizing experiences at their place of employment. However, whether they recognize it or not, most nurses have also been on the "doing end" of consultation.

Consultation is fundamentally a process of working with individuals or groups to help them solve work-related problems. Nurse consultants address work-related problems that more specifically relate to the health status of individuals or groups and to health care delivery processes. Nursing consultation then, means *working with individuals or groups to help them resolve actual or potential problems related to the health status of clients or to health care delivery.*

Consultation skills have been recognized as a core competency for advanced practice nurses (that is, clinical nurse specialists, nurse practitioners, nurse-anesthetists, and certified nurse-midwives) as well as for nurses assuming advanced nursing roles as educators and administrators (American Nurses' Association [ANA] 1995; Fenton & Brykcynski 1989). When nurses practice consultation, their ultimate goal is to enhance patient well-being. Yet in most cases, nurses learn consultation skills through trial and error, a method that is both inefficient and potentially harmful to a client's well-being. Consultation can be harmful to a client, for example, if an assessment is incomplete or a recommended intervention doesn't address the real problem issue or if a consultant fosters dependency rather than self-reliance. Rather than continue to rely on trial and error, nurses who expect to practice consultation need to base their actions on theory. A theory-based approach to consultation helps promote successful outcomes in the widest variety of problem situations.

This book presents the theoretical concepts and pragmatic processes that are the foundation of effective nursing consultation. By implementing these concepts and processes, nurses can enhance their consultation skills and, ultimately, improve the well-being of patients.

This first chapter begins with a description of consultation and consultation relationships. It goes on to describe nursing consultation and compare it with consultation as practiced by professionals in other disciplines. Nursing consultation is then compared with the nursing process and other nursing activities. In the final section of this chapter, variables in nursing consultation are discussed.

As you read this chapter, consider the following questions:

- What types of experiences have you had with consultants? Were they positive or negative experiences? What do you think explains this?

- How have you practiced nursing consultation? What was that experience like?

- How do you envision yourself incorporating consultation into your advanced nursing role?

- What skills and assets do you have that should facilitate your practice of nursing consultation? What gaps in knowledge and skill can you identify?

Basic Consultation Concepts

One way to begin to understand the nature of nursing consultation is to examine how consultation is described by other professions in which the act of consulting has evolved into a highly developed practice and a more recognizable role.

Defining Consultation

The word "consultation" is often used ambiguously. The common element of virtually all definitions of consultation, however, is problem solving. The two definitions that follow, while drawn from disciplines or perspectives other than nursing, illustrate both the problem-solving focus of consultation and the characteristics of consultation relationships.

One team of organization development consultants (specialists concerned with helping organizations function more effectively) defines consultation as a two-way process of problem solving: "a process of seeking, giving, and receiving help. Consultation is aimed at aiding a person, group, organization, or larger system in mobilizing internal and external resources to deal with problem confrontations and change efforts" (Lippitt & Lippitt 1986).

Human resources professionals, who work in administrative or direct service roles within such settings as school systems and community social service agencies, put forth their own definition of consultation. According to one human services theorist, consultation occurs when a professional "assists a consultee with a work-related (or caretaking related) problem with a client system, with the goal of helping both the consultee and the client system in some specified way" (Dougherty 1995).

Both of these definitions reveal that consultation is a process that is intended to solve a problem and, by doing so, bring about change. The two definitions also reveal that the focus of consultation is helping individuals or groups learn to solve their own problem(s), rather than solving problems for them. Finally, these definitions indicate that consultation involves a consultant who is the professional guiding the process, the consultee or individual who is receiving the help, and other parties who hold a stake in both the consultation process and its outcomes. These ideas are explored further in the following sections.

The Characteristics of Consultation Relationships

The characteristics of consultation relationships can be grouped into three categories: the parties involved in the consultation process, the "phenomena of interest" in consultation, and the roles and responsibilities of consultants.

The Parties Involved in Consultation Consultation typically involves three parties: a consultant, a consultee, and a client. The consultant is the helper. More precisely, the consultant provides the leadership for the problem-solving efforts. The consultee is the person or group that is working directly with the consultant to learn problem-solving skills. In some cases, the consultee is the person who has asked for help on behalf of a client. In other cases, a "contact person" who is not directly involved in the problem-solving activities may have requested the consultation. For example, a hospital administrator might ask a consultant to work with selected nurse-managers (the consultees). The client is the individual, group, or organization that is the intended beneficiary or target of the consultation. In other words, the client is the party on whose behalf help has been sought. It is important to understand that clients are not usually active participants in the consultation process. Thus consultation is a tripartite (three-part) relationship that involves cooperative efforts between a consultant and consultee in order to enhance a client's well-being.

Consultation takes place within an environment called the "client system." The client system includes anyone who, in addition to the consultant, consultee, and client, may have some stake in the consultation process and its outcomes. It is important to note that these *consultation stakeholders* are neither involved in the consultation process nor a target of its results. The relationships among the parties in a consultation relationship are illustrated in Figure 1-1.

The Phenomena of Interest in Consultation A profession's "phenomena of interest" is the range of problems that gives it purpose and defines its scope of practice. Consultation has as its phenomena of interest work-related problems. Consultants help consultees resolve work-related (as opposed to personal) problems that affect client well-being and thus deal with the *issues* that are causing a problem rather than consultees' personal or emotional reactions to the problem situation.

The Roles and Responsibilities of Consultants Consultants work with consultees to help them incorporate behavioral, cognitive, attitudinal, or organizational changes that will result in problem resolution. While helping consultees make these changes, consultants attempt to empower consultees and increase their self-sufficiency. A professional goal and responsibility of a consultant then, is to become progressively

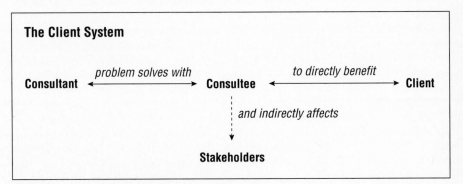

Figure 1-1. The Consultation Relationship
During the consultation process, the consultant and consultee collaborate to solve problems that are affecting a client's well-being. The client is the intended beneficiary of the interactions between the consultant and consultee. Stakeholders are other individuals who are indirectly affected by the consultation process and its outcomes. Together, these parties comprise the client system.

unnecessary (Lippitt & Lippitt 1986). Consultants accomplish this goal through a "skills transference" process that helps consultees learn to make better use of their own personal and professional resources. Hence, consultants have remedial as well as preventive responsibilities towards their consultees: They want to help consultees resolve their present problem as well as learn to respond more effectively to similar problems in the future (Zins 1993).

Consultants not only offer education and clarify situations, but they diagnose a presenting problem's likely cause and suggest problem-solving strategies (Barron 1989). Consultees, however, are always free to accept or reject a consultant's opinions and advice. In a sense then, a consultant is only an "option-giver." In other words, consultants "do not, indeed cannot tell managers [or other consultees] what to do, nor do they actually effect change, unless of course they are specifically employed to supervise a process of transition" (Windle & Boyd 1989).

Consultants are responsible for projecting the likely effects and side effects of their recommendations. For example, a consultant who recommends downsizing as a solution to an organization's financial problems has the responsibility to not only predict the effects of downsizing on the organization's budget. The consultant must also predict the effects on worker productivity and morale, quality of service, and the organization's public image. Consultants bear only limited responsibility for change in a client's status or problem resolution because change is contingent upon a consultee's implementation of a consultant's recommendations. However, they do bear responsibility for the quality of the options they present to a consultee and for informing the consultee about the limitations of any proposed problem solution.

Nursing Consultation

Consultation is not a new role for nurses. Florence Nightingale, for example, acted as a consultant during the Crimean War when she worked with British Army officials developing strategies to stem the post-battlefield mortality rate. Following the war, she consulted with nurses throughout the world on issues regarding nursing education, hospital organization, and patient care. After Miss Nightingale, consultation among nurses was so informal that it failed to receive notable publication. It was not until the 1950s, when more nurses were visible in academic settings and earning graduate degrees, that accounts of nursing consultation began to appear in the professional literature (Robinson 1982). These initial accounts described nursing consultation as a service provided primarily by nurse educators and nurse administrators. By the late 1960s, however, accounts of clinical consultation were becoming more common. The majority of the accounts at this time focused on the then-evolving clinical specialty role of psychiatric consultation-liaison nurse (to be discussed in Chapter 17).

Today consultation is formally recognized as a component of nursing practice. Patricia Benner (1984) implies that skill in consultation is a competency of expert nurses within the practice domain she calls "Organizational and Work-Role Competencies." Fenton (1985) identifies consultation as a specific practice domain for clinical nurse specialists by citing examples of how clinical nurse specialists provide "expertise and guidance, both formally and informally, to other health care providers." In addition, Brykcynski (1989) relates how nurse practitioners provide "consultation to physicians and other staff on patient management." Thus at every level of professional nursing practice, consultation skills are now a role expectation and core competency. These skills are especially important for nurses who wish to assume leadership roles in resolving current nursing and health care problems.

Nursing consultation, like other forms of professional consultation, involves a tripartite relationship (consultant + consultee + client). Nurse consultants work with consultees to help them resolve problems that affect a client's well-being. Nursing consultation is unique, however, in that patients are always the ultimate beneficiaries (or victims) of the consultation process. For example, even if the client in a nursing consultation relationship is an organization (as in a work redesign effort), it is the patients who ultimately benefit (or suffer) from the consultation process and its outcomes. In a nursing consultation relationship, patients may be either the intended beneficiary—that is, the client—or, as illustrated in the previous example, an unintended beneficiary or stakeholder.

Consultees with whom nurse consultants work include staff nurses, families, nursing faculty, and other health care providers. A nurse consultant's clients include patients, family members, work units, organizations, students, and communities. Stakeholders in the nursing consultation process may include, in addition to patients, other health care providers. For example, work redesign efforts, as mentioned above, affect patients, but may also affect physicians and personnel in other hospital departments. Client systems within which nursing consultation occurs include nursing units, hospitals, community-based health care agencies, private medical practices, academic institutions, and communities. The relationships between the parties involved in nursing consultation are illustrated in Figure 1-2. Examples of client systems, problem situations, consultees, and clients encountered in nursing consultation are described in Box 1-1.

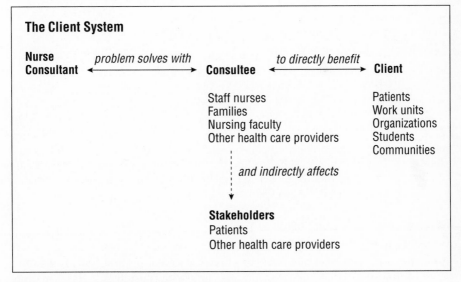

Figure 1-2. The Nursing Consultation Relationship
Like consultation that is practiced by other professionals, nursing consultation involves a tripartite relationship that occurs within the context of a client system. Nursing consultation, however, is unique in that patients are always affected—either intentionally and directly or unintentionally and indirectly—by the nursing consultation process and its outcomes. The client systems in which nursing consultation may occur include hospital units, organizations, academic institutions, private health care practices, community-based health care agencies, and communities.

Box 1-1. Nursing Consultation: Client Systems, Problem Situations, Consultees, and Clients

Following are examples of the types of problem situations in which a nurse consultant might be involved. Who would be possible stakeholders in each of these examples?

Client System	Problem Situation	Consultee	Client
Nursing unit	Complex patient with unfamiliar treatment plan	Staff nurses	Patient
Hospital	Poor results on patient satisfaction survey	Nurse managers	Hospital Patient(?)
Nursing unit	Family needs help preparing for home care needs of ill family member	Family members	Patient
Academic institution	Need to revise curriculum	Faculty	Students
Community	Meningitis outbreak	Health care providers	Community members
Private medical practice	Declining patient volume	Office staff	Medical practice

Nursing consultation has as its phenomena of interest problems related to the health status of clients or to health care delivery processes. The ultimate goal of nursing consultation is more effective patient care and, consequently, increased patient well-being. Thus nursing consultation and its phenomena of interest are an extension of nursing's concern: "the diagnosis and treatment of human responses to actual or potential health problems" (ANA 1980).

Nursing Consultation Compared to Consultation in Other Professions

A nurse consultant's roles and responsibilities are similar to those of consultants in other professions in that nurse consultants work with consultees to develop problem-solving options (Alvarez 1992). In addition, like consultants in other professions, nurse consultants seek to improve their consultees' problem-solving skills so that they are better able to respond to similar problems in the future. Advanced practice nurses who are functioning as consultants assume even more specialized roles. Consultants who are clinical nurse specialists, for example, may act as expert advisors, role models, and advocates. Working in these consultant roles, clinical nurse specialists (1) provide expert guidance and advice about patient problems both formally and informally, (2) interpret the nursing role for nursing staff in specific patient situations by identifying patient needs not apparent to less expert nurses, and (3) serve as patient advocates by broadening the staff's understanding of the experience of the patient and family, and helping staff to change their responses to the patient (Fenton 1985). Nurse practitioners function as consultants when they provide advice to physicians and other health care providers on patient management (Brykcynski 1989).

As is the case with other forms of professional consultation, the consultee in a nursing consultation relationship is free to accept or reject the nurse consultant's recommendations and opinions. The consultee then, bears the ultimate responsibility for whether or not a problem is resolved and patient well-being is enhanced. Even in situations where the client is a patient and the consultee a staff nurse, the direct responsibility for enhancing the patient's well-being rests with the consultee. The only exception to this is when a consultee's lack of skill presents a serious threat to patient well-being. In this situation, the nurse consultant has the ethical responsibility to assume direct caregiving activities on a temporary basis until the consultee or another staff nurse is able to do so.

Like other professional consultants, a nurse consultant is responsible for the effects of an intervention on a client (Barron 1989). The nurse consultant has the additional responsibility, however, of considering the effects of a recommended intervention on patients even when they are not the client. For example, work redesign may resolve a hospital's (the client's) financial problems, but its effects on patient care must also be projected and articulated by the nurse consultant.

Nursing Consultation Compared to the Nursing Process

Nursing consultation and the nursing process share a similar phenomena of interest and both work towards similar goals. Nursing consultation differs significantly from the nursing process, however, because it involves indirect rather than direct intervention. Indirect interventions such as nursing consultation are "performed away from the patient but on behalf of a patient or group of patients" and are "aimed at management of the care environment and interdisciplinary collaboration" (ANA 1995). In the nursing process, nurses usually interact directly with patients to enhance their well-being rather than on their behalf through an intermediary (such as a consultee). As illustrated in Figure 1-3, the nursing process is a dyadic helping relationship that contrasts with the tripartite relationship of nursing consultation.

Nurses involved in the nursing process often assume similar roles to those engaged in the nursing consultation process. In the nursing process, however, nurses enact these roles (teacher, coach, advisor, and so forth) directly with patients rather than through an intermediary (a consultee). In this process, the patient is both the intended and ultimate beneficiary of nursing interventions as well as a participant in them. Recall that in nursing consultation, the patient is, again, the ultimate beneficiary of the consultation process though not necessarily the intended beneficiary, nor is the patient a participant in consultation interventions.

As a final point of comparison, in the nursing process it is the nurse who is directly responsible for patient outcomes. In nursing consultation, however, the consultee bears this responsibility. The nurse consultant only maintains responsibility for the quality of options that are proposed for responding to a problem. Chapter 2 and Chapters 8–12 discuss further the differences between the nursing process and the nursing consultation process.

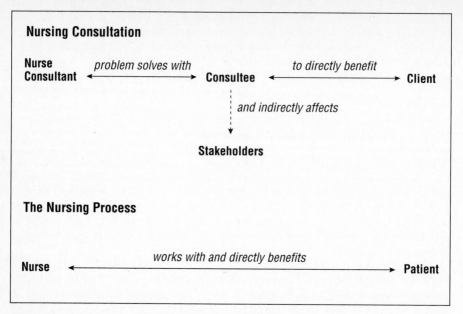

Figure 1-3. Comparison of Nursing Consultation and the Nursing Process
Despite their differences, both nursing consultation and the nursing process work towards the same goal: promoting a patient's well-being.

Nursing Consultation Compared to Other Nursing Activities

Nurses undertake a variety of activities (such as medication administration, teaching, and counseling) that are intended to promote patient well-being. Some of the activities—such as teaching—may be used as an intervention in nursing consultation. Other nursing interventions or activities (for instance, counseling) may be confused with consultation, however, and actually contradict characteristics of a consulting relationship. The following section sets forth the differences between the roles of nurses and nurse consultants in the same or similar activities.

Consultation Compared to Counseling Nursing consultation is often confused with counseling because both activities involve giving advice. Counseling is a direct service to an individual or group that is provided for the purpose of stimulating self-awareness, helping to solve problems and make decisions, and promoting emotional and personal growth (Collins 1989). The phenomena of concern in counseling are personal issues. In contrast, consultation is an indirect service to clients that focuses on work-related issues. Although a consultee may derive personal benefits from a nurse consultant's assistance, the goal of consultation is enhanced client well-being. Consider the following difference between counseling and consulting: a nurse counselor might work with nurses who are struggling with their feelings about working with AIDS patients; a nurse consultant might work with these same nurses to help them develop protocols for the care of these patients.

Consultation Compared to Teaching When teaching is used in the nursing process, it is a direct patient care intervention—for instance, a nurse teaching a newly diagnosed diabetic how to administer insulin injections. Nurse consultants frequently use teaching as an intervention when working with consultees as well, though in the nursing consultation process, teaching is an indirect patient care intervention. For example, a nurse consultant might develop teaching sessions to help staff (the consultees) in a long-term care facility learn how to keep patients with dementia (the clients) safe in a restraint-free environment.

The teaching role in nursing also differs from teaching during consultation, specifically in terms of the nature of the relationship between those involved. Formal teaching is an unequal relationship to the extent that it incorporates evaluation and the giving or withholding of rewards (for example, hospital discharge for the diabetic patient). Because a nurse consultant works with consultees as peers, the evaluation that occurs during the nursing consultation process is intended to promote professional growth and problem solving rather than form the basis for reward or punishment.

Consultation Compared to Managing and Supervising Nurse consultants incorporate supervisory and managerial activities into the consultation process when they direct problem-solving activities. For example, a nurse consultant might manage the logistics of a needed skills-training session. The practice of these activities in nursing consultation is different, however, from enacting a formal supervisory relationship. Whereas nurse supervisors are administratively responsible for their supervisees, nurse consultants and their consultees interact as peers. Lastly, supervisory relationships tend to be ongoing whereas consultation relationships are only temporary and are terminated once the consultee has learned problem-solving skills.

Consultation Compared to Collaboration Collaboration is a partnership established for the purpose of accomplishing a commonly held goal (Kyle 1995). Although nursing consultation involves a collaborative relationship between a nurse consultant and consultee, it differs from collaboration per se because the goal of a consultation relationship is specified by the consultee. Collaboration also differs from nursing consultation because it presumes joint involvement in the "action phase" of the relationship as well as joint responsibility for the outcome of the relationship. In consultation, however, both the "action" (implementation of recommended problem-solving activities) and the outcome of the relationship are the responsibility of the consultee.

Consultation Compared to Case Management Case management involves coordinating health care activities to meet an individual patient's health care needs. Nurse case managers seek to meet a patient's health care needs while balancing costs against likely outcomes (Seuntjens 1995). Nurse case managers usually interact directly with patients and have both the authority and accountability for coordinating care. This puts the responsibility for outcomes directly on the case manager. This situation is in sharp contrast to nursing consultation where the consultant does not interact directly with patients and where the consultee bears responsibility for the outcomes of the relationship.

Consultation Compared to Change Agency Change agents engage in deliberate processes to precipitate and accomplish change (Hansen 1995). Because a successful consultation accomplishes changes in behaviors, attitudes, or beliefs, consultants are often considered to be change agents. Change agency differs from nursing consultation, however, because it involves unilateral identification by the change agent of both the opportunity for change and the desired change outcomes. The need for change in nursing consultation is identified by the consultee. The nurse consultant's task is to provide options about how the desired change can be brought about. It is the consultee who establishes the goals and implements the change strategies.

Box 1-2 summarizes the differences between nursing consultation and other nursing activities.

Box 1-2. Nursing Consultation Compared to Other Nursing Activities

Nursing consultation is often confused with the following activities in which nurses engage. As you study these different helping activities, consider the following questions:

• How does the activity contradict nursing consultation?
• Who is responsible for the outcomes of the activity?
• Is the relationship to the client direct or indirect?

Activity	Focus	Goals
Nursing consultation	Work-related problems	Enhance client and patient well-being
Counseling	Interpersonal problems	Promote emotional and personal growth
Teaching	Knowledge and skill deficits	Impart new knowledge and skills
Managing	Resources (personnel, time, money)	Effective use of resources
Collaboration	Partnership	Accomplishment of mutual goals through joint action
Case Management	Cost containment, health care needs	Meet health care needs while conserving costs
Change Agency	Change	Precipitate and accomplish change

Variables in Nursing Consultation

While nursing consultation always involves a tripartite relationship within the context of a client system, the nature of a nurse consultant's relationship to the client or client system may vary. Important variables in a nurse consultant's relationship to a client or client system are insider versus outsider status and intra- and interprofessional interactions, that is, whether the interaction is with nurse consultees or with consultees who have other professional backgrounds.

Insider/Outsider Status

An internal consultant ("insider") is a member of a client system who is asked to assume a temporary and additional role as a problem solver within the system. An external consultant, on the other hand, is an outsider who establishes a temporary relationship with some members of a client system (the consultees, for example) for the express purpose of helping them to resolve a problem. Clinical nurse specialists practice internal consultation when they work with nursing staff to address problems related to the care of specific patients. These same clinical nurse specialists would be practicing external consultation if they worked with nurses in a home health care agency to address patient care problems.

Both internal and external nursing consultation relationships have advantages and disadvantages. An internal nurse consultant has the advantage of being pre-acquainted with the client system and the issues underlying the consultation problem; this often facilitates the development of rapport with the consultees. Furthermore, because an internal nurse consultant has a vested interest in successful consultation outcomes, there may be less resistance to developing an effective problem-solving relationship.

The disadvantages of practicing internal nursing consultation relate to the consultees' preconceptions, the consultant's inability to exit the client system, and the issue of fees. First, a nurse working as an internal consultant may be perceived as having less ability, credibility, and authority than an external consultant. Nursing staff tend to relate to internal nurse consultants in their "known role" (as their supervisor for instance) and often have difficulty accepting them in a role that involves a different set of tasks and responsibilities. Additionally, because internal consultants cannot completely exit the client system once the consultation relationship has ended, consultees may tend to rely too much on the nurse consultant's expertise and problem solving. This may lead to resentment and burnout on the part of the nurse consultant as well as dependency on the part of the consultee. The issue of fees can also create dilemmas for nurses practicing internal consultation. Internal nurse consultants are rarely paid a fee that is commensurate with what would typically be negotiated by an external consultant. Furthermore, nurses who are asked to take on internal consulting projects are too often expected to do so in addition to meeting their other responsibilities. The issue of fees in internal nursing consultation is discussed further in Chapter 13.

Nurses practicing external consultation enjoy certain advantages made possible by their unique role. Because they are outsiders to the client system, external consultants are more readily perceived as having expertise and credibility by consultees. External consultants tend to be less constrained by a client system's politics and internal rules so they "can ask the unaskable and suggest the unsuggestable" (Furlow 1995). Because external consultants can leave the client system at the conclusion of the consultation relationship, they generally have an easier time than do internal consultants recommending unpopular problem solutions, such as eliminating staff positions.

External consultants, however, also face distinct disadvantages. A nurse who is an external consultant will need to spend time learning how to effectively interact within a client system. Being less acquainted with the client system, external consultants run the risk of unknowingly violating a system's rules and cultural norms; this can slow down or temporarily derail consultation efforts. To gain a sense of the impact of these disadvantages, recall some of the "adjustment challenges" you may have experienced the last time you entered a new setting, during a job change perhaps, or when starting school.

Intra- and Interprofessional Interactions

Nurses practice intraprofessional consultation when their consultees are other nurses. In interprofessional consultation relationships, nurse consultants work with consultees who are from other professions. Interprofessional consultation offers the opportunity to generate a wider range of possible problem solutions because professionals from other disciplines bring different perspectives to a consultation situation. The challenge of interprofessional consultation is learning the philosophy, language, standards, and methodology of another profession.

Chapter Summary

Nursing consultation is fundamentally a problem-solving process. Consultation is not a new role for nurses but rather something that nurses have always done. Consultation is now an integral part of advanced practice nursing and advanced nursing roles. Moreover, it has been recognized as a domain of nursing practice with specific competencies. Nursing consultation shares features of consultation as practiced by other professions, and it incorporates selected activities of the nursing process and other nursing roles. Nevertheless, the collective attributes of nursing consultation distinguish it as a unique activity. Nurses who practice any form of consultation will become more effective nurse consultants by studying the concepts and processes that provide the basis for successful consultation.

Applying Chapter Content

- Explore the nursing (periodical) literature for 1975 and the present.
  What examples can you find of nursing consultation? How are the examples for these two points in time different? What do you think accounts for these differences?

- Examine how nursing consultation is practiced in your own work setting.
  What situations can you identify in your work setting that could benefit from nursing consultation?

References

Alvarez, C. (1992). Let's talk about clinical consultation. *Clinical Nurse Specialist, 6* (2), 117.

American Nurses' Association. (1980). *Nursing: A social policy statement.* Kansas City, MO: Author.

American Nurses' Association. (1995). *Nursing's social policy statement.* Kansas City, MO: Author.

Barron, A. (1989). The CNS as consultant. In A. Hamric & J. Spross (Eds.), *The clinical nurse specialist in theory and practice* (2nd ed., pp. 125-146). Philadelphia: Saunders.

Benner, P. (1984). *From novice to expert: Excellence and power in clinical nursing practice.* Menlo Park, CA: Addison-Wesley.

Brykcynski, K. (1989). An interpretive study describing the clinical judgment of nurse practitioners. *Scholarly Inquiry for Nursing Practice, 3* (2), 75-103.

Collins, B. (1989). Do you need an external consultant? A model for decision-making. *Clinical Nurse Specialist, 3* (2), 90-96.

Dougherty, A. (1995). *Consultation: Practice and perspectives in school and community settings* (2nd ed.). Pacific Grove, CA: Brooks-Cole.

Fenton, M. (1985). Identifying competencies of clinical nurse specialists. *Journal of Nursing Administration, 15* (12), 31-37.

Fenton, M. & Brykcynski, K. (1989). Qualitative distinctions and similarities in the practice of clinical nurse specialists and nurse practitioners. *Journal of Professional Nursing, 9* (6), 313-326.

Furlow, L. (1995). So what good are consultants anyway? *Journal of Nursing Administration, 25* (7/8), 13 and 15.

Hansen, H. (1995). The advanced practice nurse as a change agent. In M. Snyder & M. Mirr (Eds.), *Advanced practice nursing: A guide to professional development* (pp. 197-213). New York: Springer Publishing.

Kyle, M. (1995). Collaboration. In M. Snyder & M. Mirr (Eds.), *Advanced practice nursing: A guide to professional development* (pp. 169-182). New York: Springer Publishing.

Lippitt, G. & Lippitt, R. (1986). *The consulting process in action* (2nd ed.). San Diego: University Associates.

Robinson, L. (1982). Psychiatric liaison nursing: A review of the literature, 1962-1982. *General Hospital Psychiatry, 4* (2), 139-146.

Seuntjens, A. (1995). Case management/care management. In M. Snyder & M. Mirr (Eds.), *Advanced practice nursing: A guide to professional development* (pp. 135-152). New York: Springer Publishing.

Windle, G. & Boyd, R. (1989). Working with management consultants: Collaboration to a common end. *Senior Nurse, 9* (10), 6-8.

Zins, J. (1993). Enhancing consultee problem-solving skills in consultative interactions. *Journal of Counseling and Development, 72,* 185-190.

Additional Readings

Barron, A. (1989). The CNS as consultant. In A. Hamric & J. Spross (Eds.), *The clinical nurse specialist in theory and practice* (2nd ed., pp. 125-146). Philadelphia: Saunders. *The author provides an overview of how the consultant role can be practiced by clinical nurse specialists. Emphasis is on role implementation in a hospital setting.*

Dougherty, A. (1995). *Consultation: Practice and perspectives in school and community settings* (2nd ed.). Pacific Grove, CA: Brooks-Cole. *This comprehensive text provides an overview of the consultation process as well as its theoretical underpinnings.*

Gleason, J. & Flynn, K. (1987). The surgical clinical nurse specialist as a consultant in a tertiary care setting. *Clinical Nurse Specialist, 1* (3), 129-132. *This article illustrates how clinical nurse specialists intervene as internal consultants in one hospital setting.*

Hazelton, J., Boyum, C., & Frost, M. (1993). Clinical nurse specialist subroles: Foundations for entrepreneurship. *Clinical Nurse Specialist, 7* (1), 40-45. *This article describes how the CNS subroles of clinician, manager, educator, and researcher contribute to a CNS' ability to provide consultation and work in entrepreneurial roles.*

Jackson, R. (1994). From educator to internal consultant: Making the shift. *Nursing Staff Development Insider, 5* (1), 3-4. *The article discusses issues that arise when assuming the role of internal consultant.*

Kurpius, D. & Fuqua, D. (1993). Fundamental issues in defining consultation. *Journal of Counseling and Development, 71,* 598-600. *The authors provide and excellent summary of the nature of consultation relationships.*

Lippitt, G. & Lippitt, R. (1986). *The consulting process in action* (2nd ed.). San Diego: University Associates. *This text is an in-depth discussion on the practice of process consultation in organizational settings.*

Monicken, D. (1995). Consultation in advanced practice nursing. In M. Snyder & M. Mirr (Eds.), *Advanced practice nursing: A guide to professional development* (pp. 135-152). New York: Springer Publishing. *This chapter presents an overview of the consulting role of advanced practice nurses.*

Ulschak, F. & SnowAntle, S. (1990). *Consultation skills for health care professionals.* San Francisco: Jossey-Bass. *This text details the theory and process of internal consultation in health care settings.*

2

The Nursing Consultation Process

The consultation process is the "science" of consultation....
As with a person learning a new skill, the initial task
is to learn the basics. The next transition is to move from
the "science" or technique of the consultation process to
the "art" of the process. (Ulschak & SnowAntle 1990)

Key terms: entry, assessment, formative evaluation,
summative evaluation, ownership

Introduction

When nurses rely on the steps of the nursing process to guide their interactions with patients, they increase the likelihood that nurse-patient interactions will both meet a patient's needs and enhance a patient's well-being. In the same way, nurse consultants who follow the five steps or phases of the nursing consultation process increase the likelihood of a successful consultation outcome.

In Chapter 1, nursing consultation was described as a collaborative interaction between a nurse consultant and consultee that occurs on behalf of a client and takes place within an environment called the client system. The nursing consultation process more specifically, is a systematic and scientific approach to problem solving that a nurse consultant carries out with a consultee or group of consultees for the purpose of enhancing client well-being. The process involves five sequential and ongoing phases that provide a framework for nursing consultation relationships.

This chapter introduces the phases of the nursing consultation process and discusses the tasks or activities that characterize each phase. (Chapters 8-12 explore these phases in greater detail.) The chapter concludes by considering some of the potential problems encountered in implementing the nursing consultation process. As you read this chapter, consider the following questions:

- How is the nursing consultation process different from the nursing process?

- What specific tasks or activities seem to occur on a more or less continual basis throughout the nursing consultation process?

- Will completing the activities of the nursing consultation process always ensure a successful consultation outcome? Why or why not?

The Nursing Consultation Process: An Overview

The nursing consultation process consists of five interrelated phases (see Figure 2-1):

Gaining entry
Problem identification
Action planning
Evaluation
Disengagement

Each phase in the nursing consultation process has its own purpose, tasks, concerns, and potential problems. The essential tasks of each phase must be completed in order to achieve a successful consultation outcome. Omitting a phase or failing to complete the tasks associated with a specific phase may cause a nurse consultant to miss gathering essential information, overlook intervention opportunities, or rush the consultee to proceed prematurely with problem solving.

Each phase of the nursing consultation process is essential to the consultation relationship, yet the associated tasks and activities of each phase need to be implemented with a flexibility that allows for the unique characteristics of each problem-solving situation. Some activities of the nursing consultation process, while they begin or are

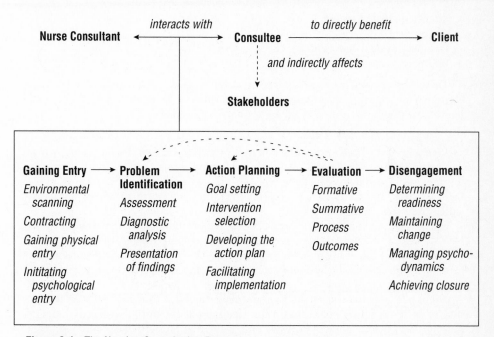

Figure 2-1. The Nursing Consultation Process
The nursing consultation process represents the interaction between a nurse consultant and consultee. The process consists of five phases, each of which has its own tasks. Note that there is a certain amount of back-and-forth movement or recycling between these phases. Recycling should occur when new information is uncovered or a proposed problem solution is either unacceptable to the consultee or is unsuccessful. Recycling allows refinement of the action plan for a problem solution and increases the likelihood that the consultation will be successful.

most important during a specific phase, occur to some degree throughout all phases of the process. A nurse consultant, for example, engages in a continual process of assessing, diagnosing, intervening, evaluating, and working to develop a trusting relationship with the consultee and other members of the client system.

Sometimes the phases of the nursing consultation process overlap, leading to a kind of back-and-forth movement or recycling between phases. For instance, a nurse consultant may find that as a consultation relationship progresses, new information about a problem situation makes necessary the repetition of previously completed phases of the process. Repeating phases of the nursing consultation process as needed increases the likelihood that the consultation problem will be resolved.

The nursing consultation process provides a necessary guide for achieving a successful consultation outcome. The manner in which a nurse consultant completes the tasks of the process, however, is just as important as performing the tasks themselves. The human processes and technical skills a nurse needs to bring to a consultation relationship are discussed in Chapter 4.

Gaining Entry

The gaining entry phase of the nursing consultation process centers around relationship building and defining. The specific tasks that need to be accomplished during this phase are:

Environmental scanning
Contracting
Gaining physical entry into the client system
Initiating psychological entry

These tasks or activities get underway at the time of initial contact between the consultee (or contact person) and the nurse consultant. Different ways in which initial contact might occur are described in Chapters 3 and 8.

Environmental Scanning Environmental scanning is the informal assessment or "scouting" process that a nurse consultant begins at the time of initial contact with a consultee. During this process, a nurse consultant gathers information and forms impressions in order to determine whether there is a fit between the needs, skills, interests, and personality ("chemistry") of the nurse consultant and those of the consultee and problem setting.

Because environmental scanning occurs before a nurse consultant and consultee have agreed to a contract, the nurse consultant is usually limited to gathering data through indirect observation and informal interviews. Publicly available information about a client system—such as mission statements and news reports—can also help a nurse consultant form impressions about the system's needs, values, and personality.

The nurse consultant uses the information gathered during environmental scanning to decide whether to continue a consultation relationship. The goal of scanning activities here is to learn about the need for, rather than to sell, consultation services. In fact, if a nurse consultant determines that involvement in a problem situation would not be mutually beneficial, the consultant is obligated to help the consultee see that their needs would be better met by someone else. Box 2-1 highlights the questions a nurse consultant may have during the environmental scanning process.

Contracting If environmental scanning results in a mutual decision by the nurse consultant and consultee to enter into a problem-solving relationship, the second task of the gaining entry phase—contracting—gets underway. Contracting is the process of identifying "mutual wants" (Dougherty 1995), the result of which is a formal agree-

---

Box 2-1. Questions for Environmental Scanning

The purpose of environmental scanning is to determine the fit between the needs, skills, interests, and personality of the nurse consultant and the consultee and client system. The following are typical questions a nurse consultant tries to answer during environmental scanning:

Questions about the problem situation:
What problem "symptoms" are bothering the consultee?
How long have the symptoms been present?
What attempts have been made to resolve the problem?
What prompted the consultation request? That is, why does this problem seem particularly bothersome now?

Questions about the consultation outcome:
What is the desired (stated) outcome for the consultation?
Does the consultee seem to have any hidden agendas?

Questions about the client system:
Who does the client system consist of?
Who will I be working with?
What is the nature of the relationship between the person requesting the
   consultation and (a) the consultee, (b) the client, and (c) the consultation
   fee payer?
Are the appropriate people involved in preliminary discussions about this
   problem and the need for consultation?
What is the level of administrative support for solving this problem?
What is the level of motivation and readiness to change within the client system?
Is the client (or contact person) leveling with me?
Are the values of the client system compatible with my own? What about
   other compatibility issues such as work and communication styles.

Questions about the consultant's skills and interests:
Is there something I can do to help resolve this problem? Do I have the skills to
resolve the problem?
Can I achieve a favorable outcome within the time frame the consultee is
   requesting?
Are there political considerations I need to think about in terms of continu-
   ing (or not continuing) involvement in this situation?
Am I interested in working on this project?

---

ment or "contract" between the consultant and consultee. A contract sets forth the purpose and goals of the nursing consultation relationship and delineates tasks, relationships, responsibilities, expectations, accountability, and the anticipated timeline for the consultation project. The contract should state the nurse consultant's expectations for evaluation of the consultation process and spell out how the nurse consultant's and consultee's personal and professional needs will be met throughout the process. Examples of nursing consultation contracts are included in Chapter 13.

Gaining Physical Entry The third task associated with gaining entry in the nursing consultation process is gaining physical entry into the client system. This task usually begins when the consultee or contact person formally introduces the nurse consultant to members of the client system. An important part of gaining physical entry (especially in organization-wide consultation situations) is administrative-level sanctioning of the consultation relationship and activities. Clearly articulated support at the administrative level can largely determine the speed at which change occurs. In a smaller-scale consultation scenario such as a clinical nurse specialist providing consultation to one or two staff nurses about a patient care issue, the consultee/staff nurse (who likely initiated the consultation relationship) might facilitate physical entry by introducing the clinical nurse specialist to other nurses on the unit and, perhaps, the patient's physician.

On the nurse consultant's part, physical entry into the problem setting can be accomplished by establishing the parameters of availability (such as work space and work hours) as well as by meeting or mingling with members of the client system on their own turf. For example, a clinical nurse specialist consulting with staff on a particular hospital unit, may gain physical entry by working each of the unit's shifts in order to spend time with nurses. Additional activities that can be used to gain physical entry are discussed in Chapter 8.

Initiating Psychological Entry The final task associated with gaining entry—initiating psychological entry—is an activity that continues throughout the entire nursing consultation process. Put simply, psychological entry involves "engaging the consultee" (Ross 1993). The nurse consultant accomplishes this task by engaging in actions that are intended to establish the nurse consultant's credibility and promote a sense of trust on the part of the consultee.

An important aspect of psychological entry is clarifying the consultant's roles and correcting distorted expectations. For example, clinical nurse specialists who provide consultation to staff nurses about problematic patient situations may need to correct the expectation that they, rather than the nursing staff, will be providing direct care to the patient. Consultation involves working with staff so they can learn to provide more effective care on their own; it means "doing with" rather than "doing for."

The outcome of psychological entry is decreased resistance to problem-solving activities and the establishment of a relationship of mutual respect and cooperation between a nurse consultant and consultee. Box 2-2 illustrates how the gaining entry phase of the nursing consultation process might take place in an external consultation scenario.

Problem Identification

The goal of the problem identification phase is to determine the cause of the "symptoms" or presenting problem. The tasks associated with the problem identification phase are:

Assessment diagnostic analysis

Presentation of findings

Assessment Assessment activities begin to take place while the nurse consultant is initiating psychological entry into a client system. Because assessment and information gathering conveys interest in the client system, this activity can actually facilitate psychological entry. To conduct an assessment of a client system, a nurse consultant systematically collects data from multiple sources using a variety of methods. This assessment is more intensive than that conducted during the gaining entry phase (environmental scanning) because here, the nurse consultant and consultee have

---

Box 2-2. Gaining Entry in an External Consultation Scenario: The Merger, Part 1

Under pressure to avoid costly duplication of services, two competing air ambulance services decide to undergo a merger. As a result of the proposed merger, some current members of the two flight teams may lose their jobs; others will be forced to assume new roles and learn new ways of doing things. Faced with increased staff anxiety, low morale, and increased absenteeism, and realizing that a successful merger is dependent on staff acceptance and commitment to the changes in service operation, a nurse consultant is contacted. The specific consultation request is, "Help us make this work."

Following this consultation request, the nurse consultant immediately begins **environmental scanning.** Informal conversations and a review of recent news articles reveal that competition between the two services has not always been friendly, and that both services have been losing money. The nurse consultant arranges for a meeting with the contact person. Getting answers to the following questions is particularly important:

Who will I be working with? What do they know about the merger and its implications?

What do you *really* want me to do? For example, will I be expected to make any personnel decisions?

What is the timeline for the merger?

Following this meeting, the nurse consultant decides the situation is a "good fit." Another meeting is scheduled for the purpose of **developing a contract.** The nurse consultant agrees to work with the client system at least until the merger is finalized, with need for continued services to be established at that time.

Physical entry gets underway when the service's chief operating officer introduces the nurse consultant to the staff of each of the merging services. The nurse consultant gains further physical entry by spending time with the staff of the two services (on all shifts)—including going on some actual flights. This latter activity also helps establish the nurse consultant's credibility and therefore initiates **psychological entry.** Psychological entry is further facilitated when the nurse consultant shares personal experiences of working as a flight nurse and working with other merging health care services.

---

established a contract. The contract both legitimizes a nurse consultant's data gathering activities and facilitates access to restricted information such as financial records or results of patient satisfaction surveys.

Information obtained during the assessment phase provides a foundation on which to design strategies for resolving the consultation problem. Examples of the issues a nurse consultant explores during assessment are presented in Box 2-3. Frameworks for conducting assessment are discussed in depth in Chapter 9.

Assessment activities assume primary importance during the problem identification phase, but occur to some extent throughout the entire nursing consultation process. The nurse consultant uses the information gained through ongoing

---

Box 2-3. Issues to Explore During Assessment

The purpose of the assessment activities that take place during the problem identification phase is to identify the cause of the problem and factors that can affect
the problem-solving process. Issues to explore during assessment include:

Issues related to the consultation problem:
What is the consultee experiencing as a result of the problem?
What is the client experiencing as a result of the problem?
Who are the stakeholders affected by this problem? How are they affected?
How do consultee attitudes, beliefs, and behaviors affect this problem?
What features of the problem setting might contribute to this problem?
What factors in the external environment might contribute to this problem?

Issues related to planning problem solutions:
What supports and blocks are there to the problem-solving process? Do these
   come from within the client system or are they external to the client system?
   What is the relative strength of each?
What assets does the consultee bring to the problem-solving process?
What will be gained and lost by solving this problem?
How will solving this problem affect the consultee? The client system?
   The stakeholders? Who stands to win or lose by solving this problem?

References: Barron (1989), Price & Reiss-Brennan (1989)

---

assessment to confirm that problem-solving activities are proceeding in the right
direction.

Diagnostic Analysis   Diagnostic analysis is the process of attaching meaning to
assessment findings and drawing conclusions about the cause of a nursing consultation problem. During this process the nurse consultant must determine the scope of
a problem—that is, how much of the client system is affected and how many factors
in the client system contribute to the problem.

Nursing consultation outcomes will only be successful if diagnostic analysis results
in an accurate problem definition on which both the consultant and consultee agree
(Kurpius, Fuqua, & Rozecki 1993). Therefore, part of diagnostic analysis is creating
"ownership" of the problem, or getting consultees to "buy into" a problem's cause and
agree to assume their share of responsibility for its solution. This is facilitated by
involving the consultee in the diagnostic analysis process.

Presentation of Findings   Presenting assessment findings and diagnostic conclusions
is an important task because it creates an awareness of a problem and its causes as
well as motivates those in the client system to give support and input regarding problem-solving strategies. The challenge of presenting assessment findings is in packaging them effectively for different audiences. Findings need to be translated into familiar language and diagnostic conclusions should be confirmed with the audience.

A nurse consultant should make an effort to reframe diagnostic conclusions and
present them as opportunities for change and improvement rather than as problems
(Cohen & Murri 1995). Take for example the case of a nursing unit unable to meet

---

Box 2-4. Problem Identification in an External Consultation Scenario: The Merger, Part 2

The nurse consultant working with the merging air ambulance services begins the **assessment activities** of the problem identification phase at the same time efforts are being made to establish psychological entry. Conversations and meetings with the members of the flight teams provide the nurse consultant with the opportunity to gather information about the team members' feelings and concerns about the merger. Additional information is gained from the administrators of the two services about how exactly the merger is likely to affect the flight teams (number or positions to be lost, new procedures to be instituted, and so forth).

Assessment reveals a high level of administrative support for the merger but a low level of support among the flight nurses. All of the nurses do, however, express commitment and motivation to "give it a good try." The services themselves are willing to commit adequate time and resources to facilitate the merger process.

Based on these assessment findings, the nurse consultant identifies anxiety and fear among the nursing staff as the major problem threatening a successful merger. A lack of information about what exactly the merger will involve on a day-to-day personal level is identified as a major **cause of the problem.**

The **assessment findings and diagnostic conclusions are presented** separately to the administrators and flight nurses of each facility. All parties concur with the diagnosis. "Ownership" of the problem is indicated by their agreement to address the issues that are contributing to the problem.

---

established patient discharge timelines. Rather than presenting the problem as the result of inefficiency on the part of staff nurses, a nurse consultant may reframe the problem as a need to explore factors on the nursing unit that, if changed, might facilitate meeting discharge timelines. Note how reframing the problem "depersonalizes" the problem's cause and creates a situation that challenges the nursing staff to find more effective ways of delivering care rather than blames them for the problem.

Box 2-4 illustrates how the problem identification phase might unfold in an external nursing consultation situation.

Action Planning

During the action planning phase of the nursing consultation process, the nurse consultant and consultee identify specific goals for the nursing consultation relationship, select interventions for achieving those goals, and develop an action plan for implementing the interventions. Also during this phase, the nurse consultant puts into place supports that will facilitate implementation of the action plan.

Goal Setting The goal setting task is characterized by a statement of desired consultation outcome, or a goal statement. In a situation where a clinical nurse specialist is providing consultation to nursing staff about a patient care issue, the goal statement would describe exactly how patient outcomes are expected to improve as a result of the nursing consultation: increased satisfaction with care, fewer complications, lower cost of care, and so forth.

Meaningful goals are based on what is both feasible and desirable in a consultation outcome. Thus when goals are being established, needs of the client, consultee, and stakeholders need to be considered; resources and constraints imposed by the client system also need to be kept in mind as goals are formulated. It might be desirable, for example, that a nursing consultation relationship results in a decreased incidence of decubiti among long-term care patients. This goal, however, might not be feasible if the problem setting lacks the financial resources to purchase needed skin care supplies, changes the staffing ratio so that nurses have time to implement new procedures, or implement any other possible problem-solving strategy.

Selecting Interventions   Most nursing consultation goals can be achieved through more than one intervention. Intervention selection begins by brainstorming about various strategies or interventions that could be used to achieve a goal. Once potential interventions are identified, each is evaluated in terms of its "fit" with the needs and resources of the client system. Strategies for decreasing the incidence of decubiti among long-term care patients might include a new turning protocol, dietary changes, or new dressing techniques. In order to determine which of the interventions would work best in the client system, the nurse consultant and consultee would need to consider such factors as financial resources, number of staff and their capabilities, and desired timeline for goal achievement.

Developing the Action Plan   The best predictor of success for a consultation relationship is an accurate problem definition that is owned by the consultee. The next best predictor is selection of the correct set of interventions that also are owned by the consultee (Kurpius, Fugua, & Rozecki 1993). Collaborative development of a detailed action plan is one way of creating ownership of goals and interventions. Even though a nurse consultant is not responsible for implementing the recommended interventions, it is necessary to help a consultee explore ways of doing so. An action plan provides this direction.

The nursing consultation action plan should identify the specific steps involved in carrying out a recommended intervention as well as the resources needed to implement each step. The nurse consultant should also check resources needed against those of the consultee (knowledge, skill) and the problem setting (time, money, equipment) to make sure that proposed interventions are feasible. The nurse consultant also needs to explore any consultee objections to the action plan and determine whether they reflect valid objections or represent resistance to change (Mendoza 1993). The final action plan should be practical, workable, and mutually agreed upon. Characteristics of effective action plans are summarized in Box 2-5.

Facilitating Implementation of the Action Plan   Even though a consultee is free to accept or reject a nurse consultant's recommendations, and implementation of the action plan is not the nurse consultant's responsibility, part of the action planning phase involves putting supports in place to facilitate implementation of the action plan. Two sets of strategies that are frequently used by nurse consultants to facilitate implementation of the action plan are team building and transition management. The goal of team building is to create cohesiveness and effective working relationships among a group of consultees. Transition management strategies focus on helping consultees anticipate and cope with the ways in which an action plan will affect them on a personal level. Both team building and transition management are discussed in depth in Chapter 10. Box 2-6 describes how the problem identification phase might occur in an external consultation scenario.

Box 2-5. Creating an Effective Action Plan

- Action plans are most likely to be effective when they are characterized by:
- Collaborative development
- Clear specification of the sequence in which interventions need to occur
- Identification of resources needed for each intervention
- Verification of the availability of needed resources
- Acknowledgment and exploration of consultee objections to the plan

---

Box 2-6. Action Planning in an External Consultation Scenario: The Merger, Part 3

After the administrators and flight nurses of the merging air ambulance services agree that communication issues are the cause of anxiety among the flight nurses, and threaten a successful merger, they work with the nurse consultant to **establish goals, select interventions, and develop an action plan.** One of the goals they establish is increased communication between administration and the flight nurses.

After brainstorming ideas for interventions and considering the needs and resources of the two flight services, it is agreed that a biweekly newsletter and weekly staff meetings will be initiated as strategies for increasing communication. The action plan details responsibilities for contributing to and producing the newsletters as well as for arranging and facilitating the meetings.

Collaborative development of the action plan served as a **team building** strategy. To help with **transition management**, the nurse consultant agrees to be a participant in the first four staff meetings and to contribute columns to the newsletter about managing change.

Evaluation

Evaluation activities in the nursing consultation process have a multidimensional focus. Developed during the action planning phase, the evaluation plan outlines the areas to be evaluated, meaningful and credible evaluation criteria, relevant information sources, and the timing of the evaluation activities. (Chapter 11 provides a more detailed discussion of developing an evaluation plan.) Evaluation focuses on more than just the outcomes of the nursing consultation process; it also considers consultee reactions to how the nursing consultation process was carried out. Information obtained from the evaluation of consultation outcomes—summative evaluation—can indicate success or can point to the need for additional interventions (in the case of an unresolved or newly developed problem, for instance).

Even though evaluation activities are most important during the fourth phase of the nursing consultation process, evaluation occurs during the other phases of the process as well. Evaluation of the nursing consultation process as it is unfolding—formative evaluation—provides a nurse consultant with the opportunity to make mid-course corrections, thereby increasing the likelihood that the consultation will be successful. As an example, evaluation of the problem identification phase might reveal a lack of consultee acceptance of the diagnostic conclusions about the consul-

---

**Box 2-7. Evaluation in an External Consultation Scenario:
The Merger, Part 4**

The nurse consultant, along with the staff and administration of the merging
air ambulance services, decides to gather two different types of evaluation data.
First, an evaluation of the perceived effectiveness of both the nurse consultant
and the consultation process itself will be obtained. This information will be
collected by means of anonymous surveys distributed to the participants once
the nurse consultant has left the client system. Since the administrators of the
services believe that meaningful indicators of the consultation's success would
be reasonable staff turnover rates and sick days, plans are made for these data
to be collected six months after the completion of the merger.

---

tation problem's cause. Based on this information, the nurse consultant can gather
additional data and reformulate the problem diagnosis in order to increase its acceptability before proceeding to the action planning phase. Evaluation activities that
might take place in an external consultation scenario are presented in Box 2-7.

Disengagement

The final phase in the nursing consultation process—disengagement—is a series of
strategically planned activities designed to increase the likelihood that problems
resolved as a result of nursing consultation remain resolved after the nurse consultant leaves the client system. The four specific tasks of the disengagement phase are:

   Determining readiness to disengage
   Maintaining change
   Managing the psychodynamics of disengagement
   Achieving closure

Often, the onset of the activities of the disengagement phase coincide with summative evaluation activities.

Determining Readiness to Disengage The activities of the disengagement phase should
not get underway until both the nurse consultant and consultee agree that it is appropriate to terminate the nursing consultation relationship. In most situations, the criteria for beginning the disengagement phase include evaluation findings that indicate a
consultee's ability to proceed with the action plan. In other cases, disengagement
needs to begin when it becomes clear that a successful outcome to the consultation is
unlikely. Additional indicators of readiness to disengage are considered in Chapter 12.

Maintaining Change A nurse consultant's second task in the disengagement phase
involves developing change maintenance strategies. These strategies should support
the consultee in maintaining changes that have occurred as a result of the consultation process. This is referred to as putting "continuity supports" into place (Lippitt &
Lippitt 1986).
   Reducing contact with a consultee while still being available for troubleshooting
and follow-up is one strategy that can be used to encourage a consultee to assume
ongoing responsibility for problem solving. Another strategy for maintaining change
is to work with consultees on developing a regular schedule of self-evaluation that
will monitor whether goals established during the action plan continue to be met,
and whether desired changes in behavior continue.

Box 2-8. Disengagement in an External Consultation Scenario: The Merger, Part 5

The nurse consultant's disengagement from the merger scenario begins by **decreasing contact** with the client system. More specifically, a daily presence within the client system ends, and the nurse consultant limits contact with the client system to attendance at the weekly staff meetings. During this "weaning period," the nurse consultant remains available for troubleshooting as needed.

Disengagement also involves **developing continuity supports** within the client system to help maintain the outcomes of the consultation relationship. One type of continuity support that often is developed by nurse consultants is training one of the staff nurses to act as an internal nurse consultant. In support of this strategy, the administrators of the services create a position for a clinical nurse specialist.

The nurse consultant anticipates increased anxiety and morale problems as disengagement (and the merger) become a reality. To **address this possible emotional response to disengagement**, the nurse consultant writes a series of articles on coping with change for use in the staff's newsletter.

To celebrate the completion of the merger, the air ambulance service plans an open house of its new facility and has a contest to design a new logo. These activities help **bring closure** to the consultation relationship. As another closure strategy, the nurse consultant writes a "closing memo" to both the staff and the administrators of the service. This memo summarizes the initial problem, the consultation activities that were carried out, the nurse consultant's impression of the current status of the initial problem, and suggestions for future actions. The nurse consultant considers the "case closed" when a return letter of thanks and acknowledgment and the final portion of the consultation fee are received.

Managing the Psychodynamics of Disengagement Disengagement activities may cause consultees to feel abandoned and inadequate. Often, as disengagement gets underway, consultee dependency and conflict seem to increase. Anticipating and managing these psychodynamics, or emotional reactions to disengagement, helps prevent a consultee from becoming overwhelmed and consequently regressing to old patterns of behavior. Providing evidence to consultees about their readiness to disengage as well as reframing disengagement as a vote of confidence are two ways in which a nurse consultant might address the psychodynamics of disengagement.

Achieving Closure A nurse consultant's final task in the disengagement phase (and in the nursing consultation process) is to achieve closure. The purpose of closure activities is to leave both the nurse consultant and the consultee with a sense of satisfaction about what they have accomplished. In organization-wide consultation situations, closure is often achieved when the nurse consultant submits a final report. A variety of symbolic rituals such as celebrations can also be used to signify closure. Clinical nurse specialists providing consultation to staff nurses might achieve closure by simply thanking the consultee for the consultation opportunity and offering to be of service in the future. Further examples of closure activities are provided in Chapter 12. Box 2-8 illustrates how disengagement might take place in an external consultation scenario.

Potential Problems in Implementing the Nursing Consultation Process

Problems that a nurse consultant might encounter while implementing the nursing consultation process can originate either with the consultee and client system or with the nurse consultant.

Problems that Originate with the Consultee or Client System

Several consultee characteristics can cause problems during the nursing consultation process. These may include denial about the need for change, a lack of a sense of shared responsibility for problem solving, or not being ready to enter into a change effort. When nurse consultants interact with a group of consultees, they may discover that not everyone in the group is ready to become involved in problem solving at the same time. Another common setting-based or consultee-based problem is misunderstanding about the identity of the client (the patient or the organization, for example) or about which outcomes (patient well-being or cost-containment) ought to drive goal setting. Finally, a consultee might put pressure on the nurse consultant to skip steps in the consultation process in order to save time and money. The risks of rushing the consultation process—solving the wrong problem, developing an unworkable action plan, and causing disorder and frustration—need to be pointed out to consultees when this pressure occurs.

Problems that Originate with the Nurse Consultant

Other problems that can complicate the nursing consultation process originate with the nurse consultant. Sometimes nurse consultants mistakenly assume that the problem presented by the consultee or contact person is the real problem. Failing to gather assessment data to validate the nature of a problem can lead to irrelevant, unworkable, and possibly harmful interventions. A related problem is trying to use the same package of interventions to solve all problems in all client systems. Lastly, nurse consultants may take on the consultee's responsibilities in the problem-solving process. A nurse consultant may, for example, implement a recommended intervention rather than give the consultee this responsibility. Should this occur, future problems that arise in the client system may be blamed on the nurse consultant because the client system has not been given the opportunity to develop its own problem-solving skills. Box 2-9 summarizes problems that can interfere with effective implementation of the nursing consultation process.

Most of the problems that potentially impede the nursing consultation process can be avoided or overcome by completing the necessary phases and tasks of the process, being clear about the purpose of each phase, and attending to issues that arise throughout the process. Continual monitoring of both progress in problem solving and consultee reactions to the consultation relationship can help a nurse consultant identify these problems before they threaten to derail the entire consultation process.

Chapter Summary

The nursing consultation process is the systematic approach to problem solving that is enacted with consultees in order to enhance client well-being. While the activities of the nursing consultation process occur in a progressive or forward-moving sequence, there is some degree of back- and-forth movement between phases. In fact, some

---

**Box 2-9. Potential Problems in Implementing the
          Nursing Consultation Process**

Problems that originate with the consultee or client system:
Consultee lacks self-awareness or denies the need for change
Consultee lacks a sense of shared responsibility for problem solving
Consultee is not ready to enter into a change effort
Different levels of readiness to problem solve among members of a
    consultee group
Misunderstanding about who the client is in the situation
Misunderstanding or conflict about goals
Pressure to rush through the consultation process

Problems that originate with the nurse consultant:
Failure to validate the nature of a consultation problem
Relying on the same interventions for all problem situations
Assuming problem-solving responsibilities that belong to the consultee

---

activities occur continually throughout the entire process. Following the phases of the nursing consultation process and completing its tasks offers the nurse consultant the best chance that a consultation relationship will be successful. Implementing the tasks of the process with a flexibility that acknowledges the uniqueness of each consultation problem and client system helps to ensure that problem solutions will be relevant, feasible, and long-lasting.

Applying Chapter Content

- Analyze two nursing consultation efforts in which you have been involved, one of which you would label "successful" and the other "unsuccessful." Which components of the consultation process were present and which were absent in each of these situations? How do you think this contributed to their success or failure? What could have been done differently in the unsuccessful situation? Differentiate how the nursing consultation process might need to be adjusted for internal versus external nursing consultation. Why do you think these adjustments might need to occur?

- How would you implement the evaluation and disengagement phases of the nursing consultation process if the action plan was rejected by the consultee?

References

Barron, A. (1989). The CNS as consultant. In A. Hamric & J. Spross (Eds.), *The clinical nurse specialist in theory and practice* (2nd ed., pp. 125-146). Philadelphia: Saunders.

Cohen, W. & Murri, M. (1995). Managing the change process. *Journal of AHIMA, 66* (6), 40-41.

Kurpius, D., Fuqua, D., & Rozecki, T. (1993). The consulting process: A multidimensional approach. *Journal of Counseling and Development, 71,* 601-606.

Lippitt, G. & Lippitt, R. (1986). *The consulting process in action* (2nd ed.). San Diego: University Associates.

Mendoza, D. (1993). A review of Gerald Caplan's *Theory and practice of mental health consultation. Journal of Counseling and Development, 71*, 629-635.

Price, J. & Reiss-Brennan, B. (1989). Consulting telesis: A systems approach. *Nursing Management, 20* (11), 80A-80F.

Ross, G. (1993). Peter Block's *Flawless Consulting* and Homunculus Theory: Within each person is a perfect consultant. *Journal of Counseling and Development, 71*, 639-641.

Ulschak, F. & SnowAntle, S. (1990). *Consultation skills for health care professionals.* San Francisco: Jossey-Bass.

Additional Readings

Badger, T. (1988). Mental health consultation with a surgical unit nursing staff. *Clinical Nurse Specialist, 2* (3), 144-148.
The case study presented in this article clearly illustrates the consultation process.

Beare, P. (1988). The ABCs of external consultation. *Clinical Nurse Specialist, 2* (1), 35-38.
The author provides guidelines for implementing the consultation process as an external consultant.

Dougherty, A. (1995). *Consultation: Practice and perspectives in school and community settings* (2nd ed.). Pacific Grove, CA: Brooks-Cole.
Section 2 of this text provides an in-depth discussion of the consultation process, including its theoretical underpinnings.

Kurpius, D., Fuqua, D., & Rozecki, T. (1993). The consulting process: A multidimensional approach. *Journal of Counseling and Development, 71*, 601-606.
The authors describe a 6-phase consultation process.

Lippitt, G. & Lippitt, R. (1986). *The consulting process in action* (2nd ed.). San Diego: University Associates.
Chapter 2 in this text presents the authors' perspective of the consultation process. Chapter 14 provides scenarios that illustrate the consultation process.

Monicken, D. (1995). Consultation in advanced practice nursing. In M. Snyder & M. Mirr (Eds.), *Advanced practice nursing: A guide to professional development* (pp. 183-195). New York: Springer Publishing.
The author presents an overview of the consultation process that is based on the work of Lippitt and Lippitt.

Ross, G. (1993). Peter Block's *Flawless Consulting* and Homunculus Theory: Within each person is a perfect consultant. *Journal of Counseling & Development, 71*, 639-641.
This article describes a 5-stage consultation process. The author emphasizes the need for authenticity in carrying out the process.

Schein, E. (1988). *Process consultation, volume I: Its role in organization development* (2nd ed.). Reading, MA: Addison-Wesley.
Chapters 10-16 in this text describe the consultation process and provide examples of its implementation in organization-wide consultation situations.

Ulschak, F. & SnowAntle, S. (1990). *Consultation skills for health care professionals.* San Francisco: Jossey-Bass.
Chapter 3 of this text describes an 8-stage consultation process for internal consultation situations.

~

3

Interaction Patterns for Nursing Consultation

The time to be aware of the choice among models is at that moment in a relationship when one party says to another: "Can you give me some help?" or "I don't know what to do with this problem I've got," or, simply, "What should I do?" (Schein 1988)

Key terms: interaction pattern, content variables, process variables, process consultation

Introduction

Just as nurses interact with patients in different ways to provide nursing care (through team nursing and primary care nursing, for example), nurse consultants interact with consultees in different ways to solve problems. Different nursing care delivery patterns describe the specific tasks (for instance, team leader versus direct care provider) a nurse must carry out in a patient care relationship. Similarly, a nursing consultation interaction pattern describes the actions and tasks of a nurse consultant and consultee in a problem-solving relationship. In nursing consultation, "interaction pattern" refers to the approach to problem solving that a nurse consultant uses in a specific situation. An interaction pattern can be thought of as a "model of delivery" for consultation services or a "style" of carrying out the nursing consultation process.

An interaction pattern provides guidelines that help determine what consultation activities are appropriate for a specific problem situation. This is valuable because the nature of help that a nurse consultant provides when a particular interaction pattern is used has a powerful influence on almost every aspect of the nursing consultation process. If an interaction pattern fits poorly with a consultee's beliefs, values, real and perceived needs, skills, and preferences, the nursing consultation relationship will likely fail.

Because a single interaction pattern will not work in all problem situations, nurse consultants need a working knowledge of a variety of interaction patterns. Nurse consultants who are familiar with and able to selectively apply different interaction patterns are more likely to be helpful to their consultees because they are better able to individualize the nursing consultation process.

This chapter describes the three interaction patterns that predominate in nursing consultation: providing a solution, prescribing a solution, and facilitating a solution. While these interaction patterns are derived from classic models of organization consultation (Schein 1988), they are equally useful in selected nursing consultation situations. Also considered in this chapter are the task implications of each interaction pattern for the consultee and nurse consultant, as well as each pattern's advantages and disadvantages. The final section of this chapter discusses factors to consider when selecting an interaction pattern and combining interaction patterns. As you read this chapter, think about the following questions:

- What are the distinguishing features of the different interaction patterns?
- How do nursing consultation roles and skills vary with each pattern?
- How would you choose which pattern to use?
- What challenges would you face implementing each of these interaction patterns as an internal and external nurse consultant?
- Which interaction pattern seems most "comfortable" to you? How might this affect your practice of nursing consultation?

Providing a Solution: The Purchase of Expertise Interaction Pattern

"Purchase of expertise" describes a model of organization consultation in which a consultant provides services that have been requested by a consultee (Schein 1988). The interaction pattern represented by this consultation model is likewise applicable to selected nursing consultation situations.

The Interaction Framework

In a typical purchase of expertise scenario, a consultee identifies a specific need and contracts with a consultant for the provision of specific services. The consultee in this scenario identifies the problem, its cause, and the desired solution. However, despite wanting the problem solved and knowing how the problem should be solved, the consultee may lack the time, skill, or interest needed to solve the problem alone and thus hires a consultant. The following scenarios are examples of nurse consultants applying a purchase of expertise interaction pattern:

A nurse-educator is asked to develop a survey and collect and analyze data for a small community hospital. The hospital wants to learn about the general health status of the community so that it can develop programs the community needs and values.

An acute care nurse is asked by a psychiatric facility to develop protocols for managing medical emergencies.

A high school is alarmed about a reported high incidence of sexual activity among its students. The principal asks a nurse practitioner to teach a class on sexually transmitted diseases to students.

A nurse manager is asked to develop staffing patterns for a renovated mother-baby unit.

The common thread in these scenarios is that the consultee identifies both the problem and the desired solution. Each scenario is characterized by a request for nursing consultation something like, "I've found this problem that I can't solve on my own. Fix it for me and bring me the bill." Note that part of this interaction pattern is the expectation that the nurse consultant will provide the problem solution. As discussed in Chapter 2, providing the problem solution or implementing the intervention is not typically a part of the nursing consultation process. Note also that the purchase of expertise interaction pattern is "content-oriented." That is, it focuses on the "what variables" in the problem situation—what the problem is and what needs to be done to resolve it.

Task Implications

The purchase of expertise interaction pattern implies tasks that both the consultee and nurse consultant must complete in order to obtain a satisfactory nursing consultation outcome. The consultee's tasks center around purchasing the "right" expertise for the problem solution. The nurse consultant's tasks focus on verifying the need for the purchased services and providing the problem solution.

The Consultee's Tasks The purchase of expertise interaction pattern is unlikely to be effective unless the consultee successfully carries out four important tasks. First, the consultee is responsible for correctly identifying the problem. Moreover, the consultee needs to accurately identify what is causing the problem and what needs to be done to resolve it (Rockwood 1993). If the consultee identifies the wrong problem and the wrong solution, the consultation process is unlikely to produce satisfactory results.

Consider the first scenario in the preceding examples. A nurse-educator is asked to provide research expertise to a hospital. The implied problem is that the hospital needs (or wants) to offer community education programs but doesn't know where to start. The consultee's assessment is that more information is needed about the health status of the community in order to develop these programs. The consultee also believes that a survey is the best way of gathering this information. The implied cause of the not knowing where to start is lack of knowledge. However, if the real problem is not a lack of knowledge about the community's needs but rather a lack of knowledge about the "how-to's" of putting together and offering programs, the consultation process is heading in the wrong direction and will likely be unsuccessful.

The consultee's second task in the purchase of expertise interaction pattern is to correctly assess the consultant's ability to solve the problem. In the previous example, if the nurse-educator who has been hired to conduct the desired survey lacks data analysis skills, the problem-solving effort will have an unsatisfactory outcome (even though the consultee has correctly diagnosed the problem).

Third, the consultee must accurately communicate to the nurse consultant the nature of the perceived problem and its desired solution. Again, using the previous scenario, if the consultee fails to clarify the exact population to survey or that the nurse consultant is expected to analyze as well as collect the data, the consultee's needs will go unmet and the problem will remain unresolved.

Finally, the purchase of expertise interaction pattern is unlikely to result in a satisfactory outcome unless the consultee acknowledges and accepts the time and resources that will be needed to implement the proposed solution, as well as any temporary side effects, such as decreased productivity. The consultee also needs to plan for possible long-term effects of the proposed consultation services. Consultees often overlook resources such as time, money, equipment, and personnel needed to solve a problem. In our working example, the resources required to conduct the desired survey might include postage costs, staff time (to administer the surveys), and a computer with data analysis capabilities. The possible long-term effects of this project on the client system might include hiring an additional staff person or remodeling a facility to accommodate the community education programs. In the purchase of expertise interaction pattern, it is the consultee's responsibility to identify any constraints that might affect the nurse consultant's ability to offer the desired service.

The Nurse Consultant's Tasks At first glance, it appears that the consultee bears all of the responsibility for a successful outcome when the purchase of expertise interaction pattern is used to guide the nursing consultation process. The nurse consultant's task is often interpreted as simply providing the contracted service and leaving. However, the nurse consultant must do more than just perform the requested service if the desired consultation outcome is to be achieved (Kurpius & Fuqua 1993).

The nurse consultant's tasks in the purchase of expertise interaction pattern can be described as verification and validation activities. The nurse consultant's first task is to verify that the consultant has correctly identified a problem's cause and is proposing a solution that will resolve the problem. In our working example, the nurse consultant would be responsible for verifying that what the hospital really needs in order to start offering education programs is more information about the community's health status. The nurse consultant would also verify that the proposed solution—gathering information through a survey—is in fact the best solution.

Secondly, in a purchase of expertise interaction pattern, the nurse consultant needs to verify that the consultee has chosen the right consultant for the problem situation. As discussed in Chapter 2, if a nurse consultant realizes that there is a lack of fit between the consultant's skills and those needed for a consultation project, the nurse consultant is responsible for helping the consultee see the need for a different consultant. Consultant skills in instrument design and data analysis would be imperative for a successful outcome in the example scenario. A nurse consultant lacking these essential skills would be responsible for referring the consultee to someone who could better meet their needs.

The nurse consultant's third task in a purchase of expertise interaction pattern is to verify that the consultee is communicating what is intended to be communicated. The nurse consultant must actively listen and ask questions so that a consultee's problems, desires, and needs are accurately understood. Again, using our working example, the nurse consultant would be responsible for verifying exactly what services the consultee wants—the exact population to survey, the nature of data analysis desired, and so forth.

The nurse consultant's final task in a purchase of expertise interaction pattern is to verify that the consultee has thought through the possible consequences of carrying out the proposed problem solution. This responsibility is a part of effective action planning (discussed in Chapters 2 and 10). In our working example, the nurse consultant would verify that the consultee has the resources needed to complete the consultation process. In addition, the nurse consultant would help the consultee think about possible long-term consequences of the consultation project. For example, what if the survey suggests a need for education about workplace hazards present in the community's major industry—could this need really be addressed or would community politics force the issue "under the table" and leave survey respondents frustrated because their needs are not addressed?

Box 3-1 summarizes the tasks that the consultee and nurse consultant need to complete if the purchase of expertise interaction pattern is to result in a satisfactory consultation outcome.

Advantages and Disadvantages

A purchase of expertise interaction pattern is attractive to consultees because it allows them to temporarily turn a problem situation over to the consultant. In situations where the proposed intervention would have negative effects, such as job losses, a purchase of expertise interaction pattern allows the consultee to maintain an appearance of detachment from the problem solutions, while the consultant takes the "heat" for any adverse side effects of the consultation. A purchase of expertise interaction pattern can also be attractive to consultants in that the consultation relationship tends to focus on a very specific problem and tends to be relatively short term in nature. The nurse consultant can perform the contracted service and leave the

---

Box 3-1. Task Implications of the Purchase of Expertise Interaction Pattern

In order for the purchase of expertise interaction pattern to result in a satisfactory nursing consultation outcome, the following tasks must be completed:

Consultee Tasks	*Nurse Consultant Tasks*
• Correctly identify the problem	• Verify the consultee's diagnosis of the problem and appropriateness of problem solution
• Choose the right consultant	• Verify one's own abilities to help with problem solving
• Communicate clearly and accurately with the consultant	• Verify what the consultee is communicating; listen, question, and clarify
• Identify and accept the possible costs and side effects of solving the problem	• Verify that the consultee has thought through the consequences of proceeding with problem solving
	• Develop the action plan
	• Implement the problem solution

---

client system without the added burden of needing to develop a long-term working relationship with the consultee.

The disadvantages of a purchase of expertise interaction pattern arise because of the consultant's limited role in initially defining the problem and in identifying interventions. The nurse consultant can be put in the difficult position of discovering that the wrong problem is being addressed or that the desired intervention is unsuitable. How should a nurse consultant respond, for example, if it becomes apparent the problem solution proposed by the consultee will only resolve the problem on a temporary basis or may actually be an avoidance tactic? A consultee's request for team building, for instance, will not likely resolve (on a long-term basis) morale problems within a work unit if those problems are occurring as a result of the management style being practiced. In a situation such as this, the nurse consultant is faced with the choice of either exiting the consultation relationship or changing the interaction pattern with the consultee in order to solve the problem in a different way. Another disadvantage of the purchase of expertise interaction pattern is that the consultee, in turning over the problem-solving task to the nurse consultant, does not learn problem-solving skills for future use.

Box 3-2 summarizes the advantages and disadvantages of the purchase of expertise interaction pattern.

Indications for Use

As suggested in the preceding discussion, a purchase of expertise interaction pattern, when misused, can become a means of avoiding a persistent problem and applying only a "band-aid" solution. This is more likely to occur when the consultation problem involves complex human relations issues, such as burnout and low morale, rather than technical issues. Therefore, a purchase of expertise interaction pattern is most appropriate when a consultee's problem is straightforward and the requested expertise is for help with problems of a technical nature.

Box 3-2. The Purchase of Expertise Interaction Pattern:
        Advantages and Disadvantages

Advantages
- Consultee can turn the problem situation over to the nurse consultant
- Consultee can appear detached from a problem solution that may have adverse side effects
- Nurse consultant can avoid the burden of needing to establish long-term problem-solving relationships

Disadvantages
- Nurse consultant may discover consultee is trying to solve the wrong problem
- Nurse consultant may discover consultee's desired problem solution will not solve the problem
- Consultee may not learn problem-solving skills for future use

---

Prescribing a Solution:
The "Doctor-Patient" Interaction Pattern

Nurse consultants can also address consultation problems by interacting with consultees in a prescriptive interaction pattern. A prescriptive interaction pattern—derived from the "doctor-patient" model of consultation—describes a content-oriented consultation model in which the consultant diagnoses and prescribes what is needed to solve a problem (Schein 1988).

The Interaction Framework

A "doctor-patient" or prescriptive interaction pattern gets its name from the way in which the typical consultation scenario unfolds: the consultee senses something is wrong (experiences a symptom) and seeks help for both a diagnosis and prescription. A typical consultation request would be something like, "Something is wrong. Find out what it is and tell me what to do." The consultee wants to learn about the problem and its cause, as well as what to do about it. This contrasts with a purchase of expertise interaction pattern in which the consultee identifies both the problem and the desired solution before seeking consultation.

Task Implications

In a "doctor-patient" interaction pattern, the consultee's tasks are analogous to behaviors associated with being a "good patient." The nurse consultant's task, in turn, is to be a "good doctor."

The Consultee's Tasks In order to achieve a satisfactory outcome using a "doctor-patient" interaction pattern, the consultee must successfully complete a series of five tasks (Dougherty 1995; Rockwood 1993). First, the consultee needs to correctly identify where in the client system the problem exists. To understand the importance of identifying the problem sources in a nursing consultation scenario, consider the example symptom of "increased use of occupational health services" at a hospital.

The consultee needs to isolate the part of the client system in which this problem is arising. For example, is this "symptom" occurring among all personnel or only among a specific employee group? Is it related to illness or to injuries? Correctly identifying the location of the problem helps the consultee determine what kind of consultant to bring in—a nurse consultant with expertise in epidemiology or one with expertise in occupational safety hazards for instance. The location of the "symptom" also helps the nurse consultant determine where to focus assessment activities; in the preceding example, this focus would be on behaviors of the nursing staff such as hand washing, or on safety conditions throughout the entire hospital.

The consultee's next two tasks are founded on a relationship of trust between the consultant and the consultee. First, the consultee must be willing to divulge the information that the nurse consultant needs to accurately diagnose the cause of the problem. To continue with the preceding scenario, the consultee would need to provide the nurse consultant with information about the nature of the visits made to the hospital's occupational health services. Second, the consultee must accept the consultant's diagnosis of the problem's cause; in the example, the diagnosis may be increased on-the-job injuries due to poor body mechanics among the nursing staff.

Once the consultee has accepted the nurse consultant's diagnosis, the fourth task involves accepting and complying with the consultant's problem solution, or "prescription." In our working example, if the nurse consultant recommends in-service education on body mechanics, "complying with the prescription" would mean implementing the class and ensuring that it is attended by all staff members.

The consultee's final task in a "doctor-patient" interaction pattern is to want to "remain healthy" after the nurse consultant leaves the client system. That is, the consultee must be willing to engage in activities aimed at preventing similar problems in the future. In our working example, successfully completing this task would mean that the consultee demonstrates problem prevention behaviors such as offering ongoing in-service education or back care exercise classes.

The Nurse Consultant's Tasks The nurse consultant must complete four tasks in the "doctor-patient" interaction pattern if a nursing consultation relationship is to result in a satisfactory outcome. These tasks entail direct involvement in both problem diagnosis and intervention selection. Note that this is in contrast to the purchase of expertise interaction pattern, where the nurse consultant's tasks center around verifying the appropriateness of a problem diagnosis and problem solution generated by the consultee and implementing the desired intervention.

The nurse consultant's first task in a "doctor-patient" interaction pattern is to gather enough assessment data to arrive at a problem diagnosis. This requires establishing a relationship of trust with the consultee. It also means gathering information from multiple sources using a variety of data collection strategies. In the working example—increased use of occupational health services—data sources might include nursing staff, maintenance personnel, and administration; data collection strategies might include interviews, observation, and record reviews.

The nurse consultant's second task in the "doctor-patient" interaction pattern is to correctly interpret the assessment data and make an accurate and acceptable diagnosis. As discussed in Chapter 2, nursing consultation outcomes will only be successful if a consultee "buys into" a problem's cause. Thus a nurse consultant needs to carefully consider the ways in which the wording and presentation of a problem's cause will affect its acceptability. Think, for example, of the possible differences in consultee reactions to attributing an increase in back injuries among nursing staff to "inattention to body mechanics" rather than "poor body mechanics." A diagnosis of "poor body mechanics" suggests that a lack of knowledge might be contributing to the

Box 3-3. Task Implications of the "Doctor-Patient"
        Interaction Pattern

The following tasks must be completed if the "doctor-patient" interaction pattern
is to result in a satisfactory nursing consultation outcome:

Consultee Tasks
- Correctly identify the source of
  the problem
- Provide the nurse consultant with
  adequate and accurate information

- Accept the consultant's diagnosis
  of the problem
- Comply with the recommended
  problem solution

- Be willing to engage in problem-
  prevention activities

Nurse Consultant Tasks
- Gather enough information to
  arrive at a diagnosis
- Correctly interpret data; formulate
  an accurate and acceptable
  diagnosis
- Develop acceptable problem-
  solving interventions
- Provide consultee with adequate
  support and direction to
  implement the intervention

problem. In contrast, a diagnosis of "inattention to body mechanics" suggests that the
nurses know what they are supposed to be doing but just aren't doing it. This diagnosis might be interpreted as implying carelessness and laziness as the cause of
increased back injuries, connotations that could cause defensiveness among the nursing staff.

The third task that a nurse consultant must complete in the "doctor-patient"
interaction pattern is to prescribe interventions that will be acceptable to the consultee and other members of the client system. The client system, of course, must
have the abilities and resources needed to comply with the "treatment plan." To
continue with our working scenario, prescribing in-service education as the problem solution might not make sense if the client system lacks someone who could
provide the classes. Of course, the nurse consultant could switch to a purchase of
expertise interaction pattern and contract with the consultee to provide these in-
service classes.

The nurse consultant's final task in the "doctor-patient" interaction pattern is to
provide the consultee with enough support and direction to implement the recommended intervention. The nurse consultant in our example would want to outline
content and teaching strategies, as well as provide resources (pamphlets, videotapes,
and so forth) that would enable the client system to offer the recommended in-service classes.

Box 3-3 summarizes the tasks that the consultee and nurse consultant must complete if a "doctor-patient" interaction pattern is to be effective in resolving a nursing
consultation problem.

Advantages and Disadvantages

The primary advantage of the "doctor-patient" interaction pattern is that it enables
problems to be resolved in a relatively short period of time. This is because the interaction pattern is consistent with "doing for" rather than "doing with" the consultee.

Box 3-4. The "Doctor-Patient" Interaction Pattern: Advantages and Disadvantages

Advantages
- Problems can be solved relatively quickly
- Enables an "exhausted" consultee to turn a problem over to someone else

Disadvantages
- Can foster consultee dependency
- Little opportunity for consultee to learn long-term problem-solving skills

---

In other words, the consultee is expected to contribute information, but is not generally involved in the decision-making aspects of the nursing consultation process.

The chief disadvantage of this interaction pattern is that it can foster consultee dependency. This problem is likely to occur because the nurse consultant fixes the problem for a consultee rather than involves the consultee in the problem-solving process.

Box 3-4 summarizes the advantages and disadvantages of the "doctor-patient" interaction pattern.

Indications for Use

The "doctor-patient" interaction pattern is useful in two types of problem situations. First, because the interaction pattern enables problems to be resolved quickly, it is useful in crisis situations in which a timely problem resolution is of utmost importance. It is also useful in situations where consultees are at their "wits' ends" and have exhausted their skills and energy trying to resolve a problem on their own; the model is useful in these scenarios because the "doctor-patient" interaction pattern allows a consultee to turn problem-solving responsibilities over to the consultant.

The "doctor-patient" interaction pattern could be utilized in the following problem situations:

increased incidence of hepatitis B among hospital workers
decreased revenues at a nurse practitioner clinic
decreased enrollment in a nursing program

In each of these scenarios, the nurse consultant has been presented with a troublesome "symptom" that needs both a diagnosis and a prescription that will resolve the problem in a relatively short period of time.

Facilitating a Solution: The Process Consultation Interaction Pattern

"Process consultation" is a consultation model concerned with long-term organization development and effectiveness (Schein 1988). Process consultation emphasizes the process rather than the content variables in a problem situation (the "how" opposed to the "what"). A nurse consultant using the process consultation interaction pattern is most interested in discovering how problems and problem-solving tasks are accomplished and affected by interactions between the consultee and other members of the client system (Rockwood 1993).

The Interaction Framework

When a process consultation interaction pattern is used to guide the nursing consultation process, the nurse consultant and consultee function as "co-problem solvers." The chief difference between the process consultation interaction pattern and the content-oriented consultation patterns discussed earlier in the chapter, is that the nurse consultant and consultee work together to identify a problem's causes and develop satisfactory problem-solving strategies. In this interaction pattern, the nurse consultant assumes the role of facilitator in the nursing consultation relationship.

A consultee request of "I need help fixing this problem" (rather than "fix this problem for me") indicates that a process consultation interaction pattern might be the best way to approach the nursing consultation process. In a typical process consultation scenario, the consultee senses something is wrong but does not know what is wrong, why it is wrong, or what to do about it. However, the consultee expresses desire to be involved in the problem-solving process. A nurse administrator might, for example, initiate a process consultation interaction pattern with a request such as, "We've noticed a lot more absenteeism and staff turnover lately and aren't sure why. We'd like someone to help us figure out what is going on and how to handle it."

Task Implications

In a process consultation interaction pattern, the nurse consultant's primary responsibility is to facilitate development of a consultee's problem-solving abilities. The consultee's responsibility, in turn, is to be a "good student."

The Consultee's Tasks A process consultation interaction pattern will only be effective to the extent that the consultee accomplishes three tasks. First, the consultee must be willing to take responsibility for or "own" the consultation problem. When consultees own their problems, the resistance and resentment to changes resulting from problem-solving efforts is likely to decrease. In the preceding example regarding concern about staff absenteeism and turnover, the consultee must accept the possibility that workplace conditions are contributing to the problem.

The consultee's second task in the process consultation interaction pattern is to want to learn how to solve the problem. This means the consultee must have an open mind about what the actual problem solution might be. In the working example, the nurse administrator, or consultee, must be willing to consider problem solutions ranging from changes in the current salary and benefits package to changes in personnel and education needs.

Finally, when using the process consultation interaction pattern, the consultee must be willing to be an active participant in the problem-solving process. Consultees are expected to be involved in gathering assessment, formulating a problem diagnosis, generating possible solutions, developing the action plan, and evaluating the nursing consultation process; in this interaction pattern, consultees "learn by doing." The nurse administrator in our example would need to be personally involved in every phase of the nursing consultation process.

The Nurse Consultant's Tasks A nurse consultant needs to accomplish two tasks in order to achieve a successful consultation outcome using the process consultation interaction pattern. The first task is cognitive in nature—the nurse consultant must believe that consultees are the experts in terms of knowing their own strengths, weaknesses, needs, abilities, and preferences. In a process consultation interaction pattern, the nurse consultant deliberately "taps into" the consultee's expertise and incorporates the consultee's insights and opinions into the diagnostic conclusions and action plan. Note how this contrasts with the purchase of expertise interaction

---

Box 3-5. Task Implications of the Process Consultation Interaction Pattern

If a process consultation interaction pattern is to be effective, the following tasks must be accomplished:

Consultee Tasks	*Nurse Consultant Tasks*
• Be willing to "own" the consultation problem	• Believe that consultees are the experts in terms of knowing their own strengths, weaknesses, abilities, and preferences
• Have a desire to learn problem-solving skills	
• Actively participate in problem-solving activities	• Actively involve consultee in problem-solving activities

---

Box 3-6. The Process Consultation Interaction Pattern: Advantages and Disadvantages

Advantages
• Consultee learns problem-solving skills
• Increased likelihood of problems remaining resolved

Disadvantages
• Can take longer to carry out problem-solving process

---

pattern where the consultee brings insights and preferences to the consultation relationship at the outset, and the nurse consultant has the task of verifying their accuracy and appropriateness.

The nurse consultant's second task in the process consultation interaction pattern is to actively involve the consultee in each step of the nursing consultation process. This is done by assuming the roles of teacher, guide, role model, mentor, and facilitator.

Box 3-5 summarizes the tasks that the nurse consultant and consultee need to complete when using a process consultation interaction pattern.

Advantages and Disadvantages

The primary advantage of using a process consultation (rather than a content-oriented) interaction pattern to guide the nursing consultation process is that problems are more likely to be resolved on a long-term basis. This interaction pattern leaves the consultee with problem-solving skills that can be used at the first sign of problem recurrence.

The main disadvantage of this interaction pattern is that it often takes longer to implement than do content-oriented interaction patterns. This is because of the teaching and learning that characterizes this interaction pattern. The problem-solving process may be further prolonged if the consultee initiated the process having only limited pre-existing problem-solving skills. Note that increasing the length of time to complete the problem-solving process can have negative financial implications for the client system.

Box 3-6 summarizes the advantages and disadvantages of the process consultation interaction pattern.

Indications for Use

Because a process consultation interaction pattern facilitates the development of a consultee's problem-solving skills, its use is particularly appropriate when the problem is one that is likely to recur. This interaction pattern is also effective when the presenting problem is related to nontechnical issues such as the attitudes, beliefs, and culture of a client system that could be difficult for an external nurse consultant to diagnose alone, without consultee insight. On the other hand, because it often takes longer to implement, this interaction pattern is less appropriate as an approach in urgent situations. A process consultation interaction pattern would be appropriate to consider in the following problem situations:

> A nurse practitioner is asked by the family of a client with schizophrenia to help them learn strategies for responding to the client's behavior changes and for encouraging treatment compliance.
>
> A nurse-educator is asked by the faculty at another school of nursing to help them revise their curriculum.
>
> A nurse-manager is asked to develop plans for combining the nursing staff of two merging clinics.

These problem situations are all non-urgent in nature, involve nontechnical issues such as culture, beliefs, and attitudes, and are likely to recur in one form or another. The consultee would, therefore, derive long-term benefits from new skills learned through participating in the nursing consultation process.

Matching the Interaction Pattern to the Consultee

The preceding sections of this chapter have linked the different interaction patterns to the nature of the consultation problem and the nature of a consultee's request for help. Another set of factors that can be used to determine which interaction pattern is most likely to be effective in a given problem situation is a consultee's willingness and ability to change. Taking into account these consultee characteristics reflects applying the principles of situational leadership (Hersey & Blanchard 1982) to the selection of problem-solving strategies and a nursing consultation interaction pattern.

A consultee's ability to change is reflected by the amount of direction required during the problem-solving process. Some consultees may need to be told what to do as well as when and how to do it, or may need direction in setting goals and defining roles. A consultee's willingness to change is indicated by the amount of support and encouragement needed to carry out problem-solving activities (Haffer 1986).

Consultees are described as having a low willingness and ability to change when they are unsure, insecure, incompetent, unwilling, and unable to solve their own problems (due to exhaustion, time constraints, lack of skills, and so forth). These consultees need "telling"—specific directions plus generous amounts of encouragement—if they are to resolve their problems (Haffer 1986). This style of interaction with consultees is most consistent with prescribing a solution, or using the "doctor-patient" interaction pattern.

Providing a solution or using a purchase of expertise interaction pattern is a good fit when consultees are willing to change, but are unable to do so on their own because they lack time, self-confidence, or skill. These consultees will benefit from "selling"—being provided with knowledge and a demonstration of problem-solving skills (Haffer 1986). These consultant behaviors are consistent with the purchase of expertise interaction pattern.

Box 3-7. Choosing an Intervention Pattern for a Nursing Consultation Relationship

Characteristics of the consultation problem and client system that a nurse consultant can use to guide the selection of an interaction pattern include the nature of the request for help, the nature of the problem, time and timing issues, and a consultee's willingness and ability to change.

Characteristic	Purchase of Expertise Interaction Pattern	"Doctor-Patient" Interaction Pattern	Process Consultation Interaction Pattern
Consultation Request	"Solve this problem for me"	"Tell me what my problem is and how to solve it."	"I don't know what I need but I need help."
Nature of Problem	Technical and straightforward	Technical and straightforward	Centers around human relations issues
Time and Timing	Consultee is in a hurry	Crisis situation Consultee is at wits' end or exhausted	Non-urgent problem
Willingness and Ability to Change	Willing to change but unable to do so alone	Low willingness and ability to change	Motivated to change and has some problem-solving skills

---

Other consultees will have pre-existing problem-solving skills as well as some degree of motivation and willingness to engage in change efforts. These consultees will respond to an interaction pattern that is supportive, nondirective, and participatory in nature (Haffer 1986). The interaction pattern that would best fit this nursing consultation situation is the process consultation interaction pattern.

Box 3-7 summarizes the factors to consider when selecting an interaction pattern for a nursing consultation relationship.

Combining Interaction Patterns

Consultants in other professions are beginning to question whether the interaction patterns used in consultation are as mutually exclusive as they have traditionally been presented (Dougherty 1995; Rockwood 1993). Because technical and human relations issues are often interrelated, the nursing consultation process may need to address both sets of issues in order to be most effective. If a combined interaction pattern is used to guide the nursing consultation process in a given problem situation, the question the nurse consultant needs to ask becomes, "When should I use which model?" rather than, "What model should I use?"

One approach to combining nursing consultation interaction patterns is to start out with a process consultation approach (Rockwood 1993). The advantage of this strategy is that the consultee's involvement in the activities of the problem identification phase helps the nurse consultant learn the culture of the problem setting. Consultee involvement increases the likelihood that the problem solutions developed through the consultation process will be feasible and acceptable to the consultee.

In other situations, a nurse consultant might want to begin the nursing consultation process using the purchase of expertise or "doctor-patient" interaction pattern and then change to a process approach once the initial "crisis" aspects of the problem have been resolved. A consultee often has more energy to devote to learning problem-solving skills and is more willing and able to learn once the most troublesome "symptoms" of a problem have been resolved.

Chapter Summary

Nursing consultation interaction patterns reflect different ways of interacting with consultees to help them solve problems. For nurse consultants, an interaction pattern provides a guide for approaching the nursing consultation process in a way that will prove most effective in a given situation. The interaction patterns that have been presented in this chapter differ in terms of their emphasis on the content ("what") or process ("how") issues of a problem situation. They also differ in terms of "working for" versus "working with" a consultee to solve problems.

A nurse consultant's selection of an interaction pattern should be based on the perceived needs and abilities of a consultee, including the consultee's willingness and ability to be involved in problem-solving activities. Problem situations in which nurse consultants are likely to be involved are often complex and rarely limited to only content or process issues. Therefore, nurse consultants need a working knowledge of a variety of interaction patterns as well as the ability to apply these interaction patterns if they are to be effective problem solvers.

Applying Chapter Content

Think of a consultation situation in which you have been involved. Identify the interaction pattern that was used. Was it a good fit for the situation? Why or why not? Speculate on how this same consultation experience might have been different if another interaction pattern had been used.

Identify the nursing consultation interaction pattern described in each of the following articles. Critically analyze its "fit" for the situation.

Badger, T. (1988). Mental health consultation with a surgical unit nursing staff. *Clinical Nurse Specialist, 2* (3), 144-148.

Huddleston, J. (1992). Family and group psychoeducative approaches in the management of schizophrenia. *Clinical Nurse Specialist, 6* (2), 118-121.

Infection control consultant. (1993, January). *Hospital Infection Control,* 7-9.

Kjervik, D. (1990). Law and ethics consultation. *Journal of Professional Nursing, 6* (4), 193, 246.

References

Dougherty, A. (1995). *Consultation: Practice and perspectives in school and community settings* (2nd ed.). Pacific Grove, CA: Brooks-Cole.

Haffer, A. (1986). Facilitating change: Choosing the appropriate strategy. *Journal of Nursing Administration, 16* (4), 18-22.

Hersey, P. & Blanchard, K. (1982). *Management of organizational behavior: Utilizing human resources* (4th ed.). Englewood Cliffs, NJ: Prentice Hall.

Kurpius, D. & Fuqua, D. (1993). Fundamental issues in defining consultation. *Journal of Counseling and Development, 71,* 598-600.

Rockwood, G. (1993). Edgar Schein's process versus content consultation models. *Journal of Counseling and Development, 71,* 636-638.

Schein, E. (1988). *Process consultation, volume I: Its role in organization development* (2nd ed.). Reading, MA: Addison-Wesley.

Additional Readings

Berger, M., Ray, L. & Del Togno-Armanasco, V. (1993). The effective use of consultants. *Journal of Nursing Administration, 23* (7/8), 65-69.
   The authors emphasize the need for a fit between organizational needs and a consultant's approach to problem solving.

Brack, G., Jones, E., Smith, R., White, J., & Brack, C. (1993). A primer on consultation theory: Building a flexible worldview. *Journal of Counseling and Development, 71,* 619-628.
   This article discusses the different world views that are reflected in different models of consultation. The authors emphasize the need for flexibility in one's approach to problem solving.

Dougherty, A. (1995). *Consultation : Practice and perspectives in school and community settings* (2nd ed.). Pacific Grove, CA: Brooks-Cole.
   Chapter 9 includes a discussion of Edgar Schein's models of organizational consultation.

Fuqua, D. & Kurpius, D. (1993). Conceptual models in organizational consultation. *Journal of Counseling and Development, 71,* 607-618.
   This article provides an overview to the different theoretical frameworks that underlie organizational consultation. The article also provides a useful discussion about choosing and integrating models.

Haffer, A. (1986). Facilitating change: Choosing the appropriate strategy. *Journal of Nursing Administration, 16* (4), 18-22.
   The author applies Hersey and Blanchard's situational leadership model to choosing change agent strategies.

Mendoza, D. (1993). A review of Gerald Caplan's *Theory and practice of mental health consultation. Journal of Counseling and Development, 71,* 629-635.
   This article provides an overview of how the consultant's role varies according to the model of consultation used.

Schein, E. (1988). *Process consultation, volume I: Its role in organization development* (2nd ed.). Reading, MA: Addison-Wesley.
   Chapter 3 describes the three classic models of organizational consultation.

4

Nurse Consultant
Roles and Skills

*Things rarely, if ever, go in textbook fashion. Equal
attention should be paid to both what you are doing and
how you are doing those things.* (Dougherty 1995)

Key terms: task-oriented role, process-oriented role,
universal role, competency, professionalism

Introduction

Nurse consultants, like nurses in general, adopt multiple roles when they work
with consultees. The tasks associated with each phase of the nursing consultation process should readily suggest what some of these roles might be. As you may
suspect, each role that a nurse consultant needs to assume is characterized by a set of
competencies that reflect a skills base, a knowledge base, and a set of personal attributes. As Figure 4-1 reveals, the choice of an appropriate consultation role that is supported by an appropriate set of competencies helps to facilitate a successful outcome
for the nursing consultation process.

This chapter explores some of the role choices and competencies involved in nursing consultation. The chapter begins with a description of the roles most commonly
assumed by nurse consultants. It goes on to discuss the factors related to role choice
as well as the skills, knowledge, and personal attributes needed to be an effective
nurse consultant. The final section of this chapter considers strategies for developing
the needed competencies for effective nursing consultation. As you read this chapter,
consider the following questions:

- Which roles described in this chapter are most likely to be used in each phase of
  the nursing consultation process?
- How might these roles and their associated competencies differ for internal and
  external nursing consultation situations?
- Which nurse consultant roles are most compatible or incompatible with your personal skills and attributes?
- How are the roles and competencies required for a nurse consultant similar to and
  different from traditionally recognized nursing roles and skills?

Nursing Consultation Roles

The roles that nurse consultants adopt most frequently in the course of the nursing
consultation process can be clustered into three categories: task-oriented roles, process-
oriented roles, and "universal" roles. Task-oriented roles are traditionally associated
with technical expertise and tend to be directive in nature. Process-oriented nursing
consultation roles are comparatively nondirective and more facilitative in nature

(Lippitt & Lippitt 1986). Universal roles tend to occur throughout the nursing consultation process and are often superimposed on other roles. It is rare that any nursing consultation role is enacted in isolation. It is more common for the nurse consultant to enact several roles, during any phase of the nursing consultation process, albeit in varying degrees.

Box 4-1 describes the three types of nursing consultation roles in greater detail.

Task-Oriented Consultation Roles

Task-oriented nursing consultation roles tend to have a technical focus. These roles require specialized knowledge and skills and reflect the "technical work," or tasks, that must be accomplished to satisfactorily complete the phases of the nursing consultation process. (Note how the task-oriented roles in Box 4-1 "match" the tasks of the nursing consultation process identified in Chapter 2.)

Task-oriented roles are generally used when a consultee needs direction with problem-solving activities due to either the urgent nature of the problem or to the consultee's limited problem-solving abilities. Task-oriented roles are particularly apparent when prescriptive, content-oriented interaction patterns (purchase of expertise and/or "doctor-patient") are used to guide the nursing consultation process. Although many task-oriented roles exist, six are most commonly enacted in the nursing consultation process.

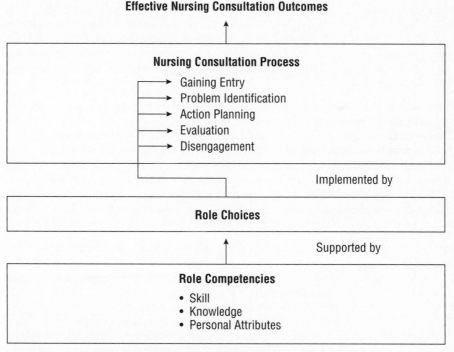

Figure 4-1. Components of Effective Nursing Consultation

Effective nursing consultation relies on carefully selecting the roles needed to implement each phase of the nursing consultation process. Role competencies are the foundation of a nurse consultant's role choice. The nurse consultant may need to adopt a new role for each phase of the nursing consultation process.

Box 4-1. Types of Nursing Consultation Roles

Task-Oriented Roles

Fact-finding

Diagnosing

Advocacy

Directing solution implementation

Educating

Coordinating resources

Process-Oriented Roles

Joint problem solving

Process counseling

Universal Roles

Providing expertise

Presenting information

Role-modeling

Providing leadership

Fact-Finding One of the most frequently enacted nursing consultation roles is that of fact-finder (McDougall 1987; Monicken 1995). Fact-finding activities predominate during the problem identification phase of the nursing consultation process. However, fact-finding takes place during other phases of the nursing consultation process as well, because nurse consultants must constantly gather information to confirm that the consultation relationship is progressing satisfactorily. As a fact-finder, the nurse consultant must know how, when, and from whom to obtain the data needed to clarify problems and identify meaningful goals and workable interventions. The following scenario illustrates a nurse consultant using the fact-finding role: A clinical nurse specialist (CNS) is asked to function as an internal consultant to determine why patient satisfaction ratings for a hospital's mother-baby unit are showing a steady decline. The CNS conducts phone interviews with former patients, spends time observing the unit, and gathers information from nursing staff and physicians.

Diagnosing The nursing consultation role of diagnostician is closely linked to the role of fact-finder. Diagnosing entails analyzing, synthesizing, and attaching meaning to data in order to draw conclusions about the cause of a consultation problem. The role of diagnostician is also used when the nurse consultant is drawing conclusions about the feasibility and effectiveness of a potential problem-solving intervention. The preceding example can be extended to illustrate the following diagnostician role:

The CNS analyzes the data gathered from multiple sources and draws conclusions about likely explanations for the decline in patient satisfaction ratings. The CNS concludes that a public relations campaign is unlikely to be an effective problem solution.

Advocacy When engaged in advocacy, a nurse consultant tries to persuade a consultee to take a specific course of action. Advocacy is based on a desire to protect the interests of those who are unable (because they lack skill, knowledge, or energy) to protect their own interests (Dougherty 1995). Advocacy takes different forms depending on the particular interaction pattern being used to guide the nursing consultation process. When a content-oriented interaction pattern (purchase of expertise or "doctor-patient") is being applied, the focus of advocacy is encouraging a consultee to take a specific course of action. This is known as "solution advocacy." This type of advocacy is appropriate because the nurse consultant is bringing objectivity and a broader perspective to a problem situation that is characterized by a sense of urgency and consultee frustration. In a process consultation interaction pattern, the focus of advocacy is encouraging the consultee to be an active participant in the problem-solving process. With this type of advocacy, known as "process advocacy," the consultee can benefit from learning problem-solving skills that can be applied to future problem situations. Following are examples of these two variations of advocacy.

Solution advocacy A nurse consultant is asked to improve patient flow in a family planning clinic. The clinic is losing money because of staff overtime and the fact that long waits often cause patients to leave without being seen. The clinic has already attempted to resolve flow problems through physical renovation of the facility. The nurse consultant persuades the clinic to revise both its appointment scheduling process and the tasks assigned to the clinical support staff.

Process advocacy A nurse consultant is asked to work with the staff of a family planning clinic to solve concurrent problems of prolonged waiting times for patients, "slow" times for the nurse practitioners, and consistent staff overtime. The nurse consultant persuades the clinic administrator to allow clinic staff to be involved in data gathering activities and brainstorming about possible problem solutions.

Directing Solution Implementation When directing solution implementation, a nurse consultant delegates specific problem-solving tasks to the consultee. The role of director varies according to which nursing consultation interaction pattern is being applied. For instance, if a purchase of expertise interaction pattern is in use, the nurse consultant may direct the consultee to assist with specific components of the intervention. (Recall that in this interaction pattern, it is the nurse consultant who implements a specific problem solution.) In contrast, with both the "doctor-patient" and process consultation interaction patterns, directing solution implementation means providing the consultee with specific directions about how to implement the action plan. (Remember also that in a "doctor-patient" interaction pattern, delegation decisions are made unilaterally by the nurse consultant; in a process consultation interaction pattern, the nurse consultant and consultee work together to decide how to delegate each task.) In these two interaction patterns, the nurse consultant directs solution implementation during the development of the problem solution action plan. The following scenarios illustrate the nurse consultant directing solution implementation.

A nurse consultant accepts a contract to develop and produce promotional materials for a telephone health information service. The nurse consultant directs the consultee to gather promotional materials that similar services in other cities are using.

A telephone health information service is concerned about its low utilization rate. A nurse consultant develops an action plan for marketing the service. The plan includes different public relations assignments for various members of the client system.

A telephone health information service is concerned about its low utilization rate. The nurse consultant and consultee work together to develop an action plan for surveying the community's needs related to the service. Together the nurse consultant and consultee decide which members of the client system are best suited for different activities in the survey project.

Educating Nurse consultants assume the role of educator when they create learning experiences for a consultee. Typically, these learning experiences are directed at helping a consultee change their level of knowledge, understanding, or functioning. A nurse consultant's ultimate goal in providing education is to develop a consultee's ability to respond to a problem situation that is likely to recur.

Like other nurse consultant roles, the role of educator changes its focus when different consultation interaction patterns are being used. In a purchase of expertise interaction pattern, a consultee may contract with a nurse consultant to provide a specific education service. In a "doctor-patient" interaction pattern on the other hand, a nurse consultant might teach a consultee how to follow through with the prescribed action plan. Because the focus of the process consultation interaction pattern is to help a consultee develop problem-solving abilities, here the nurse consultant may informally enact the role of educator throughout the nursing consultation process. The following examples illustrate different ways in which a nurse consultant may enact the role of educator.

A nurse consultant is hired to teach a group of nurse-managers about the principles of delegation.

A nurse consultant develops an action plan that includes instructions (education) about what specific tasks should be delegated to unlicensed assistive personnel.

A nurse consultant helps a consultee apply delegation principles to the development of a policy about assigning tasks to unlicensed assistive personnel.

Coordinating Resources   When enacting the role of resource coordinator, the nurse consultant finds resources that a consultee needs in order to be able to implement a problem solution. Coordinating resources is a part of the action planning phase of the nursing consultation process. Resource coordination may entail accessing needed resources on the consultee's behalf, as is the case in a content-oriented interaction pattern. When the nursing consultation process is guided by a process consultation interaction pattern, coordinating resources means working with the consultee to both identify needed resources as well as how to obtain them. Coordinating resources is illustrated in the following examples.

A nurse consultant accesses phototherapy equipment that a home health care agency needs in order to implement a phototherapy home care program.

A nurse consultant works with the staff of a home health care agency to help them identify needed equipment and possible equipment vendors for a phototherapy home care program.

Process-Oriented Consultation Roles

In contrast to task-oriented nurse consultant roles, process-oriented roles are more facilitative than directive in nature. Process-oriented nurse consultant roles focus on helping consultees accept and take responsibility for problem situations and for ongoing problem-solving activities. These nurse consultant roles are most apparent when the nursing consultation process is being guided by a process consultation interaction pattern. However, there are two process-oriented nurse consultant roles that can be identified in almost all nursing consultation relationships.

Joint Problem Solving   Nurse consultants who are engaged in joint problem solving combine their expertise and professional resources with those of the consultee to respond to a problem situation. In this capacity, a nurse consultant both acknowledges the insight and information a consultee can contribute to the nursing consultation process as well as encourages a consultee to identify alternative problem explanations and solutions. In a purchase of expertise interaction pattern, the nurse consultant acts as a joint problem solver by verifying a consultee's assessment of the problem situation. Thus joint problem solving is incorporated into diagnostic analysis and intervention selection activities. When a "doctor-patient" interaction pattern is being applied, joint problem solving is most apparent during assessment activities when the nurse consultant relies on information from the consultee to formulate a valid problem diagnosis. Joint problem solving occurs on a more continual basis when a process consultation interaction pattern is being applied.

Process Counseling   Process counseling involves helping a consultee perceive, understand, and act on interpersonal and intergroup behaviors that are contributing to a problem situation (Lippitt & Lippitt 1986). The goal of a nurse consultant who is engaged in process counseling is to support the improvement of human relationships within a problem setting. To achieve this aim, the nurse consultant helps consultees clarify the meaning of their words and explore the factors that contribute to problematic behavior. The following scenario illustrates process counseling:

Consultee: "The nurses on this unit aren't performing as effectively as they were before we restructured."

Nurse consultant: "What do you mean by 'not as effectively'?" (Clarifying communication)

Consultee: "Well, I mean they don't help each other out. It's like everyone is only interested in their own tasks. There's no teamwork."

Nurse consultant: "How has restructuring affected their work roles? Can you think what this behavior might mean?" (Helping consultee explore reasons for intergroup behavior)

Universal Consultation Roles

Providing expertise, presenting information, role-modeling, and providing leadership are four "universal" roles that occur throughout the nursing consultation process. These roles often occur at the same time that other nursing consultation roles are being enacted.

Providing Expertise In many ways, "expert" is viewed as synonymous with "consultant." It is no surprise then, that providing expertise is superimposed on most other nurse consultant roles; if a nurse consultant is not perceived as having specialized knowledge or skills, it is unlikely a consultee would request the consultant to help in solving a problem. As the different interaction patterns for nursing consultation illustrate, consultees seek content as well as process expertise from nurse consultants.

The nurse consultant's role in providing expertise deserves particular qualification because novice nurse consultants can be easily seduced by the label of "expert" as well as the authority and social and professional prestige that tends to accompany that label. Furthermore, some consultees may be lulled into a false sense of security or complacency by a consultant's "aura of expertise." As useful as this perception may be for facilitating the acceptance of a nurse consultant's recommendations, relying on the role of expert to the exclusion of all others can foster dependency on the part of the consultee rather than facilitate the development of problem-solving skills. The nurse consultant needs to be aware that while consultation, by its very nature, incorporates the expert role, actually providing expertise is only appropriate to the degree that doing so helps a consultee learn to resolve the problem situation. The limitations of expertise as a source of power for a consultant are discussed in Chapter 5.

Presenting Information The task of presenting information, like providing expertise, occurs in all phases of the nursing consultation process. A nurse consultant must continually present and share information so that a consultee can be an active participant in the problem-solving process. Typical situations in which nurse consultants are presenting information include:

presenting information that has been gathered during fact-finding

presenting conclusions about a problem's cause that have been developed while enacting the role of diagnostician

presenting information while providing education

presenting problem-solving alternatives that have been brainstormed during the process of joint problem solving presenting impressions about a group's interactions when engaged in process counseling.

Role-Modeling   Effective nurse consultants consciously and unconsciously role-model throughout the nursing consultation process. In a sense, role-modeling can be considered educating. Role-modeling includes demonstrating the skills and qualities needed for successful problem-solving. As a form of "teaching by showing," role-modeling can be a powerful strategy for teaching problem-solving skills because it enables consultees to see how specific actions, such as different ways of collecting and presenting information, influence reactions and problem-solving results.

Providing Leadership   The fourth universal nurse consultant role is providing leadership in problem solving. Nurse consultants provide this leadership by ensuring that the phases and tasks of the nursing consultation process are completed and, if necessary, repeated. Providing leadership also entails ensuring that the consultant and consultee carry out the tasks that need to occur if a specific nursing consultation interaction pattern is to be effective. It is important to recognize that providing leadership does not mean "taking over" the nursing consultation process. Rather, providing leadership can be thought of as a "total quality management" strategy for ensuring that the consultee's needs are met and the consultation problem has the best chance of being resolved.

Choosing Among Consultation Roles

Effective nurse consultants are able to choose the appropriate role for each step of a problem situation and implement those roles in a way that respects the norms and standards of the consultee and client system. Most nurse consultants, while aware of many consulting roles, have preferred ways of solving problems. Nurse consultants who work repeatedly and successfully with a limited range of problem issues may be tempted to implement roles in a similar fashion in all problem situations. Moreover nurses may be asked to consult about a specific problem, *because* of their reputation for performing specific roles effectively. The danger of relying on personal preferences and what has worked before is that doing so overlooks the unique qualities of each consultee and problem situation. Factors that the nurse consultant should consider when choosing a nursing consultation role include the consultee's confidence and level of skill within the consultation process, time constraints, and issues related to trust, teamwork, and acceptance (Ulschak & SnowAntle 1990). These factors and their implications for role choice are summarized in Box 4-2.

Consultee Skills and Confidence   The roles that a nurse consultant enacts tend to change as the relationship with a consultee develops. At the beginning of a consultation relationship, the consultee may be in a relatively dependent relationship with the nurse consultant. During this time, more directive consultative roles will tend to produce results. As a nursing consultation relationship evolves, however, consultees acquire problem-solving skills and generally gain confidence. As this growth occurs, less directive roles may become appropriate.

Time Constraints   The urgency of a consultation problem is often a driving force behind a nurse consultant's decision to use a more or less directive role when interacting with a consultee. Because nondirective, process-oriented roles tend to require more time, these roles are generally not effective in problem situations in which time is limited. Task-oriented roles, however, are particularly appropriate for urgent situations. Consider, as an example, the scenario of a budget crisis at a "free" clinic: if funds are not secured within a week, the clinic will need to close. While enacting process-

---

Box 4-2. Choosing Among Consultation Roles

The choice of a nursing consultation role is largely determined by the consultee's level of skill and confidence, time constraints, and issues related to trust, teamwork, and acceptance.

Factor	*Role Considerations*
Consultee skills and confidence	Low skills and confidence—use a more directive role. As skills and confidence are acquired, roles can become less directive
Time constraints	Urgent situation—consider task-oriented roles Non-urgent situation—consider process-oriented roles
Trust	Nurse consultant has low trust in consultee—time factors determine whether task- or process-oriented roles should be used Consultee has low trust in nurse consultant—build trust by effectively implementing a task-oriented role or by including consultee in problem-solving activities
Teamwork	Teamwork present or desired—consider process-oriented roles
Acceptance	Not important—consider task-oriented roles. Important—consider process-oriented roles

---

oriented roles might help the consultee learn how to keep a budget crisis from recurring, these roles would likely take too long to implement to solve the immediate crisis. Instead, task-oriented, directive roles such as coordinating resources, solution advocacy, and directing intervention implementation, are indicated.

Trust The level of trust between the consultee and nurse consultant is another issue to consider when selecting a nursing consultation role. Trust is present between a nurse consultant and consultee when there is rapport and a sense of mutual respect and credibility. The absence of trust can create a "Catch-22" situation in nursing consultation.

In problem situations where the nurse consultant has a low level of trust in the consultee's problem-solving abilities or contributions to the problem-solving process, the nurse consultant may need to enact a task-oriented role such as fact-finding if any progress is to be made in resolving the consultation problem. On the other hand, if there is time to use a process-oriented role such as joint problem solving, the nurse consultant may be able to gain trust in the consultee's problem-solving abilities.

In situations where the consultee has low trust in the nurse consultant, successful implementation of a task-oriented role, such as providing education, can enhance the consultee's perception of the nurse consultant's credibility and help build trust. Once initial trust has been established, the nurse consultant can more effectively implement a process-oriented role. At the same time, however, a consultee who has little trust in a nurse consultant may become very resistant to the problem-solving process when a directive, task-oriented role such as diagnosing or advocacy is used. Enacting a process-oriented role can help the consultee build trust in the nurse consultant's intentions and abilities. Trust, therefore, should not be the only criterion used for choosing a nurse consultant role, but should be considered with other factors in the problem situation.

Teamwork A further consideration for a nurse consultant when choosing a role is teamwork, either as a norm within a client system or as a desired outcome of the nursing consultation relationship. A teamwork-oriented consultee makes it feasible for the nurse consultant to use a process-oriented role such as joint problem solving. If enhanced teamwork is a goal of the nursing consultation relationship, as is the case in many problem situations involving human relations issues, process counseling would be appropriate, either alone or in combination with another consultative role such as providing education.

Acceptance Finally, the nurse consultant needs to assess how important it is for the consultee to accept the problem solution. If the consultee's acceptance of the problem-solving strategy is not important (as in the earlier example of a clinic with a budget crisis where it is the outcome rather than how it is achieved that is important), directive and task-oriented nurse consultant roles are appropriate. On the other hand, if consultee acceptance of a problem solution is important (using position cuts or fees for service as the strategy to prevent a recurring clinic budget crisis, for instance), more facilitative and process-oriented roles are likely to be effective.

Skills Base for Nursing Consultation

Nursing consultation requires a broad skills base. Nurse consultants need technical competence to perform the task-oriented roles needed during each phase of the nursing consultation process. If these roles and technical skills are to be implemented effectively, nurse consultants also need human process and communication skills. Box 4-3 outlines the technical and human process skills base needed for effective nursing consultation.

Technical Competencies

Technical competencies are the task-oriented skills needed to complete the phases of the nursing consultation process. These competencies can be grouped into two categories: diagnostic skills and problem-solving skills.

Diagnostic Skills The diagnostic skills needed by nurse consultants include the ability to select and implement data gathering approaches that are appropriate for both assessment and evaluation purposes. Effective data gathering requires knowing what information is needed and how to access it; it also requires a broad understanding of the issues related to a presenting problem—that is, an appreciation of multicausality—so that important sources and pieces of information are not overlooked. A nurse consultant working with a consultee to improve employee morale would demonstrate competence in diagnostic skills by looking beyond the obvious cause of the problem, recent work redesign for example, and investigating such diverse issues as salary, inadequate parking, and employees' stressors at home as possible contributors to the morale problem.

Box 4-3. Technical and Human Process Skills Base for Nursing Consultation

Technical Competencies: task-oriented skills needed to complete the phases of the nursing consultation process.

Diagnostic Skills
Assessment approaches and techniques
Appreciation of multicausality
Data analysis and interpretation
Problem conceptualization
Problem-solving
Collaboration
Goal setting
Ability to establish priorities
Designing, implementing, and modeling interventions
Mobilizing resources
Motivating and instilling confidence
Political astuteness
Imagination
Risk taking

Human Process Competencies: "people-oriented" skills needed to gain consultee acceptance of the consultation process and its resultant changes.

Communication Skills
Sending messages
Receiving verbal and nonverbal messages
Formal information presentation skills
Ability to give and receive feedback
Interpersonal skills
Building, maintaining, and terminating relationships
Group management skills
Ability to manage conflict and hidden agendas
Ability to manage resistance
Ability to manage dependency
Negotiation skills

Another set of diagnostic skills needed by a nurse consultant is problem conceptualization. Skill in conceptualizing problems involves the ability to assimilate and synthesize an extensive quantity of information in order to come to conclusions about a problem's cause (Cohen & Murri 1995). Problem conceptualization requires skills in both analyzing and interpreting assessment and evaluation data.

Problem-Solving Skills Nurse consultants use problem-solving skills to help consultees formulate goals, establish priorities, and implement problem solutions. Problem solving requires proficiency with a range of interventions such as educating and team building. Effective nurse consultants are able to design, implement, and model a variety of problem-solving strategies. Chapter 10 discusses problem-solving strategies in detail.

Problem solving also requires the ability to translate an idea for a possible problem solution into practice (Cohen & Murri 1995). This means that the nurse consultant must be able to set the stage for successful implementation of a problem-solving strategy by mobilizing resources, and by motivating and instilling confidence into consultees. Effective problem solving requires a nurse consultant to be comfortable working at all levels of a client system to effect change, which, in turn, requires political astuteness. Imagination and risk taking are other useful problem-solving skills.

Human Process Competencies

Human process competencies are the "people-oriented" skills needed by nurse consultants to work effectively with individuals and groups in problem-solving situations. Human process competencies reflect the "how" component of nurse consultant-consultee interactions. Competence in human process skills facilitates consultee acceptance of the nursing consultation process and the change it produces. Process competencies include communication and interpersonal skills.

Communication Skills   Communication skills are essential for maintaining the momentum of the consultation process and sustaining consultee loyalty (Cohen & Murri 1995). Effective nurse consultants are proficient at both sending and receiving messages. When sharing assessment and evaluation findings with consultees, nurse consultants need proficiency in formal information presentation skills, that is, writing, and speaking. Throughout the nursing consultation process, nurse consultants must be skilled at listening, nonverbal attending, expressing empathy, questioning, clarifying, summarizing, and giving and receiving feedback.

Interpersonal Skills   Effective nurse consultants know how to create, maintain, and terminate relationships with both individual and group consultees. Nurse consultants must be able to put people at ease and build trust. This requires skills in establishing rapport and credibility and using humor appropriately. Specific interpersonal skills needed by nurse consultants are skills in group management and negotiation.

Group management skills needed to be an effective nurse consultant include the ability to keep group members focused on the task at hand, manage conflict, manage hidden as well as formal agendas, and balance consultee needs for autonomy and direction. Other relationship-oriented human process skills needed by nurse consultants include knowing when to confront and when to listen, understanding and managing the dynamics of resistance, and recognizing and managing excessive dependency in one's self as well as in consultees (Kurpius, Fuqua, & Rozecki 1993). These human process skills are essential for working with individual as well as group consultees.

Negotiation, the process of getting what one wants from others, is an interpersonal skill that is often needed in several phases of the nursing consultation process. Implementing process-oriented nurse consultant roles such as joint problem solving may also require negotiation skills. As an example, a nurse consultant may need to negotiate the parameters of staff nurse involvement (for instance, will they be paid) in education sessions that are to be part of a problem solution. Effective negotiation requires communication skills, understanding the consultee's point of view, flexibility, and a willingness to take risks. Effective negotiation also includes the ability to separate the consultee from the problem issue, explore the consultee's interest, focus

---

Box 4-4. Knowledge Base for Nursing Consultation

Technical Knowledge: content that promotes understanding of nursing consultation relationships and the nursing consultation process.

The nursing process

The nursing consultation process

Interaction patterns for nursing consultation

Systems theory

Organizational theories and structures

Change theory

Principles of group dynamics

Power

Leadership theory

General Knowledge: supportive content that varies according to the nursing consultation setting, the interventions selected, and the nature of the problem.

Specialized clinical knowledge

Adult learning theory

Conflict resolution

Cultural diversity

---

on common interests rather than on position, and generate multiple problem definitions and problem solutions (Fisher & Ury 1981).

Knowledge Base for Nursing Consultation

The roles that are used by nurse consultants and the skills that are needed to implement these roles suggest the need for nurse consultants to have a broad knowledge base. Nurse consultants need to know about the purposes and phases of nursing consultation. Knowledge of indirect or supportive areas is also needed for effective nursing consultation. The outline of the knowledge base for nursing consultation in Box 4-4 reflects the consensus of several writers (Barron 1989; Dougherty 1995; Monicken 1995). The technical knowledge areas that are listed in the box reflect content that is foundational to an understanding of the nature of nursing consultation relationships (for instance, change theory and group dynamics) and typical nursing consultation problem settings (for example, systems theory and organizational theories). General knowledge areas include content that supports a nurse's practice of the consultant role and the nursing consultation process in specific situations.

Personal Attributes for Nursing Consultation

Effective nurse consultants have more than technical expertise, process skills, and a broad knowledge base. They also have personal and professional qualities and competencies that enhance their implementation of the nursing consultation process. These attributes are summarized in Box 4-5.

Box 4-5. Personal Attributes for Nursing Consultation

Ability to listen and empathize

Ability to communicate warmth, acceptance, and concern

Self-direction

Flexibility

Tolerance for ambiguity

Ability to share control with others

High threshold of frustration

Charisma

Credibility

Poise

Vision

High energy level

Passion for problem solving

Ability to engage in self-examination

Professionalism

Judgmental competence

Self-awareness

Personal professional growth orientation

Respect for confidences

Clear sense of responsibilities

Respect and ability to uphold contractual obligations

Willingness to be evaluated

Personal Qualities

Nurse consultants often find themselves working with a variety of clients in a wide range of settings. Interacting effectively with individual and group consultees in diverse settings requires the ability to communicate personal qualities such as empathy, warmth, respect, acceptance, and concern (Barron 1989; Ulschak & SnowAntle 1990).

Nurse consultants also need to be self-directed and flexible. They also need to be able to tolerate ambiguity and a lack of control. In other words, nurse consultants must be comfortable in situations in which problem causes and "best" solutions are not readily apparent. They must be comfortable with sharing problem-solving and decision-making activities with consultees, even when they would rather solve the problem on their own.

Nurse consultants must be able to accept the right of the consultee to act or not act on their recommendations; this requires a high threshold of frustration and the ability to tolerate rejection. Nurse consultants who are personally charismatic and who readily demonstrate their credibility are able to construct a power base for their consultation recommendations (Cohen & Murri 1995).

Poise, vision, a passion for problem solving, and boundless reserves of energy are other personal attributes needed for successful nursing consultation (Metzger 1993). Finally, effective nurse consultants have the ability to engage in self-examination and reflection about skills and knowledge areas that need further development (Barron 1989).

Professionalism

This final set of attributes needed for effective nursing consultation enables the nurse consultant to be identified as a professional. One such attribute, judgmental competency, is the ability to make decisions about appropriate courses of action in a specific consultation relationship (Brown 1993). Another important competency of effective professional nurse consultants is having a clear understanding of their responsibilities and obligations as a nurse consultant. For example, client well-being should not be sacrificed for the sake of fostering consultee independence in problem solving.

Effective nurse consultants have a high level of self-awareness. That is, they know and respect the limits of their expertise and skills. They refer to or consult with other professionals as necessary. Effective nurse consultants also maintain a personal and professional growth orientation so that they are continually updating and expanding their expertise and repertoire of intervention skills. Effective professional nurse consultants respect confidences but are also able to make appropriate judgments about the limits of confidentiality. Professional nurse consultants recognize their responsibilities to honor contractual agreements and are willing to have their performance as a nurse consultant evaluated.

Developing Knowledge and Skills for Nursing Consultation

There exists a prevailing yet mistaken belief that a nurse can become an effective nurse consultant without any deliberate education or training. Many nurses, and consultees for that matter, believe that the only thing needed to be effective as a nurse consultant is content expertise or specialized information (Brown 1993). While it is true that consultation is a functional role into which many nurses evolve as they acquire experience, content expertise, and confidence (Monicken 1995), it is also true that the different competencies required for effective nursing consultation are best acquired through different types of learning experiences. The knowledge base needed for effective nursing consultation can be effectively acquired through didactic (classroom) learning activities. Skills base competencies can be acquired in laboratory settings and through structured application exercises such as videotaping and critiquing one's interviewing and presentation skills. The judgmental competencies needed for effective nursing consultation are best acquired through supervised fieldwork (Brown 1993).

Foundational knowledge and skills for effective nursing consultation can be acquired or enhanced through a variety of formal and informal means. Academic courses and continuing education workshops are two of the more formal or structured ways of gaining theoretical knowledge. A less formal and structured way of updating knowledge is reading in both the professional and popular press topics related to personal and organizational development, current trends in one's specialty area, and health care in general. Networking, special interest groups, and general and specialty professional organizations are additional examples of some of the opportunities available to most nurses for enhancing their knowledge base for effective nursing consultation.

Consultation skills and judgmental competencies can be expanded and refined by actively seeking out the feedback of others on one's performance as a consultant. Supervised practice experiences can often be developed in return for providing nursing consultation services on a volunteer basis, especially in community service agencies. These experiences can offer opportunities to practice and receive feedback on foundational nursing consultation skills such as problem identification, educating, giving presentations, developing action plans, interpersonal communication, and evaluation.

Lastly, self-assessment tools, self-reflection, and peer review processes can be used to develop insight into the personal and professional qualities one brings to a nursing consultation situation.

Chapter Summary

Nurse consultants interact with consultees in a variety of roles. These roles require many different skills as well as a broad knowledge base. Effective nursing consultation is built on choosing the consultative role that is most appropriate for the problem setting and applying it to the nursing consultation process. Effective nursing consultation requires personal qualities and professionalism. While some of the competencies needed for effective nursing consultation can be acquired and developed through experience and professional maturation, a variety of formal and informal learning opportunities can also be used to build and enhance the knowledge, skills base, and personal attributes needed for effective nursing consultation.

Applying Chapter Content

Review the case study presented in Chapter 2. Analyze the nurse consultant's actions in each phase of the nursing consultation process. Identify the knowledge, skills, and personal qualities underlying each role.

Read the following article. Analyze the appropriateness of consultation roles and competencies used by the nurse consultant in the article.

Badger, T. (1988). Mental health consultation with a surgical unit nursing staff. *Clinical Nurse Specialist, 2* (3), 144-148.

Review the skills, knowledge, and personal attributes for effective nursing consultation that are identified in Boxes 4-3, 4-4, and 4-5 of this chapter. Identify areas of personal weakness. Also identify strategies you might use to further develop these areas.

References

Barron, A. (1989). The CNS as consultant. In A. Hamric & J. Spross (Eds.), *The clinical nurse specialist in theory and practice* (2nd ed., pp. 125-146). Philadelphia: Saunders.

Brown, D. (1993). Training consultants: A call to action. *Journal of Counseling and Development, 72,* 139-143.

Cohen, W., & Murri, M. (1995). Managing the change process. *Journal of AHIMA, 66* (6), 40-47.

Dougherty, A. (1995). *Consultation: Practice and perspectives in school and community settings* (2nd ed.). Pacific Grove, CA: Brooks-Cole.

Fisher, R. & Ury, W. (1981). *Getting to yes: Negotiating agreement without giving in.* Boston: Houghton-Mifflin.

Kurpius, D., Fuqua, D., & Rozecki, T. (1993). The consulting process: A multidimensional approach. *Journal of Counseling and Development, 71,* 601-606.

Lippitt, G. & Lippitt, R. (1986). *The consulting process in action* (2nd ed.). San Diego: University Associates.

McDougall, G. (1987). The role of the clinical nurse specialist consultant in organizational development. *Clinical Nurse Specialist, 1* (3), 133-139.

Metzger, R. (1995). *Developing a consultation practice.* Newbury Park, CA: Sage.

Monicken, D. (1995). Consultation in advanced practice nursing. In M. Snyder & M. Mirr (Eds.), *Advanced practice nursing: A guide to professional development* (pp. 183-195). New York: Springer Publishing.

Ulschak, F. & SnowAntle, S. (1990). *Consultation skills for health care professionals.* San Francisco: Jossey-Bass.

Additional Readings

Badger, T. (1988). Mental health consultation with a surgical unit nursing staff. *Clinical Nurse Specialist, 2* (3), 144-148.
This article is a case study of internal nursing consultation.

Beare, P. (1989). Essentials of win-win negotiation for the clinical nurse specialist. *Clinical Nurse Specialist, 3* (3), 138-141.
This article provides a case study of a clinical nurse specialist negotiating with a group of physicians.

Beyerman, K. (1988). Consultation roles of the clinical nurse specialist: A case study. *Clinical Nurse Specialist, 2* (2), 91-95.
The author presents the results of a study about the consultant activities of clinical nurse specialists.

Brown, D. (1993). Training consultants: A call to action. *Journal of Counseling & Development, 72,* 139-143.
The author emphasizes the need for consultants to receive formal training rather than rely on on-the-job training.

Cosier, R. & Dalton, D. (1993). Management consulting: Planning, entry, performance. *Journal of Counseling and Development, 72,* 191-196.
The authors describe the skills needed for successful management consultation.

Dougherty, A. (1995). *Consultation: Practice and perspectives in school and community settings* (2nd ed.). Pacific Grove, CA: Brooks-Cole.
Chapter 2 describes and gives examples of various roles used in the consultation process.

Fisher, R. & Ury, W. (1981). *Getting to yes: Negotiating agreement without giving in.* Boston: Houghton-Mifflin.
This is a classic text on creating win-win situations.

Hazelton, J., Boyum, C., & Frost, M. (1993). Clinical nurse specialist subroles: Foundations for entrepreneurship. *Clinical Nurse Specialist, 1* (1), 40-45.
The authors describe how the subroles of researcher, manager, educator, and clinician are used in consultation practice.

Lippitt, G. & Lippitt, R. (1986). *The consulting process in action* (2nd ed.). San Diego: University Associates.
Chapter 4 in this text describes consultation roles in terms of a continuum of task-oriented to process-oriented and directive to nondirective activities.

Stoltenberg, C. (1993). Supervising consultants in training: An application model of supervision. *Journal of Counseling and Development, 72,* 131-138.
The author argues that different consultation knowledge and skills require different learning experiences.

Ulschak, F. & SnowAntle, S. (1990). *Consultation skills for health care professionals.* San Francisco: Jossey-Bass.
Chapter 2 in this text discusses roles and skills for internal health care consultants.

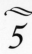

5

Understanding Organizations

*Every manager, consultant, or policymaker uses a personal
frame or image of organizations to gather information, make
judgments, and determine how best to get things done.
The more artistic among them are able to frame and reframe
experiences, sorting through tangled underbrush to find
solutions to problems.* (Bolman & Deal 1991)

Key terms: organization, theory, open system,
frame, power, culture

Entering a new setting can be overwhelming—particularly when you have a specific task to accomplish with or within the setting in a limited period of time.
Think of the last time you entered an unfamiliar setting; perhaps you were starting a
new job or returning to school. Think, too, how much easier it would have been to
enter this setting if you had some sense of what the setting was *really* like. Because all
settings are complex, ambiguous, and full of conflict, it is easy for a newcomer to
experience frustration, cynicism, powerlessness, and failure (Bolman & Deal 1991).
Nurse consultants work with, on behalf of, and within organizations and experience
these feelings every time they begin a new consultation relationship. For nurse consultants, understanding organizations can not only alleviate these feelings of frustration, but can facilitate a successful consultation outcome.

Organizations are groups of people that have been put together for a particular
purpose (Dougherty 1995). In a nursing consultation relationship, an organization
can be the consultee, the client, or the problem setting. Regardless of the role an organization plays in a specific consultation situation, understanding the characteristics,
or "personality," of the organization increases the likelihood that the consultation
relationship will be successful. Without this understanding, a nurse consultant may
attribute problems to the wrong cause, develop an action plan that is incomplete or
incompatible with the characteristics of the client system, and overlook important
evaluation information; in fact, without this understanding a nurse consultant may
never even accomplish psychological entry. Savvy nurse consultants can also capitalize on an organization's characteristics to enhance a nursing consultation relationship. For nurse consultants, the ability to understand an organization and answer the
question "What *really* is going on here?" is an essential survival skill and the adage,
"Organizations serve their masters" (Bolman & Deal 1991) holds true.

Organizational theories are sets of ideas that attempt to explain what organizations need in order to be effective. It is beyond the scope of this chapter to introduce
and develop all theories, sources, and explanations about organizations. Instead, the
purpose of this chapter is to provide enough practical information to enable nurse
consultants to function effectively and professionally with or within an organization.
This purpose is consistent with the goal of this text: to teach the specific skills of nurs-

ing consultation. Recognizing that there exists a wide variety of theories about organizations, the theories or perspectives presented in this chapter have been purposefully selected to enrich the reader's thinking and foster the development of new attitudes and ideas about how organizations work and how nurse consultants can help organizations solve their problems.

This chapter begins by presenting open systems theory as the over-arching theory that cuts across or undergirds all other organizational perspectives (Bolman & Deal 1991). Next, the concept of "frames" is introduced as an additional way of viewing and understanding organizations. The last two sections of the chapter present contemporary perspectives on power in organizations and organizational culture. As you read this chapter, think about the following questions:

- How do an organization's characteristics affect a nurse consultant's access to the organization's members, optimum ways of communication, and selection of a problem solution?

- What are your own beliefs and biases about organizations? What implications might these have for your practice of nursing consultation?

- What types of problems with a nursing consultation relationship might your beliefs and biases create? How would you address these problems?

Organizations as Open Systems

Open systems theory is a broad-based perspective on organizations that is derived from attempts to understand biological events (Dougherty 1995). Open systems theory views organizations as living organisms striving to adapt and respond to their environments, and having various degrees of success in doing so. An open systems perspective is the one used most frequently by consultants (Ridley & Mendoza 1993). The perspective cuts across all other organizational perspectives and is generally considered the best perspective available for conceptualizing an organization as a complex whole.

Components of Open Systems

Open systems are characterized by components and subcomponents. These components comprise the "personality" of a system: what it does and why it carries out its tasks the way in which it does.

Outputs Outputs are the products, services, or ideas that are a system's reason for existence (Harrison 1994). Nurse consultants generally work with organizations that have a service as their output: education, home health care, acute care, long-term care, outpatient surgery, and so forth. Nurse consultants may be asked to work with organizations to solve problems related to the quantity or quality of their outputs.

Inputs Inputs are the resources an organization obtains from its environments to create outputs. Inputs can be raw materials, people (human resources), financial resources, and equipment. Information, knowledge, and legal authorizations are other examples of inputs an organization needs in order to create its output (Harrison 1994). Some types of input are linked to the creation of outputs in more than one way. Consider, for example, the input of "people" as it relates to health care organizations. First, people (patients) are needed as the "raw material" that is acted on in order to create the system output of "healthier people." In addition, people are needed as human resources who will act on the patients to create the organization's product.

Technology A system's technology refers to the techniques used to transform inputs into outputs (Harrison 1994). Nurse consultants work primarily with systems that emphasize mental technologies such as diagnostic reasoning, physical technologies such as hands-on nursing care, chemical technologies such as drug therapy, and social technologies such as counseling and support.

Environment Systems are embedded in two "layers" of environment. The *task environment* is the external conditions that are directly related to a system's main operation and technology (Harrison 1994). The *general environment* is the more removed external conditions that have long-term or only infrequent influences on the organization and its task environment. Box 5-1 lists conditions and institutions that might constitute an organization's task and general environments.

Goals Goals are future states sought by the system's dominant decision makers (Harrison 1994). The system component of goals includes the following subcomponents:
   Mission: the system's public communication of its overall long-term purpose. A mission statement reflects what the system wants the public to believe are its goals, values, and beliefs (Kuh 1993).
   Goals: desired end states.
   Objectives: specific targets and observable indicators of goal attainment.
   Strategies: general desired or planned route to goal achievement.
   Plans: detailed course of action toward an end.

Consider how these subcomponents might be present in the system of a university wellness committee:
   Mission: to promote the holistic health (physical, mental, and spiritual) of the entire university community.
   Goal: prevent an influenza outbreak among the university community.
   Objective: the number of employee absences attributed to influenza will be 80% lower than last year.
   Strategies: increase the influenza immunization rate among students, faculty, and staff.
   Plan: offer free immunizations at common campus locations; block student's registration if they are unable to show proof of immunization.

Behavior and Processes This system component includes the prevailing patterns of behavior, interactions, and relations among a system's members. Specific activities included as subcomponents of a system's behavior and processes are identified in Box 5-2.

Culture A system's culture includes its norms as well as its nature and identity. Culture also includes the values, beliefs, assumptions, behavior, and artifacts through which a system expresses its norms and identity. Organizational culture is discussed in a later section of this chapter.

Structure The final generally recognized system component is structure. A system's structure is the enduring relations among a system's members and the means by which these relations are maintained (Harrison 1994). Subcomponents of a system's structure are identified in Box 5-3. The function of system's structure is to hold the system together and give it order. A system often depicts its structure by means of an organizational chart. Such a chart identifies the number of units, levels of hierarchy, and pattern of communication (vertical or lateral) within a system.

   Figure 5-1 illustrates how the components of an open system link to one another. Note that technology, goals, behavior and processes, culture, and structure comprise

Box 5-1. Open System Subcomponents: The Task and General Environments

Task Environment: the external conditions that directly affect a system's main operation and technology. Subcomponents of the task environment include:
- Funding sources
- Suppliers: providers of inputs, including referral sources
- Unions
- Market for product or services
- Customers or clients
- Regulators: accrediting agencies, licensing restrictions, reimbursement policies
- Competitors
- Collaborative partners: ownership, affiliation
- Availability of inputs
- Physical environment, including location

General Environment: the external conditions that exert either ongoing and long-term or infrequent effects on the system and its task environment. Subcomponents of the general environment include:
- The economy
- The legal system
- The general state of scientific and technologic knowledge
- Social institutions (such as the family)
- Social trends
- Population composition
- The political system
- Cultures within which the system operates

Reference: Harrison, M. (1994). *Diagnosing organizations: Methods, models, and processes* (2nd ed.). Thousand Oaks, CA: Sage.

Box 5-2. Open System Subcomponents: Behavior and Processes

- Cooperation
- Conflict
- Coordination
- Communication patterns
- Means of controlling behavior: rewards and punishments
- Power relations
- Problem-solving processes
- Goal-setting processes
- Information-gathering processes
- Evaluation and self-criticism
- Learning (individual members and the system as a whole)

Reference: Harrison, M. (1994). *Diagnosing organizations: Methods, models, and processes* (2nd ed.). Thousand Oaks, CA: Sage.

Box 5-3. Open System Subcomponents: Structure

- Role assignments and job descriptions
- The physical arrangement and grouping of positions within the system
- Policies and procedures
- Communication and coordination activities: meetings, memos, and so forth.
- Personnel processes: hiring, firing, evaluations, rewards
- Actual patterns of interacting and maintaining control that differ from offi-
  cially mandated ones; otherwise known as the "informal system"

Reference: Harrison, M. (1994). *Diagnosing organizations: Methods, models, and processes* (2nd ed.).
Thousand Oaks, CA: Sage.

---

a system's internal environment. These internal environmental components are linked to a system's external environments by the system's inputs and outputs.

Properties of Open Systems

In addition to having the components described above, open systems are character-ized by a set of "properties" or behavioral characteristics.

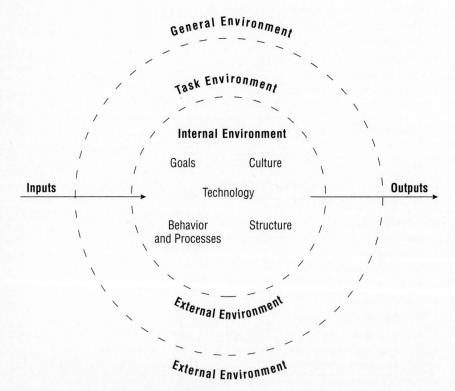

Figure 5-1 Organizations as Open Systems
A system's components define its personality, describe what the system does, and identify factors that explain its operating style.

First and foremost, the components of open systems are interrelated and influence one another (Bolman & Deal 1991; Fuqua & Kurpius 1993; Harrison 1994). This means an open system is influenced by its members and internal environments as well as by its external environments. Developments in one system component then, can have far-reaching effects. For example, new regulations (external environment) about patient care tasks that can be performed by unlicensed assistive personnel could affect a home care agency's personnel needs (human resource inputs) as well as supervisory practices (behaviors and processes) and job descriptions (structures). These changes, in turn, could alter the agency's culture.

A second property of open systems, closely related to the first, is their hierarchical arrangement (Bolman & Deal 1991; Harrison 1994). Thus every system is at once a supersystem for the systems or components it contains and a subsystem for systems in which it is embedded.

The interrelatedness of a system's components gives rise to the third property of open systems: a system is more than and different from the sum of its parts (Bolman & Deal 1991). The nature of an open system as a whole is a product of the relationships among its components and with its external environments. A nurse-managed clinic, for example, is a product of the nursing staff—their skills and personalities, the clinic's clients and their needs and resources, the community in which the clinic is located, laws governing the practice of nursing, and so on.

The fourth property of open systems is that communication among system components occurs across semipermeable boundaries. That is, an open system is selective about what it imports and exports. This property enables a system to protect itself from being bombarded by irrelevant information and other environmental factors. It also enables a system to maintain a competitive edge by withholding information about itself from the environment.

The ability to selectively communicate with its environment accounts for the fifth property of open systems: open systems are capable of negative entropy. That is, an open system can grow and survive rather than decline and die, if it is able to work out a mutually beneficial relationship with its external environments (Bolman & Deal 1991). This capacity for negative entropy is illustrated in health care when a small rural hospital responds to its community's changing demographics and needs by changing its services; adding long-term care beds, for instance, rather than closing its doors.

A sixth property of open systems is that they are constantly in a state of dynamic equilibrium. More specifically, an open system strives to maintain a steady state in an environment that is constantly changing (Bolman & Deal 1991). Open systems engage in reactive change in response to problems in their internal or external environments that are causing disequilibrium. An example would be the firing of an unsafe employee. Open systems also maintain a steady state by engaging in proactive or anticipatory change, improving internal operations or environmental relations before problems arise. An open system may, for example, provide staff inservices on new policies or technologies. Nurse consultants work with systems to solve problems that reflect actual or anticipated disequilibrium.

The final property that characterizes open systems is that of equifinality. Because systems are comprised of highly interactive components, many different paths can lead to the same result (Fuqua & Kurpius 1993). Therefore, systems have options in terms of how they achieve their goals and maintain a steady state. If it is not feasible to change one component, resource availability, for instance, it may be possible to accomplish the same goal by changing technology or some other component.

Box 5-4 summarizes the properties of open systems.

Box 5-4. The Properties of Open Systems

- The components of a system are interrelated and influence one another.
- Every system is a hierarchical arrangement of subsystems and supersystems.
- A system is more than and different from the sum of its parts.
- System components communicate across semipermeable boundaries.
- Open systems are capable of negative entropy. That is, they have a survival and growth orientation.
- Open systems strive to maintain a dynamic equilibrium.
- The property of equifinality gives a system options for achieving its goals and maintaining a steady state. That is, in an open system, many paths can lead to the same result.

Implications for Nursing Consultation

A systems perspective is useful to nurse consultants because it encourages consideration of all parts of an organization, including the relationships and interactions that occur among these parts. Because problems are viewed as part of a complex chain of possible events and interactions, a systems perspective helps the nurse consultant more accurately diagnose the cause of a consultation problem. A systems perspective then, encourages the nurse consultant to consider an organization's problem as either a symptom of a "relationship problem" with the external environment or an "operation problem" within the organization's internal environment, rather than accept the problem at face value (Harrison 1994). Box 5-5 outlines how an open systems perspective can be used to search for explanations for an organization's problems.

A systems perspective also helps a nurse consultant to develop more effective interventions for resolving a consultation problem. Because of the interaction or chain of influence that exists among a system's components, different consultation interventions may accomplish the same results. If one proposed intervention is unacceptable to a consultee or is not feasible within the client system, a systems perspective gives the nurse consultant permission to consider other interventions that might accomplish the same goal.

Furthermore, a systems perspective facilitates the development of more effective problem solutions because it forces a nurse consultant to consider how a specific problem-solving strategy will affect other parts of the system. Anticipating how a problem solution will affect other parts of a system decreases the likelihood that the consultation process will be surprised by adverse side effects to a consultation intervention. For example, a nurse consultant might propose to address the unmet support needs of families of patients in an acute care unit by developing a support group. This problem solution, because it requires both physical space and nursing staff support, will only be successful if the nurse consultant anticipates this chain of influence and develops strategies that will help the other parts of the client system adapt to demands created by the problem solution.

A final advantage of the systems perspective of organizations is that during the evaluation phase of the nursing consultation process, the nurse consultant may consider a variety of possible indicators of success for a nursing consultation relationship. Recognizing that success can be demonstrated in a variety of ways increases the likelihood that a consultation relationship will be judged a success because in many situations, a relationship will have had a positive effect somewhere in the client system, even if the original nursing consultation problem has not been completely resolved.

> ## Box 5-5. Looking for Problem Causes:
> ### An Open Systems Perspective
>
> Explanations for an organization's problems can often be identified by gathering the following information about its components:
>
> *Outputs*
> - Quantity
> - Quality
> - Responsiveness to consumer needs and desires
>
> *Inputs*
> - Availability
> - Quality
> - Access issues: timeliness, seasonal variation
> - Cost—does high price of inputs strain other parts of the system?
> - Reserves and their liquidity
>
> *Technology*
> - Cost
> - Efficiency: accidents, waste, downtime
>
> *Environment*
> - Affiliation and ownership: associated benefits and constraints
> - Physical and social surroundings
> - Recent or anticipated changes
>
> *Goals*
> - Official goal statements
> - Mission statement
> - Plans for achieving goals—are they realistic?
> - Budget patterns and their consistency with goals
> - Consistency of strategies with mission statement
>
> *Behavior and Processes*
> - Communication patterns
> - Decision-making practices
>
> *Culture*
> - Indicators of a system's identity; consistency with goals and strategies
> - Diversity versus homogeneity of culture among the system's subcomponents
>
> *Structure*
> - Arrangement of the system: divisions, units, levels of hierarchy
> - Control mechanisms: policies, procedures, rewards, punishments, communication

Other Organizational Frames

Open systems theory explains organizations in terms of interacting components. While this is one explanation for how organizations work and what makes them effective or ineffective, it is not the only explanation. In fact, viewing organizations from only an open systems perspective fails to acknowledge the other beliefs, assumptions, and motivations that can account for organizational behavior. A more complete picture of an organization can be gained by viewing it from additional vantage points or "frames" (Bolman & Deal 1991).

The major schools of organizational thought can be consolidated into four frames, each of which acknowledges a different dimension of an organization. Most organizations view themselves from the vantage point of one frame or another. Superimposing these frames on an open systems perspective of organizations increases the nurse consultant's ability to appreciate the complexity of organizational life. This, in turn, increases the likelihood that a nurse consultant will accurately diagnose an organization's problem and generate meaningful and feasible problem solutions.

The Structural Frame

The structural frame has its roots in sociology and views organizations as rational systems. The structural frame acknowledges the link between the formal roles and relationships within an organization (the structural component of an open system) and the organization's ability to achieve its goals (Bolman & Deal 1991). Organizations that view themselves through a structural frame create structures to fit the organization's environments and technology. For example, an organization may set up a division of labor, or may establish rules, policies, and management hierarchies. These organizations tend to experience problems when their structures fail to fit the situation. Their preferred way of resolving problems is "restructuring": developing new policies, procedures, and management hierarchies.

The Human Resource Frame

The human resource frame mirrors the ideas of organizational social psychologists. This frame emphasizes the interdependence between an organization and its members. It also recognizes that organizations are inhabited by individuals with unique needs, abilities, beliefs, and attitudes (Bolman & Deal 1991). Organizations that are based on a human resource frame maintain that the key to organizational effectiveness is a good fit between the needs of the organization and the needs of its members. Conversely, when there is a poor fit between the organization and its members, one or both will suffer: individuals will be exploited or will seek to exploit the organization, or both (Bolman & Deal 1991). Thus the human resource frame emphasizes the importance of the relationship between the open system components of behavior and processes and human resource inputs (including job satisfaction) on one hand, and the components of technology, goals, and structures on the other. Organizations that are based on a human resource frame try to solve their problems by changing the organization's form (behavior and processes, structure) in such a way that enables people to get their job done and feel good about what they are doing. Offering education and training, adding more personnel, and changing the system's reward structure are examples of consultation interventions that are consistent with the human resource frame.

The Political Frame

The political frame, developed by political scientists, views organizations as "arenas" where groups compete for power and scarce resources (Bolman & Deal 1991). This frame attaches particular importance to both the structural and behavior and processes components of an open system. The political frame emphasizes that conflict is a fact of organizational life because of differences in the needs and perspectives of the organization's various members. The political frame asserts that organizational effectiveness is the result of an organization's ability to effectively negotiate, build coalitions, bargain, and compromise with its members and with its environment. Organizations working from a political frame may experience problems because power is either concentrated in the wrong places, or is so broadly dispersed that nothing gets accomplished. Problems are solved by changing the power dynamics in the organization. A later section of this chapter discusses power in organizations.

The Symbolic Frame

The final frame identified by Bolman and Deal (1991)—the symbolic frame—has its roots in social and cultural anthropology and emphasizes the importance of the cultural component of an open system. The symbolic frame differs from the other frames because it asserts organizations are *not* rational and organizational leaders have only a limited ability to create organizational effectiveness through power, processes, or structures. The symbolic frame views organizations as cultures driven by images and rituals rather than by rules and authority. From a symbolic perspective, organizational problems occur when "actors play their parts badly, symbols lose their meaning, and ceremonies and rituals lose their potency" (Bolman & Deal 1991). This frame asserts that organizations can solve their problems by rebuilding their expressive or spiritual side using symbols and rituals.

Box 5-6 summarizes the key attributes of these four organizational frames.

Implications for Nursing Consultation

The capacity to view an organization through multiple frames enhances a nurse consultant's ability to accurately diagnose an organization's problems and arrive at effective problem solutions. In contrast, a single frame captures only a part of an organization's picture. Because each frame has its blind spots and biases, no single frame is comprehensive enough to make an organization truly understandable or manageable. The following examples demonstrate a nurse consultant using only a single frame to approach the problem of staff discord in a home health care agency. Note how a "single-frame approach" can limit the scope of a problem solution.

Structural frame: "As the agency has grown, nurses' responsibilities have become blurred. Frequently, it is unclear who (staff nurse, care aide, or supervisor) is responsible for what. This is causing stress and conflict. You need to restructure. Let's start by drawing a new organizational chart. Then we'll tackle policies and procedures."

Human resource frame: "You are ignoring the nurses' needs to feel autonomous and valued. Let's put together some workshops on communication and look at some sort of an incentive system."

Political frame: "The real problem is that the CEO and board have too much power and the staff nurses have too little. We need to bring these parties together to negotiate and compromise."

Symbolic frame: "Rapid growth has caused the agency to lose its identity. Its values have also become unclear—is it profit or the patients that are of primary interest? Let's try to revitalize the agency's sense of identity and purpose. We'll start by designing a new logo. Then we'll get the staff matching jackets to wear."

In contrast, the nurse consultant who uses all four frames and open systems theory to approach this problem might respond as follows:

"This is a complex problem. As the agency has grown, roles and relationships have changed. The addition of more staff has also changed the agency's culture and power structure. Old ways of doing things and relating don't work anymore. We need to make sure we address all of these problems. Otherwise, we will only put a band-aid on the problem and the band-aid will fall off in a couple of days. Let's start by meeting with the staff to find out what they identify as the key issue. Then we'll go from there…"

In summary, the nurse consultant who can view an organization through multiple frames has a more flexible and comprehensive approach to problem solving. Hence,

---

Box 5-6. "Frames": Alternative Views of Organizations

The Structural Frame

- **Theoretical roots:** Sociology
- **Emphasis:** Rules, policies, managerial hierarchy, division of labor
- **Problem explanations:** Poor fit between a system's structural components and its environment and technology
- **Preferred problem solutions:** Restructuring
- **Open systems components reflected in frame:** Structure, environments, technology

The Human Resource Frame

- **Theoretical roots:** Organizational social psychology
- **Emphasis:** Interdependence between an organization and its members
- **Problem explanations:** Poor fit between the needs of the organization and the needs of its members
- **Preferred problem solutions:** Change the organization's form (structure and processes) to meet members' needs
- **Open systems components reflected in frame:** Inputs (human resources), technology, goals, behavior and processes, structure

The Political Frame

- **Theoretical roots:** Political science
- **Emphasis:** Conflict, power
- **Problem explanations:** Power concentrated in the wrong places or too widely dispersed
- **Preferred problem solutions:** Change power dynamics: negotiate, compromise, build coalitions
- **Open systems components reflected in frame:** Behavior and processes, structure

The Symbolic Frame

- **Theoretical roots:** Social and cultural anthropology
- **Emphasis:** The symbolic rather than rational nature of organizations
- **Problem explanations:** Symbols lose their meaning, rituals lose their potency, "actors play their parts badly"
- **Preferred problem solutions:** Rebuild the expressive and spiritual side of the organization
- **Open systems components reflected in frame:** Culture, behavior and processes, structure

---

problem solutions are more likely to be meaningful and feasible and have longevity. Box 5-7 provides examples of questions a nurse consultant can use to approach an organization and its consultation problem from multiple frames.

Box 5-7. Looking for Problem Causes: Using Multiple Frames

Structure-Oriented Questions
- What is the organization's structural arrangement (division of labor, levels of hierarchy)?
- How is the organization's structure maintained?
- Is the organization's structure "in sync" with its internal and external environments?
- What effects does the organization's structure have on the organization's cohesiveness and ability to interact with its environment (procure inputs, dispense outputs)?

Human Resource-Oriented Questions
- To what extent do people feel a part of the organization?
- To what extent are members' needs met by the organization?
- How could processes and structures be changed so that needs are better met?

Political-Oriented Questions
- What are the resources that are scarce in this organization?
- How are problems related to scarce resources handled? (Conflict, compromise, negotiation)
- Who is best able to obtain scarce resources? How do they do this? What conflicts does this create?

Symbolic-Oriented Questions
- What is the organization's identity? How is this identity communicated? Is the identity clear? Is it universally shared?
- What values are reflected in the organization's identity? Are these the values really held by the organization and its members?
- How is the organization's identity reinforced (symbols, rituals, and so forth?) Are these strategies effective?
- How can the organization's structure and behavior and processes be altered to strengthen the organization's symbolic dimension?

Power in Organizations

Power can be defined as the capacity to influence someone else's behavior and attitudes (Yukl 1989) and the ability to get things done. Every member of an organization, including a nurse consultant, has some kind of power. The ability to decipher who in an organization has what kind of power helps a nurse consultant identify individuals who can either facilitate or act as barriers to a nursing consultation relationship.

Sources of Power

Generally two possible sources of power are recognized: positional and personal. These two sources or determinants of power can interact in complex ways. In many cases, it is difficult to determine the sources from which an individual derives power. Nonetheless, it is important for nurse consultants to be able to identify the nature of the power being exercised in a situation since power dynamics and reactions to them are a common cause of organizational problems.

Positional Power Positional power is derived from opportunities inherent in an individual's position or formal role within an organization (Yukl 1989). Positional power is usually associated with being a member of the "upper" organizational hierarchy. However, members of the "lowerarchy" (Bolman & Deal 1991) have their own types of positional power.

Formal authority is the most familiar type of positional power and belongs to organizational members who are in officially sanctioned leadership or management positions. Formal authority is positional power that is inherent with membership in the upper hierarchy of an organization. Individuals who have formal authority are entitled to make requests and binding decisions, as well as exercise control to the extent that those under their authority have the duty to obey. Usually this duty to obey has been internalized because of perceptions about prerogatives, obligations, and responsibilities associated with an organizational position. Because authority is not associated with an obligation to return favors, it is acceptable as a form of power for day-to-day organizational functioning. Authority is only accepted, however, when the person exercising it is perceived by members of the lowerarchy to be a legitimate occupant of his/her position of authority.

An individual's position within the organization is also associated with control over rewards and punishments. Reward power is only effective when the promised reward is actually bestowed and is perceived as fair exchange for the request that is being made. Coercive power (related to control over punishments) is effective only when it is applied to a small proportion of followers under conditions perceived to be legitimate by the majority of them (Yukl 1989).

Other specific types of power associated with being a member of an organization's upper hierarchy include control over resources and information, ecological control, and orchestration power. Information control is a particularly important type of positional power because individuals who are able to access information also have the ability to distort it and control its distribution.

Individuals in gatekeeper and boundary positions within an organization also have positional power. These individuals interact directly with the organization's environment on a day-to-day basis and therefore have a certain degree of control over resources and information. Think, for example, of the control an office receptionist has over the number of patients (resources) seen by a health care provider during any given day.

Members of an organization's lowerarchy have their own types of positional power. The lowerarchy determines whether and how tasks are actually carried out (implementation power). Members of the lowerarchy also possess "helpless power," the right to expect assistance from individuals who are in a position to render it (Friedman 1992). Patients, for example, have helpless power in that they have the socially agreed upon right to demand assistance and resources from nurses, the health care system, and the general public. Helpless power can become manipulative and problematic when the individual or system that is being asked for help is already drained of resources. Finally, members of the lowerarchy have a certain amount of reward and punishment power. For example, workers can reward their supervisors (enhance the supervisor's image) by doing good work. They can also "punish" their supervisors by giving them unfavorable evaluations.

Personal Power Personal power is derived from an individual's personal characteristics such as knowledge, special skills, persuasiveness, and the ability to establish rapport, trust, and friendships. Personal power can be possessed by members at all

---

Box 5-8. Sources of Power

Positional Power

Positional power is derived from an individual's position or role within an organization. Positional power includes the following types of power:

- Formal authority: the right to make requests and binding decisions
- Control over resources: the ability to access needed organizational resources
- Control over rewards and punishments: the ability to bestow rewards and impose punishments
- Control over information: the ability to access, distribute, and distort information
- Ecological control: control over the organization's physical environment and the organization of work
- Orchestration power: the right to organize and plan tasks
- Implementation power: the ability to determine whether and how tasks are carried out
- Helpless power: the right to expect assistance

Personal Power

Personal power can be possessed by members at any level of an organization and can substitute for, enhance, or help an individual acquire positional power. Personal power includes the following types of power:

- Expertise: power derived from the dependence of others on an individual for special advice or assistance
- Charisma: power derived from "emotional attractiveness" and persuasive skills
- Friendship: power that creates a desire of others to please
- Trust and rapport: power that facilitates coalition-building

Reference: Bolman, L., & Deal, T. (1991). *Reframing organizations: Artistry, choice, and leadership.* San Francisco: Jossey-Bass; and Yukl, G. (1989). *Leadership in organizations* (2nd ed.). Englewood Cliffs, NJ: Prentice Hall.

---

levels of an organization. Personal power is important because it can substitute for, enhance, or help an individual acquire positional power.

Expert power is personal power that is derived from an individual's possession of specialized knowledge and skills ("expertise") and the fact that others need this knowledge and skill. Expert power is effective only to the extent that it is recognized and perceived as credible and reliable by others.

Charisma is power that is derived from "emotional attractiveness" (Yukl 1989). An individual with charisma exudes vision, enthusiasm, and strong convictions, and is able to gather followers through the use of persuasive speaking skills. Charisma enables an individual to build coalitions. Charisma is also associated with the ability or opportunity to define a group's beliefs and values.

The ability to establish rapport, trust, and friendships are additional types of personal power. Friendship and trust facilitate coalition building, as well as create loyalty and a willingness in others to return favors.

Box 5-8 summarizes the different types of power associated with position and personal qualities.

Assessing Organizational Power

A nurse consultant needs to be able to identify who has what types of power within an organization. This information gives the nurse consultant the opportunity to mobilize and create partnerships with individuals in organizations who are able to gather followers and cooperation from others.

To a large extent, the nurse consultant needs to piece together information from a variety of observations and reports in order to determine who within an organization has what kind of power. Symbols of power such as office location and furnishings, or location of an individual on an organizational chart often correspond to positional power. Job descriptions and titles (associate versus assistant, for example) also are traditional symbols of positional power. However, it is a mistake to assume that the individual with the symbols of power has the true power within the organization. Task allocation, for instance, may suggest authority—but may also reflect simple tradition.

The ability to set an organization's agendas and determine what issues are addressed, may be a more accurate indicator of *real* power. Power outcomes, such as who wins or has the final say, and decision-making processes (such as consensus or compromise and who agrees with whom) also tend to be accurate indicators of who has real influence within an organization. Compromise, for example, may indicate the ability of the lowerarchy to overrule the hierarchy. Consensus reflects the ability to form coalitions and results most likely from personal rather than positional power.

Box 5-9 lists questions for assessing power in organizations.

Implications for Nursing Consultation

Recognizing and understanding power dynamics can help a nurse consultant explain many organizational problems. For example, organizational conflict can occur when a member of the lowerarchy with personal power threatens the power of those in positions of formal authority. Problems with organizational efficiency might be attributable to a person in a boundary position who is exercising inappropriate control over resources. Finally, low morale or a lack of organizational cohesiveness might be traced to problems with control of information, rewards, or punishments. The nurse consultant could respond to these problems that are related to an organization's power dynamics in the following ways:

Help the person in a position of formal authority acquire personal skills that will enhance positional power

Clarify roles and responsibilities in relation to control over resources

Enhance perceptions of the legitimacy of control over information, rewards, and punishments

An understanding of power dynamics also enables the nurse consultant to recognize and capitalize on the power associated with the consultant role. Because the nursing consultation relationship is a time-limited one, nurse consultants lack any positional power of their own. The nurse consultant's power is derived instead from a combination of personal qualities and the ability to recognize and become aligned with persons in the organization who have positional power and can legitimize the nursing consultation relationship.

Nurse consultants are most frequently asked to help solve an organization's problem because of their perceived expertise, and for this reason it is important for nurse consultants to understand the limitations of expert power. Expert power is only effective to the extent that consultees lack the knowledge and skills needed to solve a problem on their own. Thus as a nursing consultation relationship pro-

---

Box 5-9. Questions for Assessing Power in Organizations

- Who does the organizational chart identify as being in positions of power?
- Who is in boundary positions? How much control do they have over information and other scarce resources?
- With whom are traditional symbols of power associated?
- Who gives the "orders"?
- Who wins or has the final say?
- Who controls decision-making processes?
- Who sets agendas?
- Who agrees or compromises with whom?

---

gresses and consultees gain more skill in managing their own problems, expertise becomes less effective as a source of power for maintaining the nursing consultation relationship. (However, as Chapter 12 discusses, consultee skill in managing the consultation problem on their own can be a signal to begin the disengagement phase of the nursing consultation relationship.) What is more, expert power can be initially intimidating to a consultee, especially if it increases the consultee's feeling of inadequacy. Because of these limitations of expert power, a nurse consultant needs to cultivate other forms of personal power such as charisma, friendship, and trust in order to establish and maintain an effective working relationship with a client system. Finally, nurse consultants need to learn how to supplement their personal power by building coalitions with the individuals in an organization who have different types of positional power.

Organizational Culture

An organization's culture is the pattern of beliefs, values, practices, and artifacts that define for its members who they are and how to do things (Bolman & Deal 1991). These patterns reflect the values, beliefs, and assumptions that the organization has developed over time as it has learned how to interact with its environments in order to fulfill its goals. An organization's culture represents its accumulated wisdom. This wisdom is continually being renewed and re-created as the organization admits new members.

An organization's culture serves three purposes. First, culture functions as a type of behavioral control. It does this by implicitly mandating, allowing, and prohibiting certain behaviors. For example, a culture of relative formality in a clinic might dictate behaviors such as wearing a uniform rather than street clothes, and addressing patients as Ms., Mrs., or Mr. rather than by first name.

A second purpose served by an organization's culture is integration. Culture creates "buy-in" to an organization's goals and operating decisions by fostering a sense of identity and unity. An organizational culture of harmony, for instance, may foster at least superficial buy-in to a clinic's decision to decrease work hours across the board rather than "downsize." Keep in mind with this example, however, that dissension may only be forced underground unless the organization also has a cultural value of openness.

The third purpose served by an organization's culture is that it provides a framework that helps the organization's members uniformly interpret situations they encounter. As an example, an organization's culture influences the extent to which a threatening event, such as downsizing or a budget crisis, is perceived as a problem or as an opportunity for growth.

Assessing Organizational Culture

Assessing an organization's culture involves gathering clues and drawing conclusions about the cultural meaning of these clues. Because clues can have multiple interpretations and can contradict one another, it is important to validate the accuracy of conclusions about an organization's culture with its members.

Assessing organizational culture is complicated by the fact that much of an organization's culture operates on an unconscious level and is taken for granted by both the organization as a whole and its members. Consequently, the nurse consultant must rely on observation of symbolic artifacts (tangible, visible indicators of an organization's culture) for clues about the organization's beliefs, values, and assumptions (Hughes 1990; Kuh 1993). Cultural artifacts can be material, verbal, or behavioral in nature.

Material Artifacts Material artifacts are physical indicators of an organization's culture. An organization's logo or seal is one example of a material artifact. The inclusion of a cross, for example, on the logo of many health care organizations communicates the traditional association of providing health care with benevolent, charitable, and altruistic motivations (Hughes 1990). The physical layout of an organization is another material artifact. Private offices versus open gathering spaces may suggest an organizational value of privacy as opposed to openness. The dress, appearance, and behavior of an organization's members is a third example of a material artifact. This indicator may provide clues about the tolerance of diversity and individualism within an organization. Think, for example, about the dress code at your place of employment and what this communicates about the organization's values. Is this reflection of organizational values accurate or not?

Verbal Artifacts Examples of verbal artifacts include an organization's mission statement, its public written materials such as brochures, and organizational myths. An organization's mission statement is a particularly revealing verbal artifact. A mission statement is an organization's public communication of its overall long-term purposes and reflects what the organization wants the public to believe are its values and beliefs (Kuh 1993).

Myths are stories that have developed about an organization and its members that may or may not be true. Myths help to establish, maintain, and explain certain behaviors within an organization. Myths also legitimize certain behaviors, mediate contradictions, communicate unconscious wishes and conflicts, and anchor an organization to its past. For example, the myth that "attendance" is taken at an organization's social functions and considered in an employee's performance evaluation helps to ensure that these functions will be attended. This myth also expresses the organization's wish that it be perceived as "one big happy family," a perception that can serve to hide conflict from the public.

Behavioral Artifacts Behavioral artifacts include ritualistic actions as well as standard organizational practices. Rituals decrease uncertainty and anxiety among members (especially during times of transition), and socialize and stabilize an organization's membership (Bolman & Deal 1991). Rituals can also be used to communicate messages to an organization's clients. An example of a ritualistic action would be staff nurses' tendency to take their breaks in the unit lounge rather than the hospital cafeteria. This might signify, or at least attempt to communicate, a cultural value of

---

Box 5-10. Guidelines for Assessing Organizational Culture

- Observe artifacts
  Material artifacts: logo, use of physical space, furnishings, members' dress
  Verbal artifacts: mission statement, brochures, myths
  Behavioral artifacts: rituals, standard organizational practices
- Consider as many artifacts as possible since some might have more than one possible meaning or may contradict other artifacts
- Use inductive reasoning (drawing general conclusions from specific observations) to form a cultural profile of the organization
- Verify this profile with the organization's members
- Refine impressions and gather more information as needed

"patients come first" among the unit's nurses. It might also, however, be interpreted as signifying elitism. Orientation processes are another common organizational ritual and serve to introduce new members to an organization's culture as well as decrease the anxiety associated with being "the new kid on the block." An example of a standard organizational practice would be promoting from within organizational ranks rather than doing an external search. While this practice shows support for employees, it may also indicate a lack of value for diversity.

Behavioral artifacts can be evaluated in terms of their consistency with what the organization communicates to the public about itself in verbal and material artifacts, such as its mission statement and logo. When behavioral artifacts conflict with other artifacts, behaviors should be considered the more reliable indicator of the organization's culture.

Box 5-10 summarizes the guidelines for assessing organizational culture.

Implications for Nursing Consultation

Knowledge about an organization's culture provides the nurse consultant with information about what is permissible when implementing the consultation relationship. Organizations vary, for example, in terms of beliefs about how permissible it is to ask for help in solving problems. This cultural belief affects both when in the problem cycle a nurse consultant is likely to be contacted (at the prevention, early intervention, or crisis stage) and the nursing consultation interaction pattern that is most likely to be acceptable to the client system. A process consultation interaction pattern, for instance, requires a culture of openness and assuming personal responsibility for problems and solutions.

Sensitivity to an organization's culture enables the nurse consultant to tailor interventions and recommendations to the norms and values of the client system. For example, if privacy is a value, assessment and evaluation findings are not likely to be accepted if they are presented in a public forum. When a nurse consultant's interactions and interventions ignore, or are in direct conflict with, an organization's culture, they are likely to create tension, resistance, and frustration for everyone involved in the nursing consultation relationship. As a result of this, the underlying nursing consultation problem will remain unresolved.

Lastly, awareness of an organization's culture makes good "business sense" for the nurse consultant. A nurse consultant is always a guest in a problem setting, and cultural awareness and sensitivity can decrease the discomfort and feelings of awkwardness often associated with visitor status. Cultural awareness and sensitivity also facilitate gathering needed information, establishing rapport and credibility, and generating an acceptable and successful action plan.

Chapter Summary

Nurse consultants work with, on behalf of, and within organizations. How a nurse consultant looks at an organization and how much is understood about what is *really* going on within the organization determines how successful the nursing consultation relationship will be. Viewing organizations through multiple frames, including open systems theory, and acknowledging power dynamics and culture can help the nurse consultant gain entry to as well as problem-solve with an organization. Characteristics of organizations, if ignored, can act as barriers to effective nursing consultation. On the other hand, the nurse consultant who is aware of an organization's characteristics and their relationship to a specific problem situation can at least accommodate and, possibly, mobilize these characteristics to increase the effectiveness of the consultation relationship.

Applying Chapter Content

- Use an open systems perspective to diagram your work setting.
  Identify who within this system has what kind of power. What types of consultation problems are likely to arise in this system? How would the components of this system act as facilitators and barriers to the nursing consultation process?

- Consider the frames that were discussed in this chapter.
  Which frame do you think your school or work setting uses to see itself? What problems might this create? Can you identify any current problems in this setting that are related to this frame? Which frame do you find most appealing? How might this influence your effectiveness as a nurse consultant?

- Examine mission statements and printed material from several organizations. (It might be easiest to start with your school or work setting.)
  What do these materials communicate about the organization's culture? To what extent is this consistent with your knowledge of this organization?

- Identify myths from your school or work setting.
  What purpose do these myths serve? What cultural messages do they convey? How accurate are these messages?

References

Bolman, L., & Deal, T. (1991). *Reframing organizations: Artistry, choice, and leadership.* San Francisco: Jossey-Bass.

Dougherty, A. (1995). *Consultation: Practice and perspectives in school and community settings* (2nd ed.). Pacific Grove, CA: Brooks-Cole.

Friedman, M. (1992). *Family nursing: Theory and practice* (3rd ed.). Norwalk, CT: Appleton & Lange.

Fuqua, D., & Kurpius, D. (1993). Conceptual models in organizational consultation. *Journal of Counseling and Development, 71,* 607-618.

Harrison, M. (1994). *Diagnosing organizations: Methods, models, and processes* (2nd ed.). Thousand Oaks, CA: Sage.

Hughes, L. (1990). Assessing organizational culture: Strategies for the external consultant. *Nursing Forum, 25* (1), 15-19.

Kuh, G. (1993). Appraising the character of a college. *Journal of Counseling and Development, 71,* 661-667.

Ridley, C., & Mendoza, D. (1993). Putting organizational effectiveness into practice: The preeminent consultation task. *Journal of Counseling and Development, 72,* 168-177.

Yukl, G. (1989). *Leadership in organizations* (2nd ed.). Englewood Cliffs, NJ: Prentice Hall.

Additional Readings

Bolman, L., & Deal, T. (1991). *Reframing organizations: Artistry, choice, and leadership.* San Francisco: Jossey-Bass.
The authors describe the structural, human resource, political, and symbolic dimensions of organizations. This is a highly readable text that offers a comprehensive view of organizations and how they handle change.

Deal, T., & Kennedy, A. (1982). *Corporate cultures: The rites and rituals of corporate life.* Reading, MA: Addison-Wesley.
This text is a fascinating discussion of organizational culture and its impact on organizational functioning.

Dougherty, A. (1995). *Consultation: Practice and perspectives in school and community settings* (2nd ed.). Pacific Grove, CA: Brooks-Cole.
Chapter 8 of this text provides an overview of traditional organizational theories.

Friedman, M. (1992). *Family nursing: Theory and practice* (3rd ed.). Norwalk, CT: Appleton & Lange.
The discussion of family power in this text is directly applicable to groups and organizations.

Fuqua, D., & Kurpius, D. (1993). Conceptual models in organizational consultation. *Journal of Counseling and Development, 71,* 607-618.
This article presents a useful overview of open systems theory.

Harrison, M. (1994). *Diagnosing organizations: Methods, models, and processes* (2nd ed.). Thousand Oaks, CA: Sage.
This is an excellent text about assessing organizations using an open systems framework. Assessment tools are included in the text's appendices.

Katz, D., & Kahn, R. (1978). *The social psychology of organizations.* New York: Wiley.
This is a classic text about the social nature of organizations.

Kuh, G. (1993). Appraising the character of a college. *Journal of Counseling and Development, 71,* 661-667.
The author analyzes the nature of an organization. Particular attention is given to assessment and implications of an organization's mission, philosophy, and culture.

Perrow, C. (1986). *Complex organizations: A critical essay* (3rd ed.). New York: Random House.
This classic text functions as a reader of different organizational theories.

Price, J., & Reiss-Brennan, B. (1989). Consulting telesis: A systems approach. *Nursing Management, 20* (11), 80A-80E.
The authors provide a useful discussion of systems theory.

Ridley, C., & Mendoza, D. (1993). Putting organizational effectiveness into practice: The preeminent consultation task. *Journal of Counseling and Development, 72,* 168-177.
This article describes the relationship between an organization's view of itself and how it defines organizational effectiveness.

Stone, D. (1988). *Policy paradox and political reason.* Glenview, IL: Scott, Foresman.
This fascinating text explores the political nature of organizations.

Ulschak, F., & SnowAntle, S. (1990). *Consultation skills for health care professionals.* San Francisco: Jossey-Bass.
Chapter 8 of this text focuses on organizational culture.

Yukl, G. (1989). *Leadership in organizations* (2nd ed.). Englewood Cliffs, NJ: Prentice Hall.
This text includes a useful discussion about different organizational structures and different types of organizational power.

Group Dynamics

*Group behavior can be a wonder to behold, as when a
good team begins to click. More often, however, they
are anti-holistic...* (Robbins & Finley 1996)

Key terms: task roles, personal roles, counteractive influence,
groupthink, team

Being a member of a group can be stressful. "Have I been accepted?" and, "What
am I supposed to do?" are just two of the many questions that group members
frequently ask. Working with a group to help its members accomplish a specific task
can also be stressful. Nurse consultants frequently work in this capacity with groups
of consultees or on behalf of client groups. Questions that nurse consultants need to
be able to answer when implementing the nursing consultation process with a group
include, "What really is happening here?" "Why do people behave the way they do?"
and "What can I do about it?"

Working with a group to problem-solve and implement change has both advantages and disadvantages. On the one hand, groups have greater cumulative knowledge and diversity of perspective, as well as more time and energy than individuals.
Groups, therefore, can be very creative, productive, and stimulating. On the other
hand, groups have certain liabilities. They can be stagnant and conformist. Too often,
groups overrespond to social pressures or allow personal goals or needs of group
members to undermine the group's purpose (Bolman & Deal 1991). The nurse consultant working with a group must be able to understand group dynamics and intervene to facilitate effective functioning of the group if the nursing consultation relationship is to be successful.

Group dynamics have a decisive influence on the work a group is able to accomplish. The dynamics observed in groups reflect issues related to group members'
roles and functions, group norms, intragroup cooperation and cohesiveness, and the
exercise of influence within the group (Bolman & Deal 1991; Goodstein 1978). How
these issues affect both individual group members and the group as a whole can be
observed in a group's communication and decision-making processes. The above-
mentioned issues and the ways in which group members respond to these issues,
both individually and collectively, constitute a group's dynamics.

Much has been written in nursing literature about group dynamics. Most of these
discussions have either a mental health (nurse as therapist) or management (nurse as
supervisor) perspective. The nurse consultant-consultee relationship is, in contrast, a
peer relationship; this has implications for both the significance of observed group
dynamics as well as appropriate interventions.

This chapter begins with an overview of group characteristics, group behavior,
and explanations of group behavior. The discussion that follows centers around what

the nurse consultant can learn from observing a group. The chapter then focuses on two different group situations that a nurse consultant will most likely encounter: building a work group and working with an established group. The final section of the chapter discusses teams as a specific type of group. Some questions to think about as you read this chapter are:

- What is your own preferred role in a group? What implications might this have when you work with a group as a nurse consultant?

- What would be the advantages and disadvantages of working with a group of consultees as an internal and external nurse consultant?

- Does any one nursing consultation interaction pattern seem most appropriate for situations where the consultee is a group?

- What different nursing consultation roles and skills are needed for working with individuals and groups? Which of these are strengths and weaknesses for you?

Understanding Group Behavior

Understanding groups and group behavior is facilitated by an understanding of organizations. Because groups are microcosms of larger organizations, they share all of the same problems seen in larger organizations: interpersonal friction, emotional outbursts, confusion, competing agendas, power struggles, conflict, and disputes over resources and values. Groups also face the same structural issues as organizations: how to divide responsibilities and how to integrate diverse activities into a unified whole (Bolman & Deal 1991). Finally, like organizations, any group may (and usually does) serve more than one purpose at a time. In fact, a group may serve a different purpose for different group members (Sampson & Marthas 1990). Understanding a group's behavior is facilitated by understanding the forces that influence group behaviors, group functions, levels of behavior in groups, and the relationship between interactions and influence in groups.

Forces that Influence Group Behavior

Groups mirror organizations that are open systems. (Chapter 5 discusses characteristics of open systems in detail.) Groups consist of subsystems—for example, dyads and triads—and are embedded in the suprasystem or environment of a parent organization or community. A group's behavior then, is influenced by the organization or community of which it is a part, as well as by the characteristics of its members (Harrison 1994).

Consider a single clinic within a managed care network. The clinic's functioning is influenced by the characteristics of the network as well as by the characteristics of the people who work in the clinic. Characteristics of the managed care network that could influence the clinic's functioning include management style (viewing itself through a human resource rather than structural frame), size, mission and goals, and policies and procedures. Provider (group member) characteristics that might influence the clinic's behavior and functioning are the mix of workers (nurse practitioner, physician, physician's assistant, and so forth), years of work experience, and individual personalities (for example mix of type-A and type-B personalities).

Consider as a second example, how a support group can be influenced by both its environment (meeting at a hospital or another location) and group member characteristics (such as medical diagnoses). Because of the way in which a group's members interact and influence one another, a group, like a system, is more than and different from the sum of its parts. A single clinic or support group then, is something unique in and of itself and more than just a collection of individuals.

Like organizations, groups are influenced by norms and culture. As discussed in Chapter 5, culture is not always easy to identify, but it has a strong influence on the perceptions, feelings, and behaviors of a group's members. A group's culture is reflected, in part, by its norms. Norms are assumptions and expectations about behavior that is appropriate or inappropriate in a specific situation (Schein 1988). An example of norm-driven behavior would be a clinic's practice of obtaining physician orders for certain treatment plans after the plans have already been implemented independently by the clinic nurse. This practice reflects norms of trust, autonomy, and perhaps, efficiency. In a support group, referring to each member by only their first name would reflect a norm of informality.

Other group and organizational characteristics that influence, and in fact enhance, group behavior and effectiveness include the following:

- cooperation and a sense of cohesiveness among group members and between the group and its parent organization or community

- honest communication that cuts across a system's units and levels of hierarchy

- a group norm that supports productivity

- participative supervision that is both task oriented and supportive of individual effort and learning (Harrison 1994).

Cohesiveness is a group characteristic that deserves special mention because it can have both positive and negative effects on a group's behavior. When group cohesiveness is high, group members express security, solidarity, mutual liking, and positive feelings about the group's purpose as well as its routine tasks (Janis 1982). High cohesiveness is also associated with higher levels of self-esteem among individual group members, increased member participation, and increased acceptance of goals. Cohesiveness, however, can also have a "darker" side. Cohesiveness can cause group members to develop mutual dependency rather than autonomy and to emphasize preserving the group without attention to the work (such as problem solving) that is at hand (Janis 1992). This can result in the phenomenon of "groupthink." Groupthink is discussed in a later section of this chapter.

Group Functions

In order to survive and be effective, a group must accomplish its task or purpose, meet the needs of its members, and respond to its environment. "Group functions" are the sets of activities in which a group must engage to meet these three demands.

Task Functions Task functions are goal-oriented activities. Initiating is the first task function in which a group must engage. Initiating involves stating the problem and goal, making tentative proposals about how the goal might be pursued, and identifying factors such as time and money constraints that might affect goal accomplishment (Schein 1988). A group of consultees often engages in initiating before they contact a nurse consultant for help with problem solving. Initiating may also occur during initial contact with the nurse consultant, or may continue throughout the entry and problem identification phases of the nursing consultation process. Other task functions include gathering and communicating information that will facilitate problem identification and action planning.

Internal Maintenance Functions Internal maintenance functions are activities in which group members engage for the purpose of building and maintaining "group harmony" or good interpersonal relations, and repairing damaged relationships (Goodstein 1978). Maintenance functions need to occur on an ongoing basis in any group. However, because members of groups that are just forming are frequently preoccupied with their own personal needs and the process of group building, maintenance functions are often more pronounced in established groups where some "relationship repair work" needs to take place before the group can engage in task functions. If maintenance functions are not carried out, the group member who is angry or hurt or who feels left out can be lost as a resource to the group or can act to sabotage the group's activities (Schein 1988).

Boundary Management Functions Because every group exists in either an organizational or community environment, one of its key tasks is to manage its relationship to its environment (Schein 1988). Boundary management activities center on accessing information from the environment and defining the group's niche or purpose in relationship to its environment.

Specific activities related to each of a group's functions are described in Box 6-1. As you study the list of specific activities related to each group function, think how these activities might apply to a support group that a nurse consultant is facilitating for nurses who work in an organ procurement agency. (In this nursing consultation scenario, the nurses are the consultee and the support group is the intervention being used to help nurses deal with job-related stressors. The client in this situation is the organ procurement agency itself. Families of organ donors are one set of stakeholders.) Task functions that this group would need to undertake include initiating activities that center around identifying the nursing consultation problem (job stress) and possible solutions (support group, education). Before the consultees can decide on the support group as the most appropriate intervention, however, they need to gather information to more clearly identify the problem. Specifically, they need to determine whether their stress is due to a lack of information or to a lack of support. They also need to gather information and opinions about possible problem solutions. Information sharing, clarifying, and consensus testing need to follow before the support group can be decided on as the "best" problem solution.

Once the support group is established, group members' efforts focus on ensuring that the group is meeting the needs of all members. Internal maintenance activities such as gatekeeping, encouraging, harmonizing, and compromising assume primary importance. All group members need to feel able to share their concerns and ask for as well as give support.

Boundary management functions would be important to this support group because the group operates in the rapidly changing health care environment. Even if a lack of support rather than a lack of knowledge was determined to be the cause of the stress experienced by the organ procurement nurses, the nurses still need to be kept informed (through scouting, technology gatekeeping, and translating) about new policies and procedures that could affect how they perform their jobs. These changes could either increase or alleviate their stress. The nurses in this support group will engage in guarding and patrolling when they decide what information about the group to share with the organ procurement agency, who to invite to their meetings as guests, and so forth.

Levels of Behavior in Groups

Members of groups engage in both formal and informal levels of behavior. The formal level of behavior is a task-oriented level of behavior whereas the informal level

Box 6-1. Group Functions

In order to survive and be effective, a group must accomplish its purpose, meet the needs of its members, and respond to its environment. "Group functions" are sets of activities in which a group must engage in order to meet these demands.

Task Functions

These functions help a group pursue its goal:

- Initiating: stating the problem, making proposals about how it might be resolved
- Information and opinion seeking
- Information and opinion sharing
- Clarifying and elaborating: testing the adequacy of information and improving the quality of proposed problem solutions
- Summarizing: reviewing what is known (or unknown) and what has been decided
- Consensus testing: assessing readiness to make a decision

Internal Maintenance Functions

These functions focus on keeping the group intact and keeping group members happy and productive:

- Gatekeeping: ensuring that all members have an opportunity to contribute to the group
- Encouraging: ensuring that members feel included and accepted
- Harmonizing and compromising: intervening to reduce destructive disagreements
- Diagnosing, standard setting, and standard testing: remedial measures such as airing problems and looking at the group rules and processes that are used when the group appears to be breaking down.

Boundary Management Functions

These activities focus on a group's relationship with its environment:

- Boundary defining: establishing the group's identity
- Scouting: seeking information about the environment that could have an effect on the group
- Technology gatekeeping: bringing the group information it needs to be able to perform its tasks
- Translating: ensuring that information is understood
- Negotiating: ensuring the group gets the resources it needs from its environment
- Guarding: maintaining integrity of the group by determining what information it will share with its environment
- Patrolling: looking for information leakage
- Entry and exit management: bringing in and releasing members

Reference: Harrison, M. (1994). *Diagnosing organizations: Methods, models, and processes* (2nd ed.). Thousand Oaks, CA: Sage; and Schein, E. (1988). *Process Consultation, volume I: Its role in organization development* (2nd ed.). Reading, MA: Addison-Wesley.

is a personal level of behavior. The informal level of behavior is a more subtle, implicit level of behavior that focuses on group maintenance and the personal needs of group members (Bolman & Deal 1991). At any one time, group members may be working on the group's task—but never working *only* on the group's task; they are also working on whatever personal and social needs are important to them at that point in time. In groups then, individual behavior is shaped largely by a personal agenda of needs and values, such as competition, control, self-protection, and autonomy (Sampson & Marthas 1990).

Because group members are always functioning at these two levels of behavior, each group member has two roles: a task role and a personal role. A group member's task roles are assigned responsibilities that need to be carried out in order for the group to accomplish its task (Goodstein 1978). In a support group, task roles for group members might include "attender at meetings," "active listener," and "sharer of concerns." A group member's personal roles are roles that are assumed for personal comfort and satisfaction. Examples of personal roles and needs include leader, follower, listener, talker, being liked, and being valued. The right set and assignment of task roles helps a group to accomplish its task and make optimal use of each member's talents. If group members are unable to fulfill their desired personal roles, however, they will feel frustrated and unsatisfied and may be unproductive and disruptive because they are unwilling or unable to take on their task roles (Bolman & Deal 1991).

The concepts of two levels of behavior and group members' personal needs are important for nurse consultants because surface, observed behavior is often inadequate for fully understanding group interactions. For example, personal needs and agendas often help explain the way in which a group member interacts with the group leader (who is often the nurse consultant in a nursing consultation situation) and with other group members. As described in Box 6-2, how an individual interacts with the group's leader may reflect needs and issues related to authority, dependency, freedom, and individuality. Interactions with other group members may reflect needs and issues related to intimacy, sexuality, envy, giving, and privacy (Sampson & Marthas 1990).

Influence in Groups

Just as all members of an organization (including the nurse consultant) have some type of power, all group members exert influence of one kind or another over the group's functioning. This influence is a result of the way in which a member interacts with others in the group (Schoonover-Shoffner 1989). Depending on how a group member interacts with others in the group, influence can be promotive, disruptive, or counteractive.

Promotive influence is exerted when a member's behavior facilitates progress of the group toward its goals. Examples of promotive behavior include providing helpful suggestions ("In other situations, I've seen this work…"), and encouraging and participating in brainstorming. However, most groups are characterized by more disruptive than promotive interactions (Schoonover-Shoffner 1989). Disruptive influence is a result of behavior that inhibits the group's movement to a decision or its goals. Pressure tactics, giving wrong information, and drawing incorrect conclusions from information are examples of behavior that can have a disruptive influence. Counteractive influence negates or neutralizes disruptive interactions and restores a group's movement toward its goals. Exposing and correcting misinformation is an example of an interaction that would have a counteractive influence.

Box 6-2. Understanding Group Members' Behavior: Personal Agendas and Interpersonal Interactions

In any group, individuals take on personal as well as task roles. The personal roles a group member assumes reflect a personal agenda of needs and issues. Personal roles are wanted for personal comfort and satisfaction. The needs and issues that drive personal roles can often be inferred from an individual's way of interacting with the group leader and other group members.

Interactions with Group Leaders

Need or Issue	Possible Behavior
Authority	Challenges group leader's knowledge, opinions, and right to make decisions
Dependency	Unquestionably obeys group leader; tries to establish a coalition with the leader; asks for unneeded assistance
Freedom/Autonomy	Disregards task role; makes statements such as, "Let me do it my way"
Individuality	Calls attention to self through interaction with and comments to group leader

Interactions with Group Members

Need or Issue	Possible Behavior
Intimacy and Friendship	Shares personal thoughts; excessive friendship overtures
Sexuality	Provocative posturing and/or comments
Envy	Criticizes others' ideas and actions; calls attention to own ideas and actions
Giving	Offers physical and material assistance (this often seems to occur in exchange for gestures of friendship)
Privacy	Reluctance to share personal thoughts and ideas with group members

Reference: Sampson, E., & Marthas, M. (1990). *Group process for the health professions* (3rd ed.). Albany, NY: Delmar.

A nurse consultant who is working with a group needs to create an environment where group members feel safe engaging in behaviors that will have a productive or counteractive influence. The nurse consultant, as the implied group leader, also needs to role-model promotive and counteractive influence behaviors. Strategies a nurse consultant can use to exert and role-model promotive and counteractive influence are identified in Box 6-3.

Box 6-3. Promotive and Counteractive Influence Strategies for Nurse Consultants

Promotive influence strategies facilitate a group's progress toward its goals. Counteractive influence strategies neutralize disruptive group interactions and restore a group's movement toward its goals. The following strategies represent both promotive and counteractive influence strategies for nurse consultants:

- Agree upon decision-making guidelines and criteria that will be used to make decisions

- Establish norms and guidelines for brainstorming activities

- Ask for a "recheck" of questionable information

- Don't deal with the source (person) or the nature of the wrong information, assumptions, or ideas; instead, point out questionable features and ask the group to re-examine the idea's acceptability

- Point out fallacies and concerns using "I" language ("I am concerned because…")

- Be prepared to limit the interactions and contributions of disruptive group members; do this by focusing on functions or actions rather than on personal faults

- Do your homework ahead of time so that you know the issues related to the problem

Reference: Schoonover-Shoffner, K. (1989). Improving work group decision-making effectiveness. *Journal of Nursing Administration, 19* (7), 10-16.

Learning from Observing Groups

A nurse consultant can learn much about a group's norms and power structure by simple but focused observations. This information can help the nurse consultant gain psychological entry into a group and can help build coalitions for problem solving. Group communication and decision making are two of the most important and accessible processes that can be observed.

Observing Group Communication

Communication includes the spoken word as well as facial expressions, gestures, physical posturing, tone of voice, and timing. A single message can convey facts, feelings, perceptions, and innuendos. Of particular interest to a nurse consultant are the dynamics and interpersonal interactions that accompany the verbal dimensions of communication; these behaviors are most likely to reveal a group's norms and power structure. Box 6-4 summarizes questions that can be used to guide observation of a group's communication processes. Key issues and observations are discussed in depth below.

Observation #1: Who communicates? How often? For how long? Answers to these questions reveal not only who the group's informal leader is, but also reveal members' needs for inclusion, individuality, and privacy. These observations can be

---

Box 6-4. Observing Group Communication

The nurse consultant can use the following questions as a guide for observing group communication:

- Who communicates? How often? For how long?
- Who speaks but is apparently never heard?
- Who is included in the communication network?
- Who communicates with whom?
- Who talks after whom? Who interrupts whom?
- Who is never allowed to complete their thoughts?
- Does an interruption represent support ("Attaboy") or challenge ("Yes, but...")?
- Whose words seem to have especially heavy impact?
- What communication styles are observed? How do these seem to affect others in the group?
- What does the total communication picture reveal about a group's norms and values?

Reference: Schein, E. (1988). *Process consultation, volume I: Its role in organization development* (2nd ed.). Reading, MA: Addison-Wesley.

---

charted and summarized to indicate how much of the total available "talk time" is taken up by each group member (Schein 1988). Frequently, these observations reveal that members who have been labeled as quiet and nonparticipatory have actually been talking, but no one has been listening. These observations, therefore, can also answer the question, "Who speaks but is apparently never heard?"

Observation #2: Who is included in the communication network? Who communicates with whom? To make these observations, the nurse consultant must watch a speaker's body language and eyes since a target of communication is not always addressed by name. These observations can be recorded on a matrix that has the names of group members on both the horizontal and vertical axes. A check mark can be placed in the appropriate cell on the matrix grid each time a communication event occurs (Schein 1988). Often, group members will speak first to members of the group from whom they expect resistance to an idea. This enables the speaker to determine whether the "toughest hurdle" to an idea can be passed before moving on to a problem solution. The nurse consultant may want to follow this lead of who to talk to first when presenting information (especially controversial information) to the same group. These observations can also reveal subgroups and coalitions within a group.

Observation #3: Who talks after whom? Who interrupts whom? These observations provide information about perceptions of status and group norms regarding attention to status. Usually, group members of higher rank or power or those with higher perceived status feel free to interrupt a member of lower perceived status. Thus individuals who are never allowed to complete their thoughts are generally recognized as less powerful and less important by a group.

Occasionally, a group member with lower status will interrupt a member of higher status. While this is sometimes acceptable because of a group's norm of openness, it more frequently represents a challenge to the influence of the group member who has been interrupted (Schein 1988). Thus interrupting a person of higher status may indicate a strong negative reaction to that person's words and what they imply in terms of behavioral expectations. Note that never being interrupted can sometimes indicate a total disregard for a message rather than respect for power and status.

In addition to observing patterns of interruption, the nurse consultant should observe the "patterns of triggering" represented by the interruption (Schein 1988). Interruption can be supportive ("Attaboy!") or can represent a desire to undo a decision ("Yes, but..."). In general, it takes three "Attaboys" to undo the damage caused by a "Yes, but" (Schein 1988).

Observation #4: What communication styles are observed? What effects do they have? This observation focuses on tone of voice, use of gestures, and delivery styles (for example, humorous or assertive). While these behaviors tend to reveal the sender's underlying personality more than anything else, they are also important because of the effect they can have on other members in the group. For example, do group members become defensive or are they put at ease? These behaviors can also reflect the sender's personal needs for control, individuality, and/or inclusion.

Observation #5: What does the total communication picture reveal about a group's norms and values? In making this final observation, the nurse consultant considers the meaning of a group's communication processes as a whole. The nurse consultant tries to infer the following specific norms and values because of their potential influence on the nursing consultation relationship: authoritarianism versus democracy and participation, openness versus privacy, group cohesiveness versus individualism, and dependence versus self-confidence and autonomy.

Observing Group Decision-Making Processes

Group decision making involves combining the preferences of individual members into a group choice (Schoonover-Shoffner 1989). A group's decision-making processes reveal sources of influence within the group, values about individual contributions and openness, and norms about participation. More importantly for a nurse consultant, a group's decision-making processes may help explain poor morale, lack of cohesiveness, lack of group effectiveness, and other problems for which a nurse consultant may be asked to intervene.

Attainment of a group's goals is facilitated when a group's decision-making processes allow all members to have their say and argue openly for what they believe. In contrast, if there is manipulation, compromising just to settle things, smoothing over and ignoring biases and conflicting information, or the forcing of a decision by those in authority, decision-making outcomes (and group dynamics) are more likely to be negative (Goodstein 1978). The five patterns of decision making observed most frequently in groups are: decision by lack of response (or default), decision by authority, decision by minority, decision by majority rule, and decision by consensus.

Decisions by default, authority, or minority rule occur most frequently in groups that discourage openness and participation. In groups with these norms, speaking up and opposing a decision is negatively labeled as "blocking." In these groups, there are strong pressures on group members to remain silent (Schein 1988). The danger of using one of these processes for decision making is that decisions often end up being made on the basis of inaccurate or incomplete information. Admittedly, decision by authority is a highly efficient way of making a decision and is appropriate in crisis situations such as a severe and sudden drop in a clinic's income or patient load. Whether decision by authority is effective, however, depends on the extent to which adequate information about the problem and possible solutions have been solicited before the decision is made.

Decision by majority is popular because it implies a value of democracy within a group. The danger of voting and operating on the basis of majority rule, however, is that it creates coalitions of winners and losers. Unless the losers feel that they have been *really* listened to before voting, they can become preoccupied with "winning the next round" rather than implementing the group's decision.

Decision by consensus does not mean unanimity. Rather, consensus means that everyone in a group has had an opportunity to openly share concerns and influence the decision. Consensus reflects a "sense of the group" rather than voting to demonstrate majority agreement (Schein 1988). While consensus is the most time-consuming process for reaching a decision, groups that make decisions on the basis of consensus usually make higher quality decisions, because the process allows consideration of all information and all opinions. Consensus also avoids the creation of winners and losers. Groups that make decisions by consensus frequently request nursing consultation for help with the efficiency of their decision-making processes.

Issues Related to Building a Group

In this chapter, teams are considered a special kind of group. The content in this section and in the section which follows (Issues Related to Maintaining a Group) applies to naturally-occurring groups who find themselves having to work together to solve a problem as well as to teams that have been intentionally formed in order to solve a problem.

Nurse consultants often work with groups who are coming together for the first time in a working relationship. In this situation, group-building activities need to begin during the gaining entry phase of the nursing consultation process. Group-building activities can take place as the nurse consultant establishes physical entry and works to gain psychological entry into the consultee group and client system.

Building a group is a stressful process because members are simultaneously bombarded with a variety of tasks, roles, and interpersonal demands. The beginning of a group in particular, is marked by member anxiety related to uncertainty and apprehension about both individual acceptance within the group and group expectations. The question of, "How good of a group member will I be?" causes a sense of "I-ness" to prevail during the process of group building. This self-centered behavior reflects various concerns that any new group member could be expected to experience. The nurse consultant needs to attend to these concerns so that group members will be able to pay attention to each other and the task at hand.

Human Dynamics in New Groups: "I-ness"

The behavior of group members during the group-building process can be explained by the underlying emotional issues that an individual must resolve before comfort is established in any new situation. Each member of a new group needs to resolve issues related to identity, control, balancing personal and groups needs, and acceptance and intimacy (Schein 1988).

Issue #1: Identity Each group member needs to answer the question, "Who am I to be in this group?" This issue centers around determining members' task roles. Until this issue is resolved, group members demonstrate poor listening skills, anxiety, inattention, and a lack of concern for others.

Issue #2: Control, Power, and Influence This issue addresses group members' questions about, "How much power will I have and how should I express it?" Group members try to resolve these issues by testing each other and experimenting with the effectiveness of different forms of influence, such as expertise and charisma. Concerns about power can cause inconsistency in group members' behavior as they try to sort out the most effective way of relating to each other. If the nurse consultant insists on a tight task schedule and fails to allow time for power concerns to be resolved, "testing" behavior will continue and delay work on the group's task.

Issue #3: Individual Needs and Group Goals This issue concerns group members' anxieties about balancing their own needs with the needs of the group as a whole. Specifically, group members have anxiety about, "Will the group's goals meet my own needs?" Preoccupation with this issue can cause an individual to develop a "wait and see" attitude rather than be an active participant in group activities. If too many group members take this attitude, the group never gets moving.

   The danger with this issue is that the nurse consultant or another group member will try to rescue the group by using authority to set an agenda and formulate goals. This has the effect of creating dependency in the consultee group rather than fostering the development of problem-solving skills.

Issue #4: Acceptance and Intimacy The questions behind this issue are, "Will I be liked and accepted by the group?" and, "How open will we need to be with each other?" This issue is a source of tension until the group establishes working norms about intimacy and resolves concerns about acceptance. Group members often respond to these issues by exhibiting charisma and by looking for another group member with whom they can agree and form a supportive alliance. This tendency can create dependency as well as foster the development of coalitions that emphasize meeting group members' personal and social needs rather than the group's task needs.

Strategies for Nurse Consultants Because group members are preoccupied with their own feelings during the group-building process, they are less able to listen to each other and solve group problems. The nurse consultant needs to clarify and acknowledge the personal needs of group members during the group-building process and legitimize members' testing and coping behaviors. The nurse consultant also needs to help the group understand the dynamics that are occurring so that they can confront and respond to each other's concerns, rather than just react to each other's behavior. Helping group members establish group norms and resolve concerns about their identity with the group are additional strategies that are useful during the group-building process.

   The nurse consultant can decrease the anxiety of group members by helping them establish group norms ("how we want to do things") early in the group-building process. For example, the group may need help in coming to a consensus about norms and expectations for participation, listening, interrupting, confidentiality, and formality of a group's processes. Groups also need to decide on acceptable decision criteria. The nurse consultant can facilitate group members' involvement in establishing these norms by asking them how they would like to see the group operate. Developing these norms and rules can help resolve group members' concerns about power and intimacy within the group.

   Groups may also need help in resolving their concerns about identity. As a helping strategy, the nurse consultant may assist group members in identifying what specific roles and responsibilities they want to assume within the group and what contributions they think they bring to the group. A specific strategy the nurse consultant can use to help group members negotiate roles and responsibilities is responsibility charting. A responsibility chart (Bolman & Deal 1991) identifies who is going to do what tasks in a group and how the person responsible for a particular task will relate to other groups members in regards to that task. Figure 6-1 is an example of a responsibility chart for a group of nurses who are working with a nurse consultant to plan a continuing education workshop. A responsibility chart decreases group members' anxieties about what they are expected to do in a group in terms of helping that group meet its goals. If group members are active participants in developing the responsibility chart, they can address issues related to balancing their own needs with those of the group. Group involvement in developing a responsibility

Tasks	Group Members				
	Chairperson	Treasurer	A	B	C
Establish program/ agenda	R	C	C	C	C
Arrange keynote speaker	A	C	R	I	I
Make facilities arrangements	A	C	I	R	I
Publicity	C	I	I	I	R
Registration	I	R	I	I	I
Act as on-site program facilitator	R	I	C	I	I
Solicit financial sponsorship	C	I	R	I	I
Track expenses/ pay bills	A	R	I	I	I

Key:
R = Individual who is responsible for a task or decision (this person should be identified first)
A = Individuals who need to approve the actions of R
C = Individuals whom R needs to consult before making a decision
I = Individuals who need to be kept informed by R

Figure 6-1. Example Responsibility Chart for a Program Planning Consultation
This example responsibility chart illustrates tasks and responsibilities related to planning a continuing education workshop. The responsibility chart identifies who is responsible for a specific task role in a group and how other group members relate to this performance in regards to a task. The nurse consultant works with the group to identify the person designated as "R" first. The nurse consultant remains available to the group for further problem-specific consultation, but is not involved in ongoing consultation about the implementation of each task.

chart also facilitates the development of trust and cohesion early in the group-building process.

Issues Related to Maintaining a Group

To some extent, it is easier to work with an established group than with a group that is coming together to problem-solve for the first time. Established groups tend to have norms that are understood and have become integrated into the group's way of interacting. Established groups also tend to have developed ways of accommodating members' personal roles without compromising the overall functioning of the group. Because these tasks have been accomplished, the climate of an established group can be more trusting and supportive than that of a group that is coming together in a working relationship for the first time. Members of established groups tend to be less overtly anxious than members of new groups. They are also more willing to take personal and collective risks. Established groups are characterized by a sense of "we-ness" rather than "I-ness," and by collective work toward the group's goal. The disadvantage of working with an established group, however, is that the group may have developed dysfunctional and unproductive ways of interacting. If this is the case, the nurse consultant will need to undertake group-building processes before problem solving can get under way.

Nurse consultants often work with established groups of consultees to help them solve a client's health-related problem. For example, a nurse consultant might work with a group of staff nurses to help with the implementation of critical pathways (client=nursing unit). In another situation, a nurse might provide consultation to a group of teachers about meeting the health care needs of schoolchildren who have AIDS-related illnesses.

Human Dynamics in Established Groups: Groupthink

The same cohesiveness that can make working with an established group productive can also get the group into trouble. Established groups that are excessively cohesive can become careless in their boundary management and information-gathering activities. They can also develop a sense of omnipotence and overestimate their own power and morality. This tendency causes established groups to sometimes engage in excessive risk taking. Finally, excessive cohesiveness may lead a group to develop informal norms about preserving an appearance of group harmony at all costs. Whenever the group needs to make a decision, these norms may function as a hidden agenda. The potential side effects of this type of cohesiveness can result in "groupthink" (Janis 1982).

"Groupthink" is the term that has been coined to describe a deterioration of mental efficiency, reality testing, and moral judgment that can result from in-group pressures and cohesiveness. This same phenomenon has also been referred to as the "Abilene Paradox": a willingness of group members to set aside their individual preferences and opinions to accommodate the perceived majority will (Robbins & Finley 1996). When groupthink occurs, a group's drive for cohesiveness and unanimity overrides group members' judgment as well as their motivation to consider the range of possible solutions to a problem (Janis 1982). In other words, groupthink occurs when a desire for conformity saps diversity and individual judgment. Groupthink results in poor quality decisions.

Cohesiveness of the extreme type that results in groupthink is particularly likely to develop when a group perceives itself to be facing an "enemy." The first clue that this dangerous type of cohesiveness might be developing is a group's development of a stereotyped and dehumanizing image of the source of their perceived threat. An example of this would be a group of nurses blaming problems associated with work redesign (such as possible job loss) on an "insensitive corporate monster." As these groups become cohesive, they also tend to develop extreme ideas about how the threat should be handled. These ideas are more extreme and involve more risk taking than what members would be inclined to do on their own. What develops is, in a sense, a type of "mob mentality."

Group cohesiveness sets the stage for the development or operation of the other conditions also associated with groupthink. Group cohesiveness causes a group to insulate itself from its environment and miss opportunities to take advantage of information that might challenge their decisions. Leaders of tightly cohesive groups tend to become partial to group members who conform to the majority view; this has the effect of preventing minority members from expressing their doubts. Finally, cohesiveness sets the stage for groupthink by discouraging norms that require methodical procedures and criteria for decision-making tasks (Janis 1982). The outcome of groupthink is poor quality decisions. Figure 6-2 summarizes the conditions associated with groupthink.

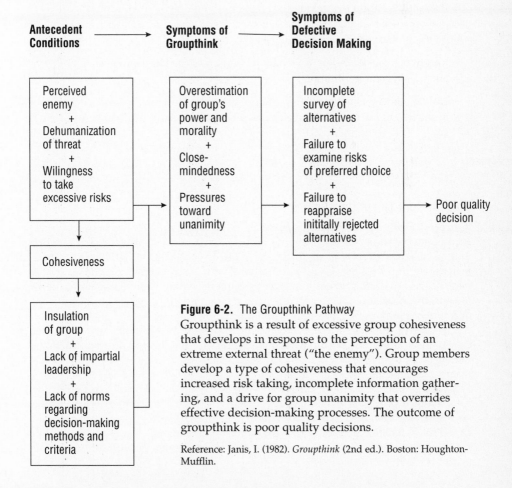

Figure 6-2. The Groupthink Pathway
Groupthink is a result of excessive group cohesiveness that develops in response to the perception of an extreme external threat ("the enemy"). Group members develop a type of cohesiveness that encourages increased risk taking, incomplete information gathering, and a drive for group unanimity that overrides effective decision-making processes. The outcome of groupthink is poor quality decisions.

Reference: Janis, I. (1982). *Groupthink* (2nd ed.). Boston: Houghton-Mufflin.

Box 6-5. Strategies for Preventing Groupthink

The following represent various strategies a nurse consultant can use to prevent groupthink:

- As the group leader, avoid stating personal preferences and try to be impartial; merely introduce the problem and the resources and limitations relevant to its solution

- Educate the group about the phenomenon of groupthink

- Establish and enforce norms regarding mutual responsibility

- Discourage the practice of trying to "score points" in a power struggle

- Role-model the solicitation and acceptance of criticism

- Assign the role of "critical evaluator" to each group member

- Assign one member the role of devil's advocate

- Break a group into several subgroups, each with its own leader

- Prevent insulation by seeking the reactions of outsiders to the group's decision; invite outsiders to meetings in order to provide another perspective on the problem and possible solutions

- Encourage consideration of the impact of the group's decision on stakeholders in the problem situation

- Hold a "second chance meeting" before implementing the decision; review problem-solving options as well as their advantages and disadvantages

Reference: Janis, I. (1982). *Groupthink* (2nd ed.). Boston: Houghton-Mifflin.

Strategies for Nurse Consultants

A key task for nurse consultants who are working with established groups in a problem-solving relationship is preventing groupthink. Nurse consultants need to work with established groups to maintain the positive aspects of cohesiveness such as increased group member security and productivity. At the same time, nurse consultants need to work to prevent cohesiveness from becoming dysfunctional by enforcing effective decision-making processes and reinforcing (or helping a group develop) norms about impartiality, listening, and information seeking.

One specific strategy a nurse consultant can help a group implement to protect against groupthink is that of developing a process for monitoring group compliance with decided upon decision-making processes. This can be done by assigning to each member the formal roles of critical evaluator and "devil's advocate" (Janis 1982). This assignation creates the expectation that group members will voice concerns they have about a proposed decision and removes the stigma that might otherwise be associated with being a critic and dissenter. Finally, the nurse consultant can role-model the behaviors of both "critical evaluator" and "impartial leader" to the group. Additional strategies the nurse consultant can use to prevent groupthink are identified in Box 6-5.

Teams: A Special Kind of Group

Teams, particularly interdisciplinary teams, have become an increasingly popular component of strategies for solving the types of complex problems that abound in today's health care environment. A team is a specific type of group that is distinguished by a collaborative effort ("teamwork") and a collective perspective. More specifically, teams are small groups of people with "complementary skills who are committed to a common purpose, performance goals, and approach for which they hold themselves to be mutually accountable" (Katzenbach & Smith 1993). In contrast, traditional work groups may be characterized by teamwork, but they lack a collective perspective. Instead, traditional work groups interact to help each individual member perform more effectively. Table 6-1 summarizes additional differences between work groups and teams.

The Usefulness of Teams

Teams are useful whenever a specific objective requires collective work and the integration of multiple skills, perspectives, and experiences. In fact, a demanding performance challenge tends to naturally create a team (Katzenbach & Smith 1993).

The usefulness of incorporating a team approach into solving complex problem situations that are likely to recur is related to several innate characteristics of teams. First, the complementary skills and perspectives of team members increases the likelihood that a problem solution will fit the client system's needs and resources. Secondly, teams tend to develop communication patterns that facilitate present as well as future problem solving. Teams also derive effectiveness from team members' trust and confidence in each others' abilities. For these reasons, teams are often the best way to integrate problem solving across structural boundaries (units and hierarchies) of an organization. A team approach fosters the development of long-term problem-solving skills that will be dispersed throughout the client system once the nursing consultation relationship has terminated. In other words, teams naturally integrate performance and learning. Last, team effectiveness is related to a sense of "safety in numbers." That is, a team is not as threatened by taking risks and changing as are individuals who are left to fend for themselves (Katzenbach & Smith 1993).

Table 6-1. Work Groups Versus Teams

Characteristic	Work Group	Team
Leadership	Strong, clearly focused	Shared
Accountability	Individual	Individual and collective
Purpose	Same as the organization's	Specific and unique to the group
Work Style	Emphasis on efficiency: discuss, decide, delegate	Characterized by open discussion and problem solving: discuss, decide, do real work together
How Effectiveness Is Judged	Influence on members	Collective work products

Reference: Katzenbach, J., & Smith, D. (1993). *The wisdom of teams: Creating the high performance organization.* New York: HarperBusiness.

Transforming Work Groups into Teams

Because teams are potentially useful in solving many nursing consultation problems, nurse consultants need to know how to create and work with teams. Transforming a work group into a team, or creating a team "from scratch," requires that the nurse consultant have a knowledge of "team basics" as well as demonstrate abilities to build team performance and function as a temporary team leader.

Team Basics   "Team basics" are the structures and processes that enable a group to function as a team. Team basics are size, skills, common purpose, common approach, and accountability (Katzenbach & Smith 1993).

Size. Teams range in size from 2 to 25 members (the ideal size is said to be 12). Teams of more than 25 members tend to get bogged down by logistics (such as meeting times) and because of difficulty reaching agreement on specifics. Larger groups also have a tendency to become hierarchical in nature and develop individual rather than collective performance goals.

Skills. Three types of skills need to be represented among team members: technical or functional expertise related to the consultation problem (such as familiarity with the needs of a certain population group), problem-solving and decision-making skills, and interpersonal skills. Team members, therefore, should be selected on the basis of their skill and skill potential, not their personality. (However, as recognized in Chapter 10, sometimes individuals need to be chosen as a team member for political reasons.) Team members with skill potential will usually develop needed skills as the team evolves.

Common Purpose. Teams are defined by a common purpose that is shaped in response to demands from actual or potential internal or external environmental changes (such as health care reform). This common purpose must be linked to specific performance goals (for example, "find ways to reduce operating costs by 10% within two months"). Clear goals help a team maintain its focus and structure small steps and "small wins" toward an overall problem solution. The achievement of small wins provides feedback to a team that is moving in the right direction.

Common Approach. Teams work only to the extent that they use a single, unified approach to making decisions while working as a group. Teams also need to agree on time commitments for both individual and group tasks.

Accountability. Teams are characterized by "mutual accountability." More specifically, team members need to hold themselves accountable for their individual contributions to the team while they hold one another accountable for members' collective contributions to the team. In addition, the team as a whole needs to hold itself accountable for the overall results.

Building Team Performance   A work group needs more than the structures and processes that comprise team basics if it is to function as an effective team. Teams also need energy, enthusiasm, and dedication to the project (achieve a 10% budget cut, for example), client needs related to the project (such as maintaining quality care), and the team itself (Peters 1987). Nurse consultants can build team performance by instilling "caring, daring, and sharing" (Peters 1987)—that is, creating an environment of mutual support and open and honest communication, encouraging risk taking and a sense of adventure, asking the "hard" questions, and creating commonly held objectives as well as a clear sense of how everyone fits in as a team member.

Specific strategies a nurse consultant can use to build team performance are identified in Box 6-6. Notice from this list that "building team performance" is a more com-

---

Box 6-6. Strategies for Building Team Performance

The nurse consultant can use the following strategies to build team performance:
- Establish the urgency and direction of the team's purpose
- Pay particular attention to first meetings and actions ("first impressions count"); be clear and attentive to members' thoughts and responses.
- Set clear standards of behavior: attendance, discussion, confidentiality, task participation, constructive confrontations, end-product orientation
- Give the team credibility by enforcing behavioral expectations
- Set upon and seize a few immediate performance-oriented goals and tasks
- Challenge the team regularly with fresh facts and information (this redefines and enriches the team's understanding of its purpose)
- Spend a lot of time together, especially at the beginning (this creates camaraderie and solidarity)
- Exploit the power of positive feedback, recognition, and reward
- Establish a measurement and reward system that fosters a sense of cohesion and unity
- Engage in ongoing team building (this facilitates discovery of personal abilities and the abilities of others as well as builds and restores trust)

Reference: Katzenbach, J., & Smith, D. (1993). *The wisdom of teams: Creating the high performance organization.* New York: HarperBusiness; and Peters, J. (1987). *Thriving on chaos: Handbook for a management revolution.* New York: Harper Collins.

---

prehensive concept than is "team building." "Team building" commonly refers to efforts to establish cooperation and comfort among the members of a group. Chapter 10 discusses team building as a "universal" consultation intervention.

The Nurse Consultant as Temporary Team Leader   Because the nursing consultation relationship is a temporary one, the nurse consultant's ultimate goal is to ensure that a team becomes either self-directed or led by one of its members. However, nurse consultants often find it necessary to assume a temporary role as team leader during the process of establishing team basics and building team performance. To a large extent, team leadership is taking a course of "disciplined action" and helping a work group adjust its attitudes and behaviors so as to develop a team perspective.

The primary task of a team leader is to keep the team's purpose, goals, and approach meaningful and relevant. Team members usually do not want leaders to go beyond this, and can become resentful if they attempt to do so (Katzenbach & Smith 1993). A team leader's other key task is to manage outside relationships on behalf of the team, including securing needed resources and removing obstacles to team functioning. To be effective as a team leader then, the nurse consultant needs to balance patience and action. Strategies for effective team leadership are presented in Box 6-7.

Challenges Related to Working with Teams

Teams are hard work. Developing and maintaining a team takes time, energy, and organizational commitment. What is more, even once teams are up and running, they can develop dysfunctional behaviors and "get stuck." In order to maximize the advantages a team approach can bring to a problem situation, the nurse consultant needs to be able to respond to two challenges: organizational biases related to teams and teams that have lost their effectiveness.

Box 6-7. Strategies for Effective Team Leadership

The following illustrate strategies the nurse consultant can use to be effective as a team leader:

- Keep the team's purpose, goals, and approach meaningful and relevant.
- Build commitment and confidence among team members (this needs to be aimed at both individual members and the team as a whole)
- Help the team strengthen its mix and level of skills by providing role modeling and task-specific training
- Manage the team's relationships with outsiders, including removing organizational obstacles to team functioning
- Create opportunities for other team members
- Do real work with the team—be a team member as well as leader
- Do not blame or allow specific individuals to fail
- Never excuse shortfalls in team performance
- Keep your leadership temporary; help the team become self-managing and/or facilitate the development of team leadership skills in a permanent team member(s)

Reference: Katzenbach, J., & Smith, D. (1993). *The wisdom of teams: Creating the high performance organization.* New York: HarperBusiness.

Organizational Biases Related to Teams Nurse consultants encounter organizational biases that can lead to both the overuse and underuse of teams. Some organizations see a team approach as the only way to solve problems. However, teams are not a solution for all problems and, if misapplied, can be wasteful (of both time and resources) and disruptive. As discussed earlier, teams are useful when solving a problem requires collective work and the integration of multiple skills, experiences, and perspectives. If a performance goal can be met through a sum of individual responsibilities and contributions, however, a traditional work group can get the job done and can often do so more effectively (Katzenbach & Smith 1993).

Organizations also have mindsets that discourage the use of teams, even when a team approach would clearly be the most effective. Many organizations, for example, intrinsically prefer individual over group accountability. These organizations often equate group accountability with "no accountability." The nurse consultant can confront this bias by educating the organization about the nature of team accountability and how it can be reinforced through a performance-oriented reward system.

Another organizational bias that can discourage the use of teams is the belief that teams are costly and time-consuming. The nurse consultant needs to confront this belief by acknowledging that while teams do take time to develop, they usually pay off in the long run. The long-term benefit of a team approach is that it will be useful for solving future organizational problems. Skills that will be used for future problem-solving situations are learned by members dispersed throughout the entire client system, rather than limited to one unit or hierarchical level in the organization.

Teams that Have Lost Their Effectiveness Teams are prone to the same dysfunctional behaviors as any other group: not listening, idea killing, personal attacks, apathy, anarchy, and groupthink (Peters 1987). When teams develop these behaviors, team functioning can break down and the team "gets stuck" (Katzenbach & Smith 1993).

Box 6-8. When Teams "Get Stuck"

Teams that have lost their effectiveness and become "stuck" frequently exhibit the following symptoms:

- Loss of energy
- Sense of hopelessness
- Lack of purpose and identity
- Cynicism and mistrust
- Finger pointing and personal attacks

The nurse consultant can use the following strategies to help a team become "unstuck":

- Revisit "team basics"—size; skill mix, level, and potential; clear and meaningful purpose, clear and unified approach; collective and individual accountability
- Go for small wins
- Inject new information and approaches
- Seek outside facilitation and help
- Change the membership of the team

Reference: Katzenbach, J., & Smith, D. (1993). *The wisdom of teams: Creating the high performance organization.* New York: HarperBusiness.

When a team becomes stuck, it loses its effectiveness. Teams that are stuck are characterized by a loss of energy, a sense of hopelessness, a lack of purpose and identity, cynicism and mistrust, and finger pointing and personal attacks.

The nurse consultant needs to respond to the challenge of a "stuck team" by first ensuring that all the team basics are present. Strategizing for small wins and providing new information can also help revitalize a team. If these efforts fail, outside facilitation or a change in membership may be needed. A change in membership (particularly adding new members) is usually considered a last resort, because it often means the team-building efforts will need to be repeated; this can create frustration for ongoing members (Katzenbach & Smith 1993). Box 6-8 summarizes symptoms of "stuck teams" and strategies for helping them become "unstuck."

Chapter Summary

Working with groups and teams can be productive and stimulating as well as confusing and frustrating. Nurse consultants are frequently asked to problem-solve with groups of consultees and form problem-solving teams. To work effectively with a group or team, a nurse consultant must understand and know how to respond to group dynamics.

Understanding both the needs of individuals within groups and the significance of observations about a group's communication and decision-making processes helps a nurse consultant avoid overreacting or underreacting to a group's behavior. Awareness of problems that can arise in groups and teams, such as groupthink and getting stuck, and the ability to address these problems are essential skills for nurse consultants. These skills facilitate effective problem solving and a successful nursing consultation relationship.

Applying Chapter Content

Make arrangements to observe two meetings of the same group or view a videotape of a meeting. (Many communities broadcast their city council meetings over cable television; this could be videotaped and viewed in class). Complete the observation guide in Box 6-9 beginning on page 104 and then answer the following questions:

What were the group's goals? Were these consistent with the group's mission?

Was the group more concerned with task, internal maintenance, or boundary management functions?

What decision-making processes did the group use? Were they effective?

Was there any evidence of groupthink?

What can you infer about group norms, personal needs of group members, and the group's power structure?

Would you describe this group as a working group or a team?

How would you interact with this group in a (nursing) consultation relationship? What strengths would this group bring to a nursing consultation relationship? What problems do you anticipate might arise?

References

Bolman, L., & Deal, T. (1991). *Reframing organizations: Artistry, choice, and leadership.* San Francisco: Jossey-Bass.

Goodstein, L. (1978). *Consulting with human service systems.* Reading, MA: Addison-Wesley.

Harrison, M. (1994). *Diagnosing organizations: Methods, models, and processes* (2nd ed.). Thousand Oaks, CA: Sage.

Janis, I. (1982). *Groupthink* (2nd ed.). Boston: Houghton-Mifflin.

Katzenbach, J., & Smith, D. (1993). *The wisdom of teams: Creating the high performance organization.* New York: HarperBusiness.

Peters, T. (1987). *Thriving on chaos: Handbook for a management revolution.* New York: Harper Collins.

Robbins, H., & Finley, M. (1996). *Why change doesn't work.* Princeton, NJ: Peterson's.

Sampson, E., & Marthas, M. (1990). *Group process for the health professions* (3rd ed.). Albany, NY: Delmar.

Schein, E. (1988). *Process consultation, volume I: Its role in organization development* (2nd ed.). Reading, MA: Addison-Wesley.

Schoonover-Shoffner, K. (1989). Improving work group decision-making effectiveness. *Journal of Nursing Administration, 19* (7), 10-16.

Additional Readings

Bolman, L., & Deal, T. (1991). *Reframing organizations: Artistry, choice, and leadership.* San Francisco: Jossey-Bass.
Chapters 5, 6, and 7 of this text provide an excellent overview of group characteristics and human dynamics in groups.

Goodstein, L. (1978). *Consulting with human service systems.* Reading, MA: Addison-Wesley.
This classic text on organizational consulting takes a systems approach to understanding groups. Chapter 4 addresses the roles of individuals within systems.

Hammer, M., & Stanton, S. (1995). *The reengineering revolution: A handbook.* New York: HarperBusiness.
The authors share strategies for using teams to accomplish radical redesign of organizational processes.

Harrison, M. (1994). *Diagnosing organizations: Methods, models, and processes* (2nd ed.). Thousand Oaks, CA: Sage.
Chapter 3 of this text presents a model for diagnosing group behavior. The appendices include suggestions for specific instruments that can be used in group assessment as well as a guide to diagnosing group behavior observed during meetings.

Janis, I. (1982). *Groupthink* (2nd ed.). Boston: Houghton-Mifflin.
This book provides fascinating examples of groupthink occurring at the national policy level. It also provides a thorough discussion of organizational and group characteristics that can precipitate groupthink.

Katzenbach, J., & Smith, D. (1993). *The wisdom of teams: Creating the high performance organization.* New York: HarperBusiness.
This is an essential handbook on creating and working with teams. Particular attention is given to the challenge of transforming work groups into teams.

Peters, T. (1987). *Thriving on chaos: Handbook for a management revolution.* New York: Harper Collins.
The author argues that self-managing teams should be the basic organizational building block. Strategies for developing these teams are presented.

Rich, B., Hart, B., Barrett, A., Marks, G., & Ruderman, S. (1995). Peer consultation: A look at process. *Clinical Nurse Specialist, 9* (3), 181-185.
This article provides an interesting case study of the human dynamics and group processes that a group of mental health nurses encountered as they worked together to establish a peer support group.

Robbins, H., & Finley, M. (1996). *Why change doesn't work.* Princeton, NJ: Peterson's.
Section 3 of this book discusses how groups can impede the change process. The idea of pushing and pulling groups toward change is presented.

Sampson, E., & Marthas, M. (1990). *Group process for the health professions* (3rd ed.). Albany, NY: Delmar.
The authors provide a good foundational text about group dynamics and strategies for working with groups.

Schein, E. (1987). *Process consultation, volume 2: Lessons for managers and consultants.* Reading, MA: Addison-Wesley.
This text consists of case studies of human dynamics in organizational consultation situations. Included are examples of effective and ineffective consultant behavior. Chapter 2 specifically addresses group processes.

Schein, E. (1988). *Process consultation, volume I: Its role in organization development* (2nd ed.). Reading, MA: Addison-Wesley.
Chapters 2-5 of this classic text focus on group dynamics. Chapter 3 provides excellent guidelines for assessing the communication behavior of groups. Chapter 4 focuses on consultation interventions for building and maintaining effective work groups.

Schoonover-Shoffner, K. (1989). Improving work group decision-making effectiveness. *Journal of Nursing Administration, 19* (7), 10-16.
This text contains useful tips for working with groups in a supervisory role as well as a good discussion of problems in group decision making and interaction and influence within groups.

Senge, P., Kleiner, A., Roberts, C., Ross, R., & Smith, B. (1994). *The fifth discipline handbook.* New York: Currency-Doubleday.
This book is a compendium of strategies for developing a learning organization and team perspective toward functioning.

Box 6-9. Group Observation Guide

Group being observed:

Stated mission of group:

Date and time of observation:

Nature of meeting observed (routine, emergency, and so forth):

Frequency of meetings:

Date of last meeting:

Agenda (attach, if available):

Composition of group (members and "official" roles):

1.   7.

2.   8.

3.   9.

4.   10.

5.   11.

6.   12.

Communication Processes (Summary):
1. Who talked the most? What was the content of their talk?

2. Who talked but was apparently never heard?

3. Who tended to speak to whom? What is the significance of this?

4. Who interrupted whom? What did these interruptions signify?

5. What was the general communication style used by this group? What effect did this have?

6. What was the total communication picture of this group?

Communication Processes

Group Member (Initiator)	Target of Communication												General Content of Talk	Communication Style	Attentiveness of Others
	1	2	3	4	5	6	7	8	9	10	11	12			
1.															
2.															
3.															
4.															
5.															
6.															
7.															
8.															
9.															
10.															
11.															
12.															

Key: √ = communication event   I+ = supportive interruption   I- = negative interruption

Group Decision-Making Processes:
1. What decision-making processes did the group use?
    Default
    Authority
    Minority rule
    Majority rule
    Consensus
2. Who appeared to be the key decision maker?

Risk Factors and Evidence for Groupthink:
1. Was there a perception of an "enemy"?
    Yes (identify):
    No
2. Was there dehumanization of the perceived enemy?
    Yes (identify label used):
    No
3. How would you describe the level of group cohesiveness?
    Low   Medium   High   Extreme
4. Was the group willing to take excessive risks?
    Yes (describe):
    No
5. Did the group overestimate its power and morality?
    Yes (example):
    No
6. Did the group seem insulated?
    Yes   No
7. What was the nature of the group's leadership?
    Partial (example):
    Impartial
8. Was there evidence of close-mindedness?
    Yes (example):
    No
9. Were there pressures toward unanimity?
    Yes (example):
    No
10. Did the group engage in a survey of alternatives?
    Yes   No
11. Was there an examination of risks related to preferred choice?
    Yes   No
12. Was there consideration of the effects of the preferred choice on stakeholders?
    Yes   No
13. Was there reappraisal of initially rejected alternatives?
    Yes   No
14. Was there a presence of critical evaluation, a devil's advocate?
    Yes   No

7

The Dynamics of Change

I often describe organizational change today as a "journey."
To many managers, it's a journey that never ends. Some
tell me the journey is leaving them breathless. My advice: learn
how to "breathe" differently and anticipate what you are likely
to experience. (Champy 1997)

Key terms: ambivalence, resistance, reluctance,
force-field analysis, vision

Introduction

Change is the only constant in health care today. Individual health care providers and organizations are faced with internal and external challenges that demand increasingly complex changes at an increasingly rapid pace. More than ten years ago, it was estimated that organizations, in general, need to "restructure" about every two years in order to keep up with the demands of the marketplace (McDougall 1987). Most likely, this time frame is even shorter for today's health care organizations. For nurses, the rapid pace of change at the organizational level means that change must also occur at the personal level: New ways of thinking and doing must be integrated into practice in order to continue providing optimum (that is, safe and satisfying) patient care. For nurses practicing in today's uncertain and challenging health care environment, a willingness to change established and comfortable habits is essential to survival (Schoolfield & Orduna 1994).

How does change fit into the nursing consultation process? First of all, nurse consultants are often asked to help solve nursing problems that arise due to an organization-wide change, such as work redesign or a merger. Secondly, nursing consultation involves working with consultees to solve actual or potential problems related to a client's health status or health care delivery issues. "Solving problems" implies needing to learn to do something differently; in other words, changing one's way of thinking or behaving. Thus change and the dynamics of change are pervasive themes in all nursing consultation relationships.

A request for nursing consultation means that either something is wrong now for a consultee or that equilibrium is threatened by environmental events. In effect, a request for nursing consultation is a request for change. Just because change is needed or desired, however, doesn't mean that it will be easy to accomplish. Furthermore, just because a problem needs to be solved (either reactively or proactively), doesn't mean that the consultee and client system will embrace the opportunity to change (Brack et al. 1993).

Change occurs on two levels: the situational/mechanical and the personal/emotional. A nursing consultation relationship will be successful only if both levels of the change experience are managed effectively. For nurse consultants then, an understanding of the dynamics of change is essential knowledge.

107

This chapter begins by discussing the "mechanics" of change, the relatively predictable evolution of change, from its first rumblings to its stabilization as the new status quo. Next, the discussion turns to common emotional responses to change and the methods used to manage these responses. The final section of this chapter presents "changemaker" skills for nurse consultants: assessing a consultee's perspective of change, actualizing change, and communicating about change. As you read this chapter, consider the following questions:

- What are your personal feelings about and typical reactions to change? What implications might these have for your practice of nursing consultation?

- How might the dynamics of change differ for organizations that operate under a structural, human resource, political, and symbolic frame?

- How might the dynamics of change differ with the use of different nursing consultation interaction patterns?

- What different advantages and disadvantages might internal and external nurse consultants have in terms of managing the dynamics of change?

The Mechanics of Change

Change is the intentional movement from a current situation (the nursing consultation problem) to a futuristic, more desirable one (the goal) (Fuqua & Kurpius 1993). Change has a predictable pattern of three stages that, while overlapping and frequently occurring very rapidly, are conceptually distinct. The "mechanics of change" are the situational events and nursing consultation tasks within each of these stages that must be accomplished if a change is to be formalized by the client system. The nurse consultant must be aware of these stages as each stage has its own set of dynamics and requires different nursing consultation roles and skills. The stages and mechanics of change that are presented in this section—unfreezing, moving, and refreezing—are based on Kurt Lewin's (1947, 1951) classic model of change.

Unfreezing

It is during the stage of "unfreezing" that a consultee first becomes motivated to change and disrupt the status quo. Unfreezing represents an awakening to a new reality and a disengagement from the past. There is a recognition that the current way of doing things is no longer acceptable (Kanter, Stein, & Jicks 1992). Unfreezing, therefore, indicates a consultee's belief that the outcome of change will be better than the present situation (Brack et al. 1993). In order for unfreezing to occur, three conditions must be met: disconfirmation, induction of guilt or anxiety, and the creation of psychological safety (Schein 1987).

Disconfirmation Disconfirmation (or a lack of confirmation) occurs when a consultee perceives that the current situation is just not good enough anymore. Disconfirmation occurs when there is evidence that expected or desired outcomes are not happening, or are threatened. An intrinsic indicator that might precipitate a hospital's decision to undergo restructuring would be a drop in census or in patient satisfaction ratings. An environmental indicator that might provide disconfirmation would be impending changes in insurance reimbursement policies. For an individual nurse, disconfirmation could come from intrinsic feelings such as decreased job satisfaction or from external information such as a poor performance evaluation. Whatever its source, disconfirmation is interpreted as a problem (either present or impending) and serves as the initial stimulus for undertaking change. This causes unfreezing to begin.

Induction of Guilt Induction of guilt is the second condition that must be in place for unfreezing to occur. The consultee must feel guilty that a goal is not being met or anxious that a value is being violated (Schein 1987). In other words, if unfreezing is to occur, the disconfirmation must be about something that is important to the consultee. Because unfreezing means a disruption of the status quo, the decision to undertake change is not made lightly, and disconfirmation must be accompanied by guilt or anxiety. For example, a one-month decline in average census at a particular clinic might not induce anxiety, but a continuation of this same downward trend for a year certainly would. For an individual nurse, evaluation comments such as "nail polish too bright" might not cause guilt, but negative comments about the nurse's quality of care probably would.

Creation of Psychological Safety Disconfirmation and the induction of guilt or anxiety are enough to get a consultee to begin to "melt" or think about making a change. However, the "big thaw" will not occur unless a third condition, the creation of psychological safety, occurs (Schein 1987). Creating psychological safety means creating an environment where "face" or self-esteem will be maintained while help is being sought. In many nursing consultation situations, by the time the nurse consultant has been contacted, the consultee has already received disconfirmation and feels anxious and/or guilty about performance or an outcome. The nurse consultant must begin to create psychological safety at the time of initial contact. Failure to create this safety can cause a consultee to freeze back up before the nursing consultation problem has been solved. As discussed later in this chapter, failure to create psychological safety is associated with resistance to change.

There is no easy formula for creating psychological safety. The key, however, is to keep the consultee from feeling personally humiliated and losing face or self-esteem (Schein 1987). The nurse consultant must help the consultee feel worthwhile even though current goals are not being met. In other words, the consultee needs to feel specific performance or outcome-related guilt in order for unfreezing to occur, but not at the risk of feeling worthless as a person. After all, the consultee knows there is a problem if help has been sought and doesn't need reminding that the problem exists but rather, needs to be given confidence that the problem is solvable.

Reassurance and supportive comments also help to create psychological safety. Consultees often need to know that their problem is within the "normal range" before they can accept responsibility for working on it. If a problem is seen as "too big" and its intervention "too complex," the "complexity syndrome" can set in and become an excuse for abandoning change efforts (Brack et al. 1993). The nurse consultant should offer reassurance that similar problems have been successfully resolved by others. When possible, former consultees with whom the nurse consultant has successfully worked on a similar problem can be asked to "give a testimonial" and provide this reassurance. Often, consultees simply need to hear that the situation is under control and is not unusual. This "saves face" by communicating that the consultee is not "abnormal" or "unusual" because of the problem.

Moving

Moving is the second stage of change (Lewin 1947, 1951). This stage signifies that change is underway and that the consultee is making the transition from what is known and comfortable to a new way of thinking and doing. Moving means embracing a vision of a new future and uniting behind the steps necessary to achieve that future (Kanter et al. 1992).

Moving requires cognitive restructuring. Cognitive restructuring can only take place, however, once unfreezing has occurred and the consultee is open to viewing a situation in different ways. Cognitive restructuring involves searching for new viewpoints or information about a situation. The two most common strategies for gathering the data needed for cognitive restructuring are identification and scanning.

Cognitive Restructuring through Identification   Identification involves becoming aligned with a role model and taking on the role model's point of view. Identification is a relatively quick way of gaining a new viewpoint and provides a certain amount of comfort to the consultee because less time is spent "in limbo" looking for a problem solution. The limitation of identification as a means of cognitive restructuring is its narrow scope: only one alternate viewpoint is accessed.

Often, consultees identify with the nurse consultant as a role model. This is most likely to happen when the purchase of expertise model is used to guide a nursing consultation relationship, or when the nurse consultant has other sources of personal power such as charisma. When identification is used as the means of facilitating cognitive restructuring, the nurse consultant should link the consultee to appropriate role models in their environment. Individuals who have successfully resolved a nursing consultation problem similar to that of the consultee are particularly appropriate choices for role models. For example, nurses involved in the implementation of a team model of nursing care delivery could be paired with nurses from a unit that has already successfully implemented this model of nursing care.

Cognitive Restructuring through Scanning   Scanning is the second strategy that consultees can use to obtain the needed information for cognitive restructuring. Because scanning involves seeking information from a variety of sources (peers, journals, workshops, and so forth), this strategy is more thorough than identification as well as more likely to produce a new perspective that really fits the consultee and the client system. However, scanning is a slower means of acquiring information and, therefore, unsuitable for urgent consultation situations.

Refreezing

Refreezing is the final stage of change. Refreezing has occurred when a new point of view has been integrated into both the consultee's self-concept and relationships with others (Schein 1987). Refreezing means that new attitudes, practices, and policies have been put into place (Kanter et al. 1992). Refreezing occurs as a result of "internal sorting." That is, the consultee discards old and inappropriate habits and attitudes, and develops and takes on new ones (Bridges 1991). The nurse consultant can facilitate refreezing by helping the consultee evaluate the effectiveness of the implemented change and by making revisions as needed. The nurse consultant can also facilitate refreezing by ensuring that system supports needed to maintain a change are in place. Examples of system supports frequently needed to support change are financial resources, vision, skills, enthusiasm, equipment, positive feedback, and reward structures. In some cases, in order to facilitate refreezing, the nurse consultant will need to help other members of the client system unfreeze in terms of their relationship to the consultee. In a work redesign scenario, for example, physicians would need to learn new ways of interacting with the nurses who are no longer bedside care providers, but rather team leaders.

The Mechanics of Change and the Nursing Consultation Process

While the theme of change permeates the entire nursing consultation relationship, the different mechanics of the change process coincide with different stages in the nursing consultation process (see Figure 7-1). Disconfirmation and induction of guilt/anxiety often precipitate a consultee's initial contact with the nurse consultant and continue throughout the gaining entry phase of the nursing consultation process. The creation of psychological safety needs to begin with initial contact and must be well under way before a nursing consultation contract is agreed upon. However, concern with creating psychological safety continues throughout the entire nursing consultation relationship and change process.

Once unfreezing has occurred, moving can get underway. The change stage of moving coincides with the problem identification and action planning stages of the nursing consultation process. Cognitive restructuring occurs during these stages as problem explanations and solutions are explored. Refreezing should be detected during the evaluation phase of the nursing consultation process and signals that it is appropriate to begin the disengagement phase. The continuity supports that are established during the disengagement phase help to ensure that refreezing will be permanent.

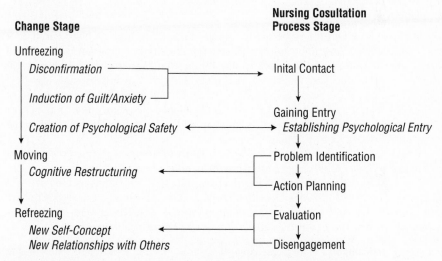

Figure 7-1. The Mechanics of Change and the Nursing Consultation Process
Change is a pervasive theme in nursing consultation relationships. The different stages of change coincide with the different stages and tasks of the nursing consultation process. The two biggest mistakes in nursing consultation and trying to facilitate change are: attempting to introduce change before unfreezing has occurred, and a lack of attention to issues and conditions needed in order for refreezing to occur.

Emotional Responses to Change

People are not inherently anti-change. Most will, in fact,
embrace initiatives provided the change has positive meaning
for them. (Robbins & Finley 1996)

Change occurs on two basic levels: the situational/mechanical level and the personal/emotional level. Lewin's description of the mechanics of change (1947, 1951), while helpful for understanding how change occurs, fails to address the emotions that occur in response to change.

"Transition" is the psychological process people go through to come to terms with the personal/emotional level of a new situation (Bridges 1991). Unless transition occurs, implementing and maintaining change can be difficult. Because the realization of change requires resources and energy from within an individual (the consultee), the nurse consultant must be able to deal consciously and constructively with the emotions and psychological transition that accompanies change (Perlman & Takacs 1990; Schoolfield & Orduna, 1994). Even when a problem solution or change is as concrete as new chart forms, it is a consultee's knowledge, attitudes, beliefs, and values that are the real targets of change (Haffer 1986). On an individual level then, change means three things: recognizing a deficit, giving something up, and learning something new. These demands can create feelings of ineffectiveness, loss of control, confusion, conflict, and loss of meaning (Bolman & Deal 1991). What change means on an individual level explains the emotional responses that tend to be associated with change: ambivalence, resistance, and grief.

Ambivalence

Ambivalence is a natural response to change (Lippitt & Lippitt 1986; Ulschak & SnowAntle 1990). Consultees might welcome the novelty of change or the improvement a change promises and be exhilarated by the challenge of change but question whether expectations are realistic and timing is right. Consultees may also feel ambivalent toward the nurse consultant as an agent of change. The nurse consultant can be seen as both necessary and hostile to the client system; as much as the client system would like their problem solved, they would also like to maintain much of the status quo (Price & Reiss-Brennan 1990).

Ambivalence causes consultees to feel alternately optimistic and pessimistic about the change process. Ambivalence often results in one of two responses: ignoring concerns and losses and rushing ahead with change, or keeping things as they are and replaying the past (Bolman & Deal 1991; Bridges 1991). Both of these responses are counterproductive to the nursing consultation process. The first ignores the need for psychological transition and the second simply abandons problem solving.

Managing Ambivalence   The nurse consultant must be able to manage ambivalence if transition and change are to be successful. The first step to managing ambivalence is bringing it out into the open and communicating its legitimacy. These actions alone can help decrease the likelihood of a counterproductive response to ambivalence (Lippitt & Lippitt 1986). The nurse consultant also needs to remain objective and avoid becoming defensive when consultees voice doubts about a proposed change. Instead, doubts and negative comments should be used as a prompt to verify the soundness of the proposed action plan.

Another strategy for responding to ambivalence is to have consultees list their questions and doubts about a proposed change in one column and their positive feelings about the change in another. The nurse consultant can then help consultees brainstorm about what can be done to respond to doubts as well as what can be done to support positive feelings (Lippitt & Lippitt 1986). In this way, ambivalence can be used as a resource for enhancing the likelihood of a more successful and long-lasting change effort. Box 7-1 summarizes strategies for managing ambivalence about change.

Box 7-1. Managing Responses to Change: Ambivalence

Ambivalence occurs because any change has costs as well as potential benefits. Strategies the nurse consultant can use to manage ambivalence include:

- *Publicize it*—"There seems to be some ambivalence..."
- *Normalize it*—"Ambivalence is a normal response to change..."
- *Use it as an opportunity to check the soundness of the action plan*—
  "What doubts do you have about this change? How could these doubts be addressed?"

Resistance

Consultees have good reason to resist change. Change is associated with the discomfort of giving up the familiar. Unlearning current ways of doing things implies doing something wrong and, therefore, threatens face (Schein 1987). Furthermore, learning something new creates a period of uncertainty, feelings of incompetence, and a temporary decrease in effectiveness. Learning something new, in other words, causes the expert to once again become a novice. In a work redesign situation, for example, the nurse who has been an expert bedside caregiver may feel like a novice as a team leader.

Resistance also occurs because change can disrupt the structural arrangements of a client system. During the moving stage of the change process, there can be a lack of clarity about who has authority, who is supposed to do what, and how to relate to each other (Bolman & Deal 1991). This creates instability and confusion, and causes feelings of powerlessness and insecurity. In a work redesign situation, for example, nurses may feel insecure and incompetent as they attempt to learn new duties, new ways of relating to patients and coworkers, and a new chain of authority.

Finally, change can be resisted for ideological reasons. Consultees may truly believe that a change is misdirected and that the current state or another alternative is better than the proposed change. They also may believe that the change violates an important personal value or organizational principle. For example, nurses involved in a redesign project may resist the proposed change because of fundamental beliefs about how care should be delivered and what nurses should do. Box 7-2 identifies other reasons for resisting change.

Managing Resistance Too often, "resistance" is used as an excuse for the failure of a consultant or manager to understand and reach out to people who are reluctant to change (Smith 1996). Because resistance (or reluctance) is an expected response to change, nurse consultants must be skilled at managing resistance if a consultation relationship is to be successful. Key stratagies for managing resistance are validating emotions, providing information and support, and dealing with bargaining.

Nurse consultants need to confront resistance by validating its underlying emotions, while still holding consultees accountable for their performance (Schoolfield & Orduna 1994). In a work redesign situation, for example, the nurse consultant can empathize with nurses about their feelings of insecurity and incompetence, but still communicate the expectation that quality nursing care will continue to be delivered. If consultees are to be held accountable for usual standards of performance while a change is being implemented, however, they need to be given what they need to feel competent and secure (Bolman & Deal 1991). Too often, the response to resistance is a "lecture" about productivity. Instead, the nurse consultant can help decrease consul-

Box 7-2. Reasons for Resistance

- Loss
- Too much uncertainty
- Surprises: no preparation or background information
- Confusion and interruption of routines
- Loss of face: looking "stupid" for past actions
- Concerns about competence to deal with the new ways
- More work: meetings, learning, and so forth
- Ripple effects: there is never only one change
- Past resentments: memories of negative change experiences
- Real threats: job loss, and so forth
- Low energy: too many changes happening too fast
- Inertia: too comfortable doing things the old way
- Uncertainty about the personal payoff versus costs of change

References: Kanter, R., Stein, B., & Jicks, T. (1992). *The challenge of organizational change.* New York: The Free Press; and Robbins, H., & Finley, M. (1996). *Why change doesn't work.* Princeton, NJ: Peterson's.

tees' feelings of powerlessness and uncertainty by using such stratagies as providing information and feedback, controlling rumors, teaching needed skills, providing needed material and psychological support, and encouraging involvement in change decisions.

Typical questions that consultees have about change are identified in Box 7-3. These questions underscore the importance of communication in overcoming resistance to change. Consider the information and supports that might be needed to overcome resistance to a proposal for work redesign: The nurses affected by the redesign could be expected to have questions and need information about job security and what new tasks they will need to take on. They might also need training in delegation skills. Resistance to work redesign might be countered by realigning and renegotiating policies, processes, roles, and reward structures so that they are supportive of the expected changes in behavior (Bolman & Deal 1991).

Bargaining is a resistance tactic that is used frequently by consultees. What consultees try to do during bargaining is offer compromises that will bargain away the proposed change. The nurse consultant needs to address bargaining by first considering that it might be a valid reaction to the nurse consultant's attempt to implement a change that would either be a poor fit with the client system and its problem, or would possibly create new problems (Brack et al. 1993). If this explanation for bargaining is ruled out, the nurse consultant should respond to bargaining by focusing on the needs of the consultee that are threatened by the change (security and feelings of competence, for example) and exploring how these needs can be met (with information or training, for example) without compromising the desired change outcome (Perlman & Takacs 1990). If bargaining is a reaction to a genuine difference in values, the nurse consultant should try to persuade the consultee to give the change a try, and then evaluate and reconsider.

Box 7-4 summarizes strategies for managing resistance to change.

Box 7-3. Typical Questions about Change

- How do we get from here to there?
- What is involved in this change process?
- Who will do what and how will they do it?
- What do we have to learn that we don't already know?
- When will we start to see results?
- How will we be kept informed of progress?
- What is expected of me?
- Is this change the only one planned, or is it just one of many?
- Is management truly committed to this idea?

Reference: Robbins, H., & Finley, M. (1996). *Why change doesn't work*. Princeton, NJ: Peterson's.

Box 7-4. Managing Responses to Change: Resistance

Consultees resist change because it is associated with feelings of incompetence, ineffectiveness, and confusion. Resistance can also occur when change conflicts with personal values. Strategies the nurse consultant can use to manage resistance include:

- Validate the underlying emotions of the resistance while still demanding accountability
- Keep communication open: listen, solicit and give feedback, provide information
- Give consultees the material and psychological support they need to feel competent and secure
- Realign and renegotiate policies and roles to make them supportive of expected new behaviors
- Explore the possibility that bargaining may indicate a proposed change is a poor fit for the system
- Respond to bargaining by negotiating a "trial" of the proposed change that will be followed by evaluation and reconsideration

---

Grief

Grief is the third common emotional response to change. Grief occurs because change involves the loss of old, established, comfortable ways as well as one's old role and identity. Because change involves loss, a grieving process needs to take place so that the past is let go of and the change can be embraced (Schoolfield & Orduna 1994). In change situations, the grief response consists of the classic grief reactions: denial, anger, bargaining, depression, resignation, openness/acceptance, and re-emergence (Perlman & Takacs 1990).

Denial and Anger The first stage of the grief response, denial, often takes the form of denying that a problem actually exists. In other cases, ambivalence and active resistance may signal denial. To some extent, denial is an unavoidable part of the unfreezing process. Just as unfreezing must occur, denial must be resolved before moving toward change can get underway.

When a consultee realizes that change is going to proceed and the status quo is going to be disrupted, anger often occurs. In this stage of the grief process, consultees tend to glorify the past and exaggerate the problems of the present. Others, the nurse consultant and management in particular, become the target of anger and are blamed for the difficulties of the change process.

Bargaining, Depression, and Resignation   Bargaining occurs as a resistance tactic once change efforts are underway or perceived as inevitable. Once the change is, in fact, underway and accompanying feelings of incompetence, ineffectiveness, and powerlessness become a reality, depression follows. When resistance tactics are recognized as being ineffective by the consultee, resignation occurs. During this phase of the grief process, there is usually compliance with a change, but no enthusiasm for it. The challenge for the nurse consultant is to transform compliance into commitment so that change will continue (refreeze) once the nursing consultation relationship has ended.

Openness/Acceptance and Re-emergence   The final stages of the grief response coincide with the refreezing stage of the change process. Openness/acceptance occurs when consultees accept the personal implications of change and rearrange their values and self-concept to accommodate the change. Re-emergence, the last stage in the classic grief response process, signifies that refreezing has occurred and the change is integrated fully into consultees' ways of interacting within the client system. Re-emergence means that the past has been let go of both emotionally and intellectually. Re-emergence (and refreezing) mean that consultees have redefined their roles and identity in relationship to the nursing consultation problem and the client system. Figure 7-2 illustrates the relationship between the grief process and the mechanics of change.

Managing Grief   Nurse consultants need to understand that completion of the grief process is necessary if change is to be successful and long-lasting. Failure to allow a grief response results in change that is only short-lived because losses have not been

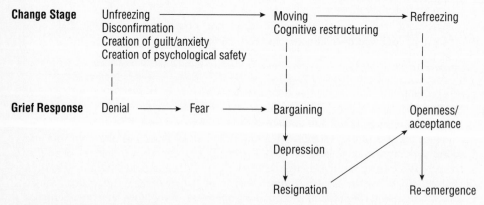

Figure 7-2. Change and Grief
Grief accompanies change because change means loss. The classic grief reactions of denial, anger, bargaining, depression, resignation, openness/acceptance, and re-emergence can be observed as the stages of change unfold.

Box 7-5. Managing the Emotions of Change: Grief

Grief is a normal reaction to change because change means the loss of comfortable habits, as well as familiar ways of interacting, thinking, and behaving. Change also means the loss of actual or symbolic roles and identities. Passage through the stages of grief is necessary if change is to be successful and long-lasting. Managing grief means facilitating passage through the stages of grief rather than trying to eliminate it. Grief management strategies for the nurse consultant include:

- Acknowledge what has been lost
- Respect the past
- Have empathy for what the loss means to those involved (consultees)
- Put supports in place to facilitate adaptation to both the loss and new identity
- Have patience
- Use rituals to bring closure to the past and recognition to the future

References: Bridges, W. (1991). *Managing transitions: Making the most of change.* Reading, MA: Addison-Wesley; and Perlman, D., & Takacs, G. (1990). The 10 stages of change. *Nursing Management, 21* (4), 33-38.

---

adapted to or acknowledged. Rather than managing grief in the sense of eliminating it, the nurse consultant needs to facilitate the consultee's movement through the various stages of grief by helping the consultee accept and adapt to the losses and role changes associated with the change. Managing grief requires acknowledgment, empathy, and patience. What the consultee has lost even temporarily as a result of change needs to be acknowledged. The past and emotions associated with this loss need to be respected. Patience and support are also needed as consultees adapt to the loss of an old identity and the taking on of a new identity. Finally, rituals can be used to help consultees achieve closure with the past and recognize the future (Bridges 1991).

Box 7-5 summarizes grief management strategies for the nurse consultant. As you review these strategies, consider how they might be used in the change scenario of work redesign. Some of the losses experienced by nurses who are involved in work redesign include loss of their traditional role as bedside caregiver (replaced by the roles of delegator and team leader) and loss of a certain type of relationship with both patients and staff. These losses require adaptation and the taking on of a new professional identity. These losses also result in a typical grief response on the part of the consultee. The nurse consultant working with the nurse consultees in this scenario needs to acknowledge these losses and put supports (such as education) in place that will promote adaptation to a new nursing role. The client system will need to be patient as the role changes for the nurses result in temporary decreases in productivity. Accomplishment of the change (implementation of the new care delivery system) could be acknowledged with rituals such as an open house or "graduation" celebration.

Changemaker Skills for Nurse Consultants

As discussed in Chapter 1, change agency is fundamentally different from nursing consultation. In order to differentiate the two, Kanter, Stein, and Jicks (1992) use the term "changemaker" to describe a consultant's role in the change process. Nurse consultants fulfill the specific changemaker roles of "strategist" and "implementor." In the strategist role, the nurse consultant identifies a problem, creates a vision, and identifies feasibility issues related to the proposed change. In the implementor role, the nurse consultant manages the day-to-day process of change and ensures that the supports needed for change are in place. The specific changemaker skills that the nurse consultant needs in order to fulfill these roles are the abilities to assess a consultee's perspective of change, actualize change, and communicate about change.

Assessing Consultees' Perspective of Change

Say the word "change" to any randomly selected group and you will
likely get three different responses. Some throw up their hands and say,
"God, not again." Others say, "Well, it's about time." The third group
will simply throw up. (Robbins & Finley 1996)

A consultee's perspective of change has implications for the roles a nurse consultant will need to assume during the nursing consultation relationship. A consultee's perspective of change also determines the types of barriers that may be encountered as change strategies are being developed and implemented. Understanding a consultee's perspective of change helps the nurse consultant anticipate the ways in which change may be experienced by the consultee. Understanding a consultee's perspective of change also helps the nurse consultant select the intervention strategies and interaction style that will most effectively facilitate problem solving and subsequent change. Change is generally viewed by consultees in one of three ways: as something needed to achieve a goal, something needed in order to solve a problem, or something that "just happens" (Hansen 1995). Box 7-6 presents questions the nurse consultant can ask to determine a consultee's perspective of change.

Change as Choice When change is viewed as a choice, it is often undertaken proactively rather than reactively; it may even be pursued aggressively. Consultees who view change as choice see change as tolerable, if not desirable. Consultees with this perspective view change as a means to achieve a goal (such as improved market positioning). They also tend to view change as a linear, orchestrated process, and therefore respond well to carefully orchestrated change activities where change can be experienced as a series of steps and stages. Since these consultees often plan change in anticipation of environmental events, they are ideal candidates for a process consultation interaction pattern.

Change Only if Necessary Consultees who view change as something that is undertaken only when a problem needs to be solved tend to view change as troublesome and unpredictable, as something they "have to do." From this perspective, a system's need to change is often triggered by input and output problems such as the inability to secure needed resources (such as patients) or to find "buyers" for its products/services (a certain kind of health care delivery, for example). The desired outcome of this type of change is increased security. For these consultees, change is often reactive and occurs under a time crunch.

The nurse consultant is likely to encounter increased resistance from consultees who have this perspective of change. Even though these consultees recognize they have a problem to solve, they perceive themselves (perhaps accurately) as having little choice in regard to change. These consultees often experience change as chaos, confusion, and panic.

Box 7-6. Assessing a Consultee's Perspective of Change

Change is generally viewed by consultees in one of three ways: as something undertaken by choice in order to attain a goal, something to become involved in only when a problem needs to be solved, or something that is an inevitable necessity and "just happens." Questions the nurse consultant can ask to determine a consultee's perspective of change include:

- What triggers change for the consultee?
    Goals?
    Problems?
    Nothing?
- How does the consultee respond to pressure about change?
    Proactively or reactively?
    Aggressively, passively, or with resistance?
    With a time crunch?
- What is valued as the outcome of change?
    Improved positioning?
    Security?
    Stability and equilibrium?
- What does change look and feel like as it is occurring?
    Steps and stages?
    Chaos, confusion, and panic?
    Patterned transition in growth?
    Lurches and stumbling?

Nurse consultants often find themselves assuming the role of troubleshooter for consultees who have a problem-oriented view of change. In these situations, the purchase of expertise or doctor-patient interaction patterns tend to be the most effective and, in fact, are sometimes necessary. A goal of the nurse consultant working with consultees who view change from this perspective is to facilitate the consultees' learning to engage in environmental monitoring and more proactive forms of change.

Change "Just Happens" The third perspective that consultees may have about change is that change is something that "just happens." Change is viewed by these consultees as inevitable and inherent to the process of a system's relationships evolving with its environments. These consultees may undertake change proactively or may seek nursing consultation and change when they are experiencing problems with equilibrium and stability (for example, issues with processes). Grief, ambivalence, resignation, and passive resistance are common responses of consultees who have this perspective of change. These consultees tend to experience change as a patterned transition in growth, but also as a process that occurs with lurches and stumbling.

Nurse consultants working with consultees who view change as an inevitable necessity need to encourage consultee involvement in the change process. In these situations, nurse consultants often find a process consultation interaction pattern to be a necessary and effective means of creating ownership of a problem solution and its resultant change.

Actualizing Change

The costs of failed change attempts are high. Loss of jobs, loss of energy, loss of trust and credibility, loss of respect, anger, increased stress, and a decreased willingness to take risks are just a few of the outcomes of change failures (Robbins & Finley 1996). Change can fail for any number of reasons (see Box 7-7), many of which the nurse consultant can prevent by attending to the dynamics of the nursing consultation process and by managing the emotional responses to change. Additional stratagies that nurse consultants can use to ensure that a proposed change is actually implemented are using force-field analysis and creating ownership of change.

Force-Field Analysis   Force-field analysis (Lewin 1951) is a strategy nurse consultants can use to help consultees identify and visualize factors in a problem situation that could act as either barriers or supporters of change. Force-field analysis can also be used to assess the "rightness" of a client system's decision to proceed with a change.

In force-field theory, an organization's current state is conceptualized as reflecting an "organizational equilibrium" in which two sets of forces are visible: restraining forces or factors that act to maintain the status quo, and driving forces or factors that encourage movement away from the status quo and support a proposed change (Lewin 1951). Driving and restraining forces can be environmental/situational or personal/emotional factors. These forces vary in their degree of intensity or importance.

Equilibrium or the status quo exists as long as these two sets of forces—the "force-field"—are in balance. According to force-field theory, there are three basic interventions a nurse consultant can use to induce change: add driving forces, eliminate or reduce restraining forces, or do some of both. Changing the balance of driving and restraining forces introduces a state of disequilibrium and provides the disconfirmation needed to get change underway ("unfreezing"). Disequilibrium remains as long as change is in progress. Once goals have been accomplished or "refreezing" has occurred, a client system returns to a state of equilibrium under new conditions.

Force-field analysis is most useful when carried out collaboratively by the nurse consultant and consultee. The consultee can help identify relevant drivers and restrainers as well as estimate their intensity. The consultee can also help identify which forces are most important and feasible to act on to encourage movement away

---

Box 7-7. Why Change Fails

- The wrong idea
- The right idea, but the wrong time
- The wrong reason
- Lacks authenticity
- Reality contradicts the change
- Loss of perspective (mission, values, and so forth)
- Wrong leader
- Change only for the sake of change
- People aren't prepared or convinced about the need for change
- People get carried away by change: "the sin of excess"
- People don't get carried away enough
- Bad luck: unforeseen environmental events

Reference: Robbins, H., & Finley, M. (1996). *Why change doesn't work*. Princeton, NJ: Peterson's.

from the status quo. Figure 7-3 depicts what a force-field analysis might look like, in this case, completed by a group of nurses involved in a work redesign situation.

Creating Ownership of Change   A second change-actualizing skill that nurse consultants need is that of creating ownership of change. To create ownership of change, the nurse consultant needs to help consultees see themselves as beneficiaries rather than victims of change (Cohen & Murri 1995). This can be accomplished by setting forth a vision of what the change will be like and engaging

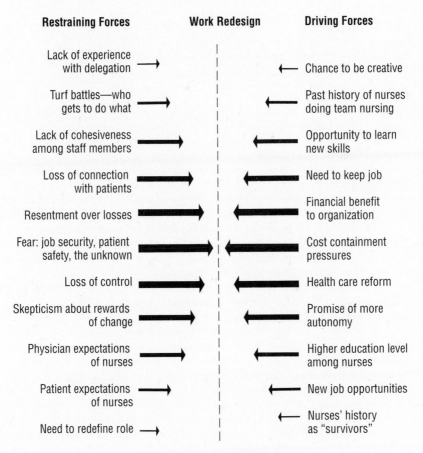

Figure 7-3. Staff Nurses' Force-Field Analysis for Work Redesign

This force-field analysis is from the perspective of staff nurses involved in a work redesign project. Management and physicians might identify different driving and restraining forces. In this force field, fear is the strongest restraining force and cost containment pressures are the strongest driving force. Cost containment pressures will most likely continue to increase on their own to further "push" for work redesign. As they increase, however, fear is likely to increase. In this scenario, the nurse consultant needs to develop interventions that will address the restraining force of fear if the change (work redesign) is to be successful. The driving force of nurses' perceptions of themselves and the nursing profession as "survivors" can also be supported to facilitate this change process.

Box 7-8. Creating Ownership of Change

Strategies the nurse consultant can use to create ownership of change include the following:

- Help consultees see themselves as beneficiaries rather than as victims of change
- Involve consultees in creating the change vision and in developing problem-solving/change strategies
- Create a sense of "we-ness" and unity about the change effort and what it involves
- Ensure administrative and emotional support for undertaking the change
- Use a pilot group to demonstrate the change; broadcast their success and let them "teach" the next group
- Be sure that proposed changes are consistent with the needs and culture of the client system

Reference: Robbins, H., & Finley, M. (1996). *Why change doesn't work*. Princeton, NJ: Peterson's.

---

consultees' imagination in further developing this vision. Ownership of change is facilitated when consultees have a strong sense of belonging to and being valued by the client system (Price & Reiss-Brennan 1990). Consultees should be encouraged to play with the problem solution or "change idea" and modify it as needed to fit both their own needs and those of the client system. Encouraging consultee involvement in this way communicates a valuing of both the consultee as an individual and the expertise they can bring to the change situation. Change (problem-solving) strategies will more likely be accepted, implemented, and long-lasting when consultees are involved in every step of the problem-solving process.

Because change is resisted less when the client system is actively engaged in the change process, establishing a sense of "we-ness" and unity ("We're all in this together") is essential for creating ownership of change. Unity and ownership of change is facilitated when consultees feel supported, both administratively and emotionally, for exposing themselves to the possible personal risks associated with change. Nurse consultants need to persuade the client system to give consultees the time and resources needed to make a change and show measurable success.

Unity and ownership of change can also be fostered by first implementing the change in a pilot group of pro-change consultees and by building supportive coalitions. Once this pilot group achieves success, their accomplishment should be broadcast throughout the client system. The pilot group can then be used to teach a second group the new behaviors and attitudes the change requires. This strategy creates unity and ownership of change by its "snowball effect" of involvement and success.

Finally, change must be consistent with the needs and culture of the client system if it is to be owned by the system and its members. Change that violates cultural norms will most likely be resisted, rejected, or sabotaged. Box 7-8 summarizes strategies for creating ownership of change.

Communicating about Change

The importance of communication in the change process has been mentioned a number of times throughout this chapter. However, communication is frequently impeded during the change process by several forces:

- Consultee belief that change is a waste of time due to previous negative change experiences

- False familiarity ("We've been through this before")

- Consultee fear

- The rumor mill

- "Sloppy execution" of communication: incomprehensibility, abstraction, complexity, and clichés (Hammer & Stanton 1995)

Facilitating change through communication demands two sets of skills: selling change and talking through the change process.

Selling Change

Change is an act of the imagination. Until the imagination
is engaged, no important change can occur. (Robbins & Finley 1996)

Until consultees are "sold" on a change, they will be resistant, or at least reluctant, to expose themselves to the personal costs associated with change. A key to selling change is creating a vision of how the change will look and feel, both while it is underway and once it is accomplished. To sell change, the nurse consultant must first "segment the audience" (Hammer & Stanton 1995). This means the nurse consultant first recognizes that different stakeholders in the change process will be affected by the change in different ways and then personalizes the change message given to each group in terms of timing, media, and emphasis. To continue with the example of work redesign used throughout this chapter, the staff nurses would need to hear that the redesign vision will mean increased autonomy and job security. In contrast, administrators may need to hear the vision of an improved profit margin and a more secure competitive edge. Selling change is also facilitated by using multiple voices and multiple channels of communication; this increases the likelihood that each listener will find a speaker to whom they can relate.

Talking through the Change Process Closely related to change-selling skills, but having a different focus, are the communication skills that the nurse consultant needs to use on an ongoing basis to guide consultees through the change process. Specific attention needs to be given to reinforcing the "core message" of the change process:

- purpose: why we must go through this; the scope and scale of the change

- process: how it will be accomplished, including the governing process for managing the change

- progress: are we on track with how we envisioned the change unfolding

- problems: setbacks that have occurred and lessons that have been learned (Champy 1997; Hammer & Stanton 1995)

This core message needs to be repeated and communicated clearly, honestly, and in tangible terms. Talking through the change process is more effective when the nurse consultant communicates with passion and enthusiasm as well as logic. The nurse consultant also needs to use communication skills to encourage, console, and express appreciation. Finally, talking through the change process requires two-way communication. Nurse consultants need to both listen and respond to what consultees have to say. Box 7-9 summarizes the skills a nurse consultant needs to communicate effectively about change.

Box 7-9. Communicating about Change

- Segment the audience; address different groups of stakeholders differently in terms of timing, media, and emphasis
- Use multiple channels of communication; supplement verbal communication with nonverbal messages in the form of memos, posters, and so forth
- Use multiple voices; different messengers will present different viewpoints (this helps to ensure that every listener will find someone with whom they can identify)
- Communicate clearly; keep in mind the essential core of the change message: purpose, process, progress, and problems
- Honesty is the only policy—"I don't know" is better than a lie
- Use emotions, not just logic; convey passion and enthusiasm about the change
- Use communication to heal, console, encourage, and express appreciation
- Communicate tangibly. Back up words with actions and evidence
- Communicate, communicate, communicate
- Listen, listen, listen

Adapted from Hammer, M., & Stanton, S. (1995). *The reengineering revolution: A handbook.* New York: Harper Business.

Chapter Summary

Because consultation is fundamentally a problem-solving process, change is inherent in all nursing consultation relationships. A request for nursing consultation is, in effect, a request for help to make a change. To be effective as problem solvers and changemakers, nurse consultants need an understanding of both the mechanics of change and the emotional responses change precipitates. To function effectively in the changemaker roles of strategist and implementor, the nurse consultant needs to be able to assess a consultee's perspective of change, as well as actualize and communicate about change.

Applying Chapter Content

Reflect on two change situations in which you have recently been involved, one of which was successful and the other unsuccessful. What factors can you identify that contributed to these different change outcomes?

Consider the following change scenarios:

- Adding a nurse practitioner to a clinic that is only staffed by physicians
- Implementing a MSN program in a nursing department that currently has only a BSN program
- Transforming a wing of a rural acute care hospital into a long-term intermediate care facility

Conduct a force-field analysis on each of these change scenarios. How could you use this information to facilitate the proposed change? Specifically, how could you use this information to sell and talk through the proposed change?

What specific sources of resistance would you anticipate in each of these scenarios? How would you attempt to address these?

What types of losses would occur with each of these scenarios? How could consultees be compensated for these losses?

How could the application of change-actualizing strategies such as building coalitions and implementing a "pilot" project change be used in each of these scenarios?

References

Bolman, L. & Deal, T. (1991). *Reframing organizations: Artistry, choice, and leadership.* San Francisco: Jossey-Bass.

Brack, G., Jones, E., Smith, R., White, J., & Brack, C. (1993). A primer on consultation theory: Building a flexible worldview. *Journal of Counseling and Development, 71,* 619-628.

Bridges, W. (1991). *Managing transitions: Making the most of change.* Reading, MA: Addison-Wesley.

Champy, J. (1997). Preparing for organizational change. In F. Hesselbein, M. Goldsmith, & R. Beckhard (Eds.), *The organization of the future* (pp. 9-16). San Francisco: Jossey-Bass.

Cohen, W., & Murri, M. (1995). Managing the change process. *Journal of AHIMA, 66* (6), 40-47.

Fuqua, D., & Kurpius, D. (1993). Conceptual models in organizational consultation. *Journal of Counseling and Development, 71,* 607-618.

Haffer, A. (1986). Facilitating change: Choosing the appropriate strategy. *Journal of Nursing Administration, 16* (4), 18-22.

Hammer, M., & Stanton, S. (1995). *The reengineering revolution: A handbook.* New York: HarperBusiness.

Hansen, H. (1995). The advanced practice nurse as a change agent. In M. Snyder & M. Mirr, (Eds.), *Advanced practice nursing: A guide to professional development* (pp. 197-213). New York: Springer Publishing.

Kanter, R., Stein, B., & Jicks, T. (1992). *The challenge of organizational change.* New York: The Free Press.

Lewin, K. (1947). Frontiers in group dynamics. *Human Relations, 1,* 5-41.

Lewin, K. (1951). *Field theory in social sciences.* New York: Harper & Row.

Lippitt, G., & Lippitt, R. (1986). *The consulting process in action* (2nd ed.). San Diego: University Associates.

McDougall, G. (1987). The role of the clinical nurse specialist consultant in organizational development. *Clinical Nurse Specialist, 1* (3), 133-138.

Perlman, D., & Takacs, G. (1990). The 10 stages of change. *Nursing Management, 21* (4), 33-38.

Price, J., & Reiss-Brennan, B. (1989). Consulting telesis: A systems approach. *Nursing Management, 20* (11), 80A-80E.

Robbins, H., & Finley, M. (1996). *Why change doesn't work.* Princeton, NJ: Peterson's.

Schein, E. (1987). *Process consultation, volume II: Lessons for managers and consultants.* Reading, MA: Addison-Wesley.

Schoolfield, M., & Orduna, A. (1994). Understanding staff nurses responses to change: Utilization of a grief-change framework to facilitate innovation. *Clinical Nurse Specialist, 8* (1), 57-62.

Smith, D. (1996). *Taking charge of change.* Reading, MA: Addison-Wesley.

Ulschak, F., & SnowAntle, S. (1990). *Consultation skills for health care professionals*. San Francisco: Jossey-Bass.

Additional Readings

Barker, E. (1990). Use of a diffusion of innovation model for agency consultation. *Clinical Nurse Specialist, 4* (3), 163-165.
The author presents a model that identifies expected patterns of responses to change. Particular attention is given to initiating and adopting change.

Bolman, L., & Deal, T. (1991). *Reframing organizations: Artistry, choice, and leadership.* San Francisco: Jossey-Bass.
Chapter 9 of this text discusses conflict and loss.

Bridges, W. (1991). *Managing transition: Making the most of change.* Reading, MA: Addison-Wesley.
This text focuses on the psychological processes that accompany change.

Burke, W. (1990). *Organizational development: A process of learning and changing.* Reading, MA: Addison-Wesley.
The author presents a model of organizational change that takes into particular consideration the effect of climate and culture on change results.

Hammer, M., & Stanton, S. (1995). *The reengineering revolution: A handbook.* New York: Harper Business.
Chapter 9 addresses "The Art of Selling Change" and includes a case study that demonstrates the application of communication techniques.

Hesselbein, F., Goldsmith, M., & Beckhard, R. (1997). *The organization of the future.* San Francisco: Jossey-Bass.
This compendium of essays presents viewpoints and strategies on how organizations must change for the future.

Kanter, R., Stein, B., & Jicks, T. (1992). *The challenge of organizational change.* New York: The Free Press.
This is a comprehensive text on instituting change in organizations. It combines theoretical insights into the change process with portraits of organizations experiencing change and strategies for implementing change.

Kotter, J. (1990). *A force for change: How leadership differs from management.* New York: The Free Press.
Unit 2 of this text offers ideas on direction-setting, aligning people, motivating, and inspiring that are helpful for the nurse consultant.

Mohrman, A., Mohrman, S., Ledford, G., Cummings, T., & Lawler, E. (1989). *Large-scale organizational change.* San Francisco: Jossey-Bass.
This text focuses on initiating change in large organizations.

Nadler, D., Shaw, R., & Walton, A. (1995). *Discontinuous change: Leading organizational transformation.* San Francisco: Jossey-Bass.
The authors offer a theoretical framework for moving organizations through complex changes. The book includes interviews with change leaders.

Perlman, D., & Takacs, G. (1990). The 10 stages of change. *Nursing Management, 21* (4), 33-38.
The authors relate change to Kubler-Ross's stages of grief.

Peters, T. (1987). *Thriving on chaos: Handbook for a management revolution.* New York: Harper Collins.
Section 5 of this book provides strategies for leading others through change. Particular attention is given to developing a vision.

Robbins, H., & Finley, M. (1996). *Why change doesn't work*. Princeton, NJ: Peterson's.
The authors examine barriers to change and offer strategies for making change successful. A highly readable book.

Schein, E. (1987). *Process consultation, volume II: Lessons for managers and consultants*. Reading, MA: Addison-Wesley.
Chapter 6 describes and expands on Lewin's theory of change.

Schein, E. (1988). *Process consultation, volume I: Its role in organization development*. (2nd ed.) Reading, MA: Addison-Wesley.
Chapter 9 discusses intragroup processes related to change.

Senge, P., Kleiner, A., Roberts, C., Ross, R., & Smith, B. (1994). *The fifth discipline fieldbook: Strategies and tools for building a learning organization*. New York: Currency-Doubleday.
The authors focus on change as a participative process and learning opportunity.

8

Gaining Entry in Nursing Consultation

Starting a relationship with a new client has
always been the real challenge for me.
(Metzger 1993)

Key terms: scanning, contracting, physical entry, psychological entry, hidden agenda

How many times have you found yourself in a working relationship that you felt was just not a "good fit"? The situation may have involved working with a patient, a student, or another nurse. As in many other helping relationships, in traditional nurse-patient relationships, nurses often have no choice about with whom they work or for whom they provide care. In most cases, nurses simply receive a patient assignment and carry out a plan of care.

The working relationship is different in nursing consultation. Nurse consultants have the opportunity and the responsibility to determine their "fit" with a consultee and client system before becoming involved in a problem-solving relationship. Nurse consultants also have the opportunity to get acquainted and begin to establish trust and credibility with a consultee before the actual work of the consultation relationship begins. These "fit-determining" and getting acquainted activities and opportunities occur during the gaining entry phase of the nursing consultation process.

Building and defining relationships is the focus of the gaining entry phase of the nursing consultation process. The specific tasks that need to be accomplished during this phase are environmental scanning, contracting, gaining physical entry into the problem setting, and initiating psychological entry with the client system. Taken together, these tasks serve a twofold purpose. First, environmental scanning provides the nurse consultant with information needed to make a decision regarding whether or not to continue the consultation relationship. Secondly, the tasks of contracting, gaining physical entry, and initiating psychological entry establish the tone and set the stage for the subsequent working phases of the nursing consultation process (Figure 8-1). Thus the work of the gaining entry phase prepares a pathway for effective consultation (Monicken 1995).

The gaining entry phase of the nursing consultation process begins at the time of a potential consultee's request for help and culminates in the initiation of deliberate problem-solving activities. Although accomplishing each task in the gaining entry phase is necessary to facilitate successful nursing consultation, the way in which each task is carried out will differ according to the unique features of each consultation situation. The tasks of the gaining entry phase may vary in their timing, degree of formality, level of complexity, and relative emphasis, depending both on the interaction pattern being used to guide the problem-solving activities and on whether the nurse is acting as an internal or external consultant.

This chapter discusses each of the tasks that comprise the gaining entry phase of the nursing consultation process, with consideration to the specific purpose of each task, strategies for carrying out each task, and potential dilemmas associated with each task. Variations in how the tasks of the gaining entry phase might be carried out are illustrated by scenarios that appear in a series of boxes throughout the chapter. As you read this chapter, consider the following questions:

- What different sets of dilemmas might internal and external nurse consultants face during the gaining entry phase of the nursing consultation process?

- Does the gaining entry phase differ when the consultee is an individual or group? If so, how? Does it differ when the client is a patient or a unit within a health care organization? If so, how?

- What are some problems that might arise later in the nursing consultation process that could indicate incomplete, unsuccessful, or careless completion of the tasks of the gaining entry phase?

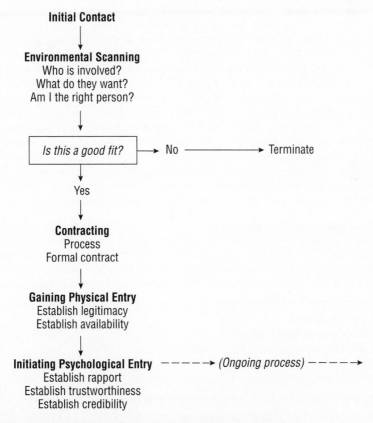

Figure 8-1. The Gaining Entry Phase of the Nursing Consultation Process
The activities of the gaining entry phase set the tone for the subsequent working phases of the nursing consultation relationship.

Environmental Scanning

Environmental scanning is the informal assessment or scouting that a nurse consultant begins at the time of initial contact with a potential consultee or the organizational contact person. During environmental scanning, the nurse consultant gathers information and forms impressions that support a decision about whether or not to enter into a working relationship with the consultee and client system. To reach this decision, the nurse consultant compares how well his/her skills, interests, resources, and work style match those needed or desired by the consultee and client system.

Strategies for Environmental Scanning

One of the challenges of environmental scanning is getting enough information to make the decision to continue or not continue a nursing consultation relationship. During environmental scanning, the nurse consultant does not have a formal contract that enables and facilitates an in-depth assessment of the client system. Consequently, a nurse consultant's information sources may be limited to those that are more or less "public property." Informal scouting and exploratory meetings are the most commonly used information-gathering strategies during the environmental scanning process of the gaining entry phase.

Scouting "Scouting" means investigating a problem and its setting by performing informal research (Metzger 1993). Scouting can include searching out news reports about the problem setting, reading the setting's mission statement in order to get a sense of its values, and conducting informal interviews with persons who know something about the problem issue or problem setting. Some problem settings such as hospitals can also be observed informally to gather clues about their personalities, cultures, availability of resources, and possible barriers to problem solving. For example, a nurse consultant might note a hospital's culture of formality or the presence of furnishings and equipment, which could imply either financial resources or a heavy debt load. Even these informal observations can give the nurse consultant some sense of degree of fit with the client system. This information might also be interpreted as indicating the importance to the client system of its public image, which might be a factor that will facilitate problem-solving activities.

Exploratory Meetings An exploratory meeting with the contact person (who may or may not be the consultee) can provide information about a client system's openness, commitment, and compatibility issues, as well as their perceptions of a problem. Exploratory meetings can be held with individual and family consultees as well as organization contact persons. Questions that a nurse consultant might ask during an exploratory meeting include:

How can I be helpful?
How did you happen to call me?
What is problematic about your situation?
How do you know this is a problem?
How would you like things to be different once the problem is resolved?

In addition to involving the contact person and the nurse consultant, it is often helpful if an exploratory meeting includes someone else from the client system such as a well-respected nurse or a family member. This person may be able to convince other members of the client system of the value in engaging in the proposed consultation relationship.

Exploratory meetings can be held either on-site or off-site. Holding an exploratory meeting on-site facilitates observation of the problem setting and reinforces the work-related (rather than social) nature of a nursing consultation relationship. On the other hand, holding an exploratory meeting at a neutral site may give the consultee a greater sense of control because they are away from the problem setting; an off-site meeting may also decrease any perceived pressure to agree to an immediate contract (Dougherty 1995).

An external nurse consultant needs to decide whether or not to charge for an exploratory meeting. While nurse consultants often consider exploratory meetings a cost of doing business, charging for these meetings can provide a test of a client system's motivation and commitment to get help (Schein 1987, 1988). Charging for an exploratory meeting also acknowledges that the consultee or contact person often gains useful information and insight from the conversation that has taken place during the meeting. Sometimes, this insight makes continuing the consultation relationship unnecessary.

Realistically, an internal nurse consultant may not be able to charge for an exploratory meeting. This because an internal nursing consultation project is usually considered to be within the nurse consultant's "usual" scope of responsibilities. The internal nurse consultant should try, however, to schedule any exploratory meetings during regularly scheduled (and paid) work hours.

Dimensions of Environmental Scanning

Environmental scanning is like going on a first date and making a decision about whether or not to go out again. As suggested by the preceding discussion of strategies for environmental scanning, the primary roles a nurse consultant assumes during environmental scanning are those of observer, questioner, and listener (Lippitt & Lippitt 1986). The specific questions a nurse consultant seeks to answer during environmental scanning are: (1) "Who is involved?" (2) "What do they want?" and (3) "Am I the right person?"

Who Is Involved? The process of identifying who is involved in the consultation relationship has two dimensions. The first involves identifying the parties that comprise the client system and how they are related to one another. The second involves identifying qualities or attitudes held by these parties that might facilitate or hinder a problem-solving relationship.

Identifying Roles and Relationships First, the nurse consultant needs to identify all of the parties involved in the problem situation (that is, who comprises the client system). This is important because there are no surer obstacles to implementing a plan of action than those presented by the parties who have been left out of the process (Monicken 1995). Secondly, the nurse consultant needs to identify the roles of the parties in the client system as well as determine how these parties are related to one another.

First, it is important to pinpoint the identity of the client. (Recall from Chapter 1 that clients are the targets or intended beneficiaries of the nursing consultation relationship but are not typically involved in the problem-solving process.) Clients in nursing consultation can be individual patients, a group of patients, students, a community, a work unit, or an entire organization. Determining the client's identity can be especially difficult in organizational consultation situations because there may be a number of parties that directly benefit from the consultation process. For example, who is the client in a nursing consultation project that focuses on work redesign or nursing staff cross-training? Is the client the group of patients who are served by the system (benefit = better, more cost-effective care) or the entire health care organization (benefit = a better organizational financial picture)? Identifying the client is important since the client's needs and welfare must be the primary concern when the consultant and consultee develop problem-solving interventions.

Sorting out relationships within the client system is another important task of the nurse consultant. The first relationship to sort out is that between the contact person and the consultee since it is the consultee with whom the nurse consultant will be directly working to solve the consultation problem. A person who is serving only as the contact person will not be involved directly in problem-solving activities and may have only a limited vested interest in the problem situation and its resolution. Questions that should be asked about the contact person and the consultee include:

   Is the contact person the consultee, a representative of the consultee, or a representative of the client?
   If the contact person is not the consultee, does the consultee know that help is being sought? (Resistance tends to be lower when consultees have a role in identifying both a problem and a need for help.)
   Is the contact person in a supervisory relationship over the consultee? (If so, the consultee may feel coerced to participate in the consultation process and the nurse consultant may encounter a higher degree of resistance.)

It is also important to determine the relationship between the contact person and the fee payer for the nursing consultation. Ideally, this is the same person since it is the fee payer who has control over the financial resources available to the nurse consultant for problem-solving activities. What is more, the fee payer's sanctioning of proposed consultation interventions (as well as sanctioning by others in positions of authority) sends a powerful message to both consultees and the nurse consultant about the legitimacy of the nursing consultation relationship. If the contact person is not the fee payer, the nurse consultant needs to make every effort to include the fee payer in any exploratory meetings that take place.

Assessing Personal Qualities and Attitudes After the nurse consultant identifies all the parties involved in the consultation relationship and the relationship between these parties, the next step involves identifying any personal qualities or attitudes within these parties that may help or hinder the problem-solving process. During this part of environmental scanning, the nurse consultant focuses on the following two questions:

   Is the consultee (and the client system as a whole) someone with whom I want to work?
   Does this situation offer the opportunity for a compatible and mutually beneficial relationship?

To answer these questions, the nurse consultant needs to examine the openness, readiness to change, and level of commitment to change of both the consultee and other members of the client system.

Openness Openness corresponds to a willingness to assume ownership for both the consultation problem and the outcomes of the consultation process. Openness has two dimensions. First, openness means that consultees are willing to share information about the perceived problem. This is necessary if the nurse consultant is to diagnose the problem accurately and formulate appropriate problem-solving interventions. Secondly, openness means consultees and other members of the client system are willing to explore a variety of problem-solving interventions. Openness in regards to problem-solving interventions helps to ensure that the interventions chosen are both appropriate and feasible. Because the consultees are usually the members of the client system who are most directly affected by the consultation process, their openness is critical to the success of the nursing consultation relationship. After all, they are the persons who are most intimately involved in the consultation process and who are being asked to change their behavior. The following consultee behaviors may indicate a lack of openness:

The consultee seems too certain about a problem and its cause.

The consultee presses the nurse consultant for a quick fix to a superficial problem.

The consultee only wants reassurance for a course of action that is already underway.

The consultee miscasts the nurse consultant as an expert who will cure all of the client system's problems.

A nurse consultant who encounters one or more of these behaviors during environmental scanning needs to confront the consultee about the discrepancy between their behavior and their professed desire for change. (Confrontational interventions are discussed in Chapter 10.) The nurse consultant who continues a consultation relationship when there is a lack of openness needs to accept the possibility of being held responsible if the consultation problem remains unresolved or recurs.

Readiness to Change Readiness to change refers to a willingness to devote the time, money, energy, personnel, and other resources needed to solve a problem. Readiness to change generally corresponds to a consultee's and client system's degree of "pain" or dissatisfaction with the status quo. In general, a consultee or client system experiencing a higher degree of pain is more likely to devote time, energy, and resources to problem solving.

Readiness to change can be explored by asking the consultee to develop a list of reasons for not pursuing a problem solution and a parallel list of reasons in favor of problem solving (Lippitt & Lippitt 1986). Readiness to change is suggested when the consultee is able to both come up with more reasons than not for proceeding with problem solving and counter the reasons given for not pursuing a problem solution.

Considering readiness to change can give the nurse consultant some idea about how a formal problem-solving relationship with the consultee and client system might unfold (Kurpius, Rozecki, & Fuqua 1993). Think, for example, about how readiness to change might be indicated in a situation in which a hospital administrator (the contact person) asks a nurse consultant to help implement a computerized charting system in order to decrease the amount of time nursing staff (the consultees) spend on charting. The ideal scenario would be that the reasons in favor of this change (such as an impending decrease in staffing) outweigh the reasons opposing it. If, however, the nurses come up with an equal list of reasons for and against the new charting system, implementation of the new system would progress slowly. If the nurses identify more reasons for *not* implementing the system, implementation efforts would most likely trigger conflict. When this latter situation occurs, the consultant needs to convince consultees of the benefits of changing their behavior. The nurse consultant can also attempt to change consultee norms and values that are inhibiting readiness to change. (These nurse consultant actions are examples of empirical-rational and normative-re-educative problem-solving approaches, respectively. Both of these approaches to problem solving are discussed in Chapter 10.)

Commitment to Change The consultee's level of commitment to change is another attribute that determines the likely success of a consultation relationship. A high level of commitment is associated with a willingness to see the consultation process through rather than rush through or skip steps. Consultees usually display a higher level of commitment when they identify the consultation problem themselves rather than when someone else (such as a contact person) tells them that a problem exists. Initially, at least, the consultee should display more commitment to and enthusiasm for the consultation relationship than the nurse consultant (Ulschak & SnowAntle 1990). Commitment is suggested by behaviors such as attentiveness and active participation at meetings. If commitment to change is low, the nurse consultant may have difficulty maintaining the relationship and may encounter efforts to undermine the consultation process. In addition, if the nurse consultant's commitment to the project is greater than the consultee's, problem solutions may be formulated without consultee input and may fail to resolve the problem situation. The nurse consultant can respond to a low level of commitment with strategies similar to those used to address a lack of readiness to change.

What Do They Want? The second question that drives environmental scanning focuses on the consultee's and client system's expectations of the nursing consultation relationship. In particular, the nurse consultant needs to be on the lookout for hidden agendas. "Hidden agendas" are unspoken reasons for seeking consultation or unspoken expectations about the consultation relationship. For instance, in the previous example of a consultation request to implement a computerized charting system, is the real purpose to free up nurses so they can spend more time providing direct patient care or is the real purpose of the project to reduce staffing? Common hidden agendas in nursing consultation include the following:

Trying to use the nurse consultant to evaluate the consultee's work performance
Using the consultation process to make decisions about terminating a consultee's employment
Using the consultation process to support a decision that has already been made
Using the nurse consultant as a "go-between" in client systems where the parties are unwilling to communicate with each other directly

Identifying where a client system is in its "lifecycle" can help uncover unvoiced consultee needs or desires (Kurpius et al. 1993). Table 8-1 identifies cues a nurse consultant can use to determine a client system's lifecycle stage. Consider a client system in an early stage of development such as a newly established nurse practitioner clinic. This client system, while it may not voice these concerns directly, may need help setting boundaries (how many patients to see, with which preferred provider plans to affiliate), establishing priorities (what equipment to buy), and resolving time management issues. Alternately, a client system in a state of decline or crisis may be looking for a "rescuer" on whom they can become dependent or for a scapegoat on whom they can blame their problems.

A nurse consultant needs to verify any suspected hidden agenda. Once verified, a hidden agenda should be put "on the table" and the nurse consultant should negotiate responsibilities regarding the unspoken issues and expectations. A decision about whether or not to continue a consultation relationship when a hidden agenda is uncovered depends on the nurse consultant's personal value system as well as an assessment of whether more good than harm (for all parties involved) will result from continuing the relationship.

Am I the Right Person? One of the most important predictors of a mutually productive nursing consultation relationship is compatibility between the nurse consultant and consultee. While these two parties don't necessarily need to like each other, they do need to level with each other about their respective needs and values. In order to answer this final question that underlies environmental scanning then, the nurse consultant must decide whether or not his/her values, preferred working style, skills, and interests are a good match for the problem situation. The consultant's decisions about each of these factors further helps to determine the "rightness" of the nurse consultant for the problem situation.

Table 8-1. Indicators of a Client System's Lifecycle Stage

A client system's lifecycle stage is more than a function of its chronological age. Lifecycle stage is also reflected by a system's energy level, creativity, tolerance of uncertainty, stability, and productivity.

Lifecycle Stage	Energy Level	Creativity	Tolerance	Stability	Productivity	Concerns
Early	High—sometimes chaos seems to reign	High—lots of openness to ideas	High—willingness to take risks	Low—rapid change, little recovery time	Initially low, but increasing	Setting boundaries and limits; harnessing energy so that it is productive
Mid	Steady—adequate to maintain productivity	Tends to come in waves	Lower—emphasis is on homeostasis	High—both a major value and a concern	Stable, peaks during this stage	Maintaining productivity while avoiding complacency
Aging	A tendency towards slowing down	Generally low, satisfied with status quo	Low—not willing to take risks	Initially high, but can decline if threatened by decreased need for products	High, but can decline if not responsive to changes in environment	Continuing to maintain productivity by responding to environment; avoiding decline

Values Being the right person for the job is largely based on the compatibility of the nurse consultant's and client system's values. Shared values that are particularly predictive of a productive working relationship are openness, participation, and mutual accountability. When these values are held by one party (for example, the nurse consultant) but not the other (in particular, the consultee), the problem situation will most likely be characterized by frustration and resentment.

Preferred Working Style A match between the nurse consultant's and consultee's working styles also influences a nurse consultant's rightness for a particular problem situation. Working style encompasses both the interaction pattern that is driving the nursing consultation relationship and the consultant's and client system's needs for inclusion and control. To get a sense of the importance of these issues, consider how difficult it would be to implement a process consultation interaction pattern if the consultee only wants to purchase content or skill expertise. Consider, also, the problems that could arise if the nurse consultant is someone who likes to have control over the situation and the consultee has this same tendency.

Skills Being the right person for a nursing consultation situation also means a nurse consultant's skills and those needed for solving a specific consultation problem match. Not only will a mismatch result in a problem remaining unresolved, the nurse consultant can be held liable for an unsatisfactory consultation outcome. Thus nurse consultants have a legal and ethical responsibility to avoid involvement in nursing consultation relationships for which they lack the appropriate skills. (Additional factors related to liability issues in nursing consultation are discussed in Chapter 14. Ethical considerations in nursing consultation are presented in Chapter 15.)

Interests The final consideration in determining whether a nurse consultant is the right person for a particular problem situation is that of interests. "Interests" includes a desire to be involved in a problem situation because of cognitive or affective reasons (the problem is perceived as interesting or worthwhile, for example) as well as more practical interests such as compatibility of the consultee's timeline for the project with the nurse consultant's other commitments. Another practical reason or interest for deciding whether or not a consultation opportunity is right for the consultant is the political implications of involvement in the problem situation. The opportunity for a favorable performance evaluation or letter of reference can be a political reason for accepting a consultation opportunity. On the other hand, accepting a consultation opportunity might adversely affect one's reputation or current position. Think, for example, of the possible risks involved in helping a family planning clinic implement abortion services.

Summarizing Environmental Scanning: Is this a Good Fit?

As mentioned earlier (and illustrated in Figure 8-1), environmental scanning provides the nurse consultant with information needed to reach a decision about continuing a proposed consultation relationship. If the nurse consultant interprets the information obtained from environmental scanning to indicate a "goodness of fit," the second task of the gaining entry phase—contracting—gets underway. If, however, the nurse consultant determines there is not goodness of fit, the relationship terminates. Box 8-1 summarizes factors that are associated with goodness of fit between the nurse consultant and a problem situation.

It is important that a nurse consultant learn to say no to a consultation request that appears, for one reason or another, to not be a good fit. Learning to turn down a consultation request is a means of self-care for a nurse consultant. Proceeding with a

---

Box 8-1. Determining Goodness of Fit: A Checklist

The presence of the following conditions suggests goodness of fit between a nurse consultant and a consultation opportunity:

☐ Clarity of roles and interrelationships among members of the client system

☐ If the contact person is not the consultee, consultee awareness that help is being sought

☐ Involvement of the fee payer in early discussions about the consultation relationship and process

☐ Openness of the consultee and client system

☐ Both consultee and client system show signs of readiness to change

☐ Both consultee and client system show signs of commitment to the consultation process

☐ Absence of hidden agendas or ability to satisfactorily negotiate responsibilities regarding hidden agendas

☐ Compatibility of values

☐ Compatibility of work styles

☐ Compatibility of nurse consultant's skills with those needed to solve the consultation problem

☐ Nurse consultant is interested in the problem situation

☐ Compatibility of consultee's timeline for the project and the nurse consultant's availability

☐ Political reasons or acceptance of the political implications of involvement in the consultation relationship

---

consultation relationship in a "poor fit" situation can result in frustration for both the nurse consultant and the consultee, and as mentioned earlier, can expose the nurse consultant to liability problems. In addition, nurse consultants who say yes to every consultation request can find themselves expected to solve every problem that comes along and therefore become overburdened. Overextending oneself as a nurse consultant can ultimately lead to burnout and ineffectiveness.

The two scenarios presented in Box 8-2 illustrate how the task of environmental scanning can vary in different consultation situations.

Contracting

If, as a result of environmental scanning, the nurse consultant decides to pursue a formal problem-solving relationship with the consultee and client system, the gaining entry phase progresses to the task of contracting. In nursing consultation, this task has two dimensions: the contracting process itself and the product, the formal contract. The purpose of the contracting process is for the nurse consultant and consultee (or other representative of the client system) to come to an agreement about how to meet mutual "wants" related to the consultation relationship. The contracting process culminates in the development of a formal contract, the tool for making explicit and protecting the wants of the parties involved in the consultation relationship. It should be noted that some nurse consultants choose to develop a series of contracts throughout the consultation process. For example, a nurse consultant might carry out separate

---

Box 8-2. Variations in Environmental Scanning

Scenario #1: External Consultation, Purchase of Expertise Interaction Pattern
In this "long-distance" consultation scenario, initial contact consists of a telephone request from a hospital-based community health educator to a university-based nurse-educator in another state. The community health educator is asking the nurse-educator to develop a survey for use at an upcoming health fair. Analysis of the survey data is also requested. The stated goal is to develop a "report card" of the community's health so that the hospital can plan relevant health programs for the community.

Environmental scanning is conducted over the telephone at the time of initial contact. The following roles and interrelationships among members of the client system are identified:

Contact person = health educator

Fee payer = hospital administrator

Consultee = nurses who will be administering the surveys; they are aware that consultation is being sought

Client = hospital

Stakeholder = community

Other key issues explored during environmental scanning are:

Possible hidden agendas: Is there an expectation that current community health services will be evaluated?

Compatibility of time line for project with the nurse consultant's other commitments

Extent of on-site support such as financial resources, copying, computer resources and expertise

---

contracting processes and develop distinct formal contracts for the problem identification and action planning phases of the nursing consultation process as well as for any involvement in the actual implementation of a problem solution.

At this point, contracting is discussed as a process and tool for gaining entry to a client system so that the problem-solving phases of the nursing consultation process can get underway. A more in-depth discussion of consultation contracts can be found in Chapter 13 of this text. Examples of contracts and a checklist of contract components are also included in that chapter.

The Contracting Process

The contracting process is a discussion between the nurse consultant and consultee or other representatives of the client system that focuses on both defining how the nursing consultation process will evolve and exploring expectations about one another's roles and responsibilities during the consultation relationship. The purpose of the contracting process is to establish formal agreement about how the consultant's, consultee's, and client system's needs and desires will be met during the nursing consultation process.

The contracting process may begin at the time of initial contact or during the exploratory meeting between the nurse consultant and consultee or contact person. Whether the contracting process can be completed in one meeting or requires a series

---

Box 8-2. Variations in Environmental Scanning *(continued)*

Scenario #2: Internal Consultation, Process Consultation Interaction Pattern

In this scenario, a mental health nurse practitioner who has a part-time position at a long-term care facility is approached by the facility's director of nursing services with a request to help staff develop skills for communicating with residents who have Alzheimer's disease.

Environmental scanning takes place during an off-site exploratory meeting with the director. The following roles and interrelationships among members of the client system are identified:

Contact person = director

Fee payer = the chief operating officer (administrator) of the facility

Consultee = nursing staff, including director; nursing staff are not aware of the consultation request

Clients = residents

Other key issues explored during environmental scanning are:

Is staff participation voluntary or mandatory?

Do staff perceive a communication problem?

Possible hidden agendas: Is there an expectation to evaluate staff performance in any way?

What type of organizational support is there for this project (money, staff time)?

Will the nurse consultant be paid extra for this project or is it considered "part of the job"?

---

of meetings depends on the complexity of the problem situation as well as on the initial compatibility and extent of agreement among the parties involved in the contracting process.

In complex problem situations such as long-standing or organization-wide problems, the contracting process typically requires more time and involves multiple discussions, in part, because a greater number of stakeholders may be affected by the consultation process. Complex problems are also more likely to require an extensive problem identification phase and the development of a multifaceted action plan. All of these characteristics of complex problems increase the number of roles, the number of wants, and the extent of responsibilities that will need to be negotiated during the contracting process.

Members of the client system who should be included in the contracting process are the contact person, the fee payer, and the consultee. The contact person should be present to clarify the consultation request and goals. The fee payer needs to be present so that resources available to support the consultation process are taken into consideration. The consultee needs to be present since it is the consultee who will be expected to carry out the tasks or change behavior to address the consultation problem. Which of these parties actually accepts or signs the contract will vary. However, it is important that whoever signs the contract assumes the responsibility for seeing that the terms of the contract are upheld.

Box 8-3 lists questions that can be used to guide the contracting process. The parties involved in contracting can respond to these questions either verbally or in writing.

Box 8-3. Questions to Guide the Contracting Process

Questions for members of the client system:

What do I want to have happen as a result of this consultation relationship?

What am I willing to do to accomplish these goals?

How much help do I want accomplishing these goals?

How much time can I devote to this project? When can I give this time?

What resources (including skills) can I bring to this project?

What constraints and limitations of resources am I aware of that could affect my involvement in this project?

Questions for the nurse consultant:

What do I want from this consultation relationship—fee expectations, other less tangible payoffs?

What am I willing to do to accomplish the goals of this consultation? Am I willing to be involved in the implementation of any recommended problem solution or do I see implementation as solely the responsibility of the consultee?

How much time am I willing to devote to this project? When do I have this time?

What resources and support from the client system do I need? How much participation from the consultees do I expect?

Responses can then be compared and differences negotiated and resolved. At the conclusion of this process, the formal contract is drawn up by either the nurse consultant or a representative of the client system.

It is important to recognize that both the nurse consultant and the consultee (as well as other members of the client system) enter the contracting process with a set of unspoken expectations about the consultation relationship (Dougherty 1995). From the consultee's perspective, this "psychological contract" reflects expectations about what will be gained from the nursing consultation relationship and what obligations such as tasks and resource commitment will be accepted. For the nurse consultant's part, the psychological contract includes expectations about what will be given (time, for instance) in the problem-solving relationship and what responsibilities or specific tasks will be taken on. It also includes expectations about what (for example, fees) is to be gained. For a formal consultation contract to be successful, these implicit wants must be made explicit during the contracting process. When the contracting process overlooks the issues of the psychological contract, the nursing consultation process can be disrupted by the resentment that builds because the involved parties' needs are not being met.

The Formal Contract

The formal contract developed as a result of the contracting process serves as a tool for protecting the interests of the parties involved in the consultation process. It does this by delineating the roles and responsibilities (including specific tasks and time lines) of the nurse consultant and consultee and by clarifying accountability issues such as evaluation, feedback, and fees. The contract further protects the interests of

---

Box 8-4. Variations in Contracting

Scenario #1: External Consultation, Purchase of Expertise Interaction Pattern
In this long-distance consultation scenario, the contracting process takes place over the telephone at the time of initial contact. The only parties involved are the contact person (a health educator at a small community hospital) and the nurse consultant (a nurse-educator in another state). The formal contract takes the form of a written letter of understanding that is developed by the nurse consultant. Two signed copies of this letter are sent to the contact person—one for the hospital's files and one that is to be returned to the nurse consultant after it is signed by both the contact person and the hospital administrator.

Scenario #2: Internal Consultation, Process Consultation Interaction Pattern
In this scenario, the contracting process takes place in a meeting at the long-term care facility (the problem setting). The contact person (who will also be a consultee), the facility's administrator, and the nurse consultant (who is a part-time employee of the facility) are present. The formal contract is developed by the facility administrator. It is a formal document with "legalese." The contract is reviewed by the contact person but signed by the administrator and nurse consultant. Both the facility and the nurse consultant retain a copy of the signed contract.

---

parties involved in the consultation process by making explicit the ground rules that will be followed for confidentiality, and terminating the consultation relationship. Chapter 13 includes a checklist of the specific components that should be included in a formal consultation contract.

The actual format of the contract will vary according to the nursing consultation situation. A brief memo may be adequate as a contract for many internal nursing consultation situations. In other situations, the consultation contract might take the form of either a written letter of understanding that is signed by one or both parties or a formal document with legal language. The format that is used for the contract generally mirrors the culture of the client system (for example, its degree of formality), the degree of familiarity between the consultant and the consultee or representative of the client system, and the working style of the person who actually develops the formal contract. The format should, however, be acceptable to both signing parties.

Box 8-4 illustrates how contracting might be accomplished in two different nursing consultation scenarios.

Gaining Physical Entry

The third task of the gaining entry phase in the nursing consultation process is to gain physical entry into the problem setting. Gaining physical entry has a twofold purpose: to establish the legitimacy of the nursing consultation relationship and to establish the parameters of the nurse consultant's involvement with the consultees and other members of the client system. Successfully gaining physical entry means that the nurse consultant is accepted as a temporary physical part of the problem setting and client system. Both the consultee (or contact person) and the nurse consultant have responsibilities in terms of facilitating physical entry into the problem setting.

Consultee Roles in Facilitating Physical Entry

The consultee or contact person typically initiates the process of gaining physical entry by formally introducing the nurse consultant and announcing the consultant's purpose and specific activities to as many of the consultees and stakeholders as possible. Ideally, this introduction occurs in person. However, memos and e-mail messages are other strategies that can be used to introduce the nurse consultant to the consultee and other members of the client system. It is especially helpful to the nursing consultation relationship when the nurse consultant and the consultant's mission are introduced by someone who is in a position of influence within the client system. For instance, this person could be the nurse-manager of a hospital unit or the head of a family. In organizational settings, administrative-level sanctioning of the nursing consultation relationship is associated with increased cooperation with problem-solving efforts (Dougherty 1995).

Another way in which the consultee can facilitate the nurse consultant's physical entry into the client system is by making available an on-site physical working space. Assigning work space further demonstrates a sanctioning of the nurse consultant's activities. It also sends a message about willingness on the part of the client system to allocate the resources needed to support the nursing consultation process.

Nurse Consultant Roles in Gaining Physical Entry

The nurse consultant gains physical entry into the problem setting by being available to the consultees. The nurse consultant demonstrates commitment to the consultation relationship by being at an assigned work space on a predictable basis. At the same time, however, the nurse consultant should mingle and meet with consultees in their own work areas. This demonstrates interest in the consultees and their experiences of both the problem and the problem-solving process. It also facilitates both psychological entry into the client system and the gathering of information about the problem situation. A nurse consultant who is working with hospital staff should make an effort to spend time with and be available to the staff on all shifts.

Box 8-5. Variations in Gaining Physical Entry

Scenario #1: External Consultation, Purchase of Expertise Interaction Pattern
In this "long-distance" consultation scenario, gaining physical entry is not required.

Scenario #2: Internal Consultation, Process Consultation Interaction Pattern
In this scenario, the contact person facilitates gaining physical entry by introducing the nurse consultant and the consultation project to all staff. This occurs at a staff meeting and through personal introductions to nursing staff who are not present at the meeting. Even though the nurse consultant is a part-time employee in the problem setting, it is important not to assume that all staff have had previous contact with the nurse consultant.

The nurse consultant's strategies for gaining physical entry consist of: (1) distributing a memo that includes information about office location and hours of availability and (2) spending time with the nursing staff on all shifts.

The nurse consultant can also facilitate physical entry and being accepted as a temporary part of the client system by minimizing interruptions and disruptions in the consultee's workday. This can be done by making every possible effort to adapt problem-solving activities to the problem setting's usual work schedule.

Box 8-5 illustrates how gaining physical entry might occur in the two consultation scenarios previously described.

Initiating Psychological Entry

The final task of the gaining entry phase is to initiate psychological entry into the client system. As mentioned in Chapter 2, efforts to gain psychological entry occur throughout the course of the nursing consultation process. The outcome of gaining psychological entry is "engaging" the consultee. Successful psychological entry decreases the chance that the consultee will resist problem-solving efforts. Psychological entry occurs by creating "buy-in" for the problem-solving process and by fostering the consultee's willingness to participate in problem-solving activities and accept the implications of the problem-solving process. Effective psychological entry occurs to the extent that the nurse consultant establishes rapport with the consultee, and the consultee perceives the nurse consultant to be trustworthy and credible.

Establishing Rapport

A nurse consultant and consultee have established rapport when their working relationship is characterized by harmony, synergy, and mutual respect. Following a client system's rules, regulations, and communication channels and patterns demonstrates respect for the client system and is one set of strategies that can be used to establish rapport. Paying attention to cultural norms in highly visible areas such as language and dress helps the nurse consultant look less like an outsider; this, too, helps the nurse consultant establish rapport. For example, an external nurse consultant who is working with nursing staff might look less conspicuous wearing a lab coat over street clothes. This simple action can facilitate staff openness and acceptance of the nurse consultant and, therefore, help establish rapport.

Establishing Trust

A nurse consultant is perceived as trustworthy when consultees feel safe and validated or accepted in their interactions with the nurse consultant. A nurse consultant can build a reputation of trustworthiness by being empathetic and demonstrating understanding of a consultee's fears and concerns about being involved in problem-solving activities. In the present health care climate, it is realistic for nurse consultees to be worried about how organization-wide problem-solving outcomes might affect their jobs. The nurse consultant who acknowledges these concerns conveys empathy, which helps establish a perception of trustworthiness. A nurse consultant also builds a reputation of trustworthiness by respecting confidences, refusing to take sides, and avoiding involvement in issues that are not a part of the consultation contract.

Establishing Credibility

A nurse consultant who has established credibility is perceived by the consultee and client system as believable. One strategy a nurse consultant can use to establish credibility is sharing relevant experiences from problem situations similar to that of the consultee. For example, a nurse consultant can share stories about how other nurses have coped (both successfully and unsuccessfully) with work redesign. A nurse

---

Box 8-6. Variations in Initiating Psychological Entry

Scenario #1: External Consultation, Purchase of Expertise Interaction Pattern
In this long-distance consultation scenario, another individual's perceptions of
the nurse consultant's trustworthiness and credibility actually precipitated the
initial contact. This reputation facilitated the development of psychological
entry. During the initial telephone conversation with the contact person, the
nurse consultant also uses the following strategies in an effort to gain psychological entry:
To establish rapport, the nurse consultant is careful to use language that was not
too "ivory tower." Research and data analysis principles are explained in a
simple and straightforward manner.
To establish trustworthiness, the nurse consultant conveys empathy for the contact person's fears that both the project will be too complex and "the hospital
won't do anything with this information." The nurse consultant also suggests
that a goal of the project might be to develop meaningful ways of presenting
the survey findings to different possible audiences.
To establish credibility, the nurse consultant shares survey techniques and data
presentation strategies that have been successful with another client system.

Scenario #2: Internal Consultation, Process Consultation Interaction Pattern
The nurse consultant in this scenario had previously established rapport, trustworthiness, and credibility with the consultees as a mental health nurse practitioner. However, psychological entry still needs to be gained so that the
nurse practitioner would be accepted in the new role as nurse consultant.
To establish rapport, the nurse consultant pays attention to the cultural norm of
"no shoptalk on breaks."
To establish trustworthiness, the nurse consultant conveys empathy for the consultees' feelings of discomfort when trying to interact with residents suffering
from Alzheimer's disease. Consultees are also assured that observations of
their interactions will not be reported to their supervisor.
To establish credibility, the nurse consultant shares a couple of simple communication techniques that can be put to immediate use and will yield immediate
positive results.

---

consultant can also establish credibility by planning problem-solving activities that
will demonstrate an immediate beneficial effect (Chapter 10 discusses this strategy
further).

Box 8-6 illustrates how psychological entry could be initiated in the two consultation scenarios discussed previously in this chapter.

Potential Difficulties in Gaining Entry

As straightforward and common sense as the process of gaining entry in nursing consultation seems, this phase is not without potential difficulties. The nurse consultant

who is aware of these potential dilemmas can monitor for their occurrence and address them before they compromise the entire nursing consultation process. The difficulties that arise most frequently during the gaining entry phase are resistance and inattention to details.

Resistance

Resistance is a common reaction to any situation that involves change. The nurse consultant needs to recognize that resistance is a survival mechanism that protects a consultee or a client system from perceived threats. Resistance that occurs during the gaining entry phase is often an emotional response a consultee is having regarding the proposed problem-solving process and change.

Consultees might be resistant to the nursing consultation relationship for several reasons. They may have an aversion to the foreseen outcome of the consultation relationship (for example, computerized charting). Consultees might also be resistant because they perceive that the costs of the proposed problem solution will outweigh its benefits. Will the time saved by computerized charting, for example, outweigh costs—such as decreased productivity and possible overtime while learning the system, as well as the cost of installing the system? Consultees can also be resistant because they believe the nursing consultation outcome will result in some sort of punishment such as job loss. Finally, consultee resistance can represent a desire to maintain things as they are in order to protect "turf" and vested interests.

When resistance is encountered during the gaining entry phase, the nurse consultant should respond by first acknowledging it as a natural part of change. The nurse consultant should also encourage the consultee to express or "vent" the concerns that are causing the resistance. Finally, the nurse consultant needs to avoid taking the resistance personally. This defensive reaction can be viewed as insecurity and can threaten the nurse consultant's credibility as a problem solver.

Inattention to Details

Both the nurse consultant and the consultee can jeopardize the entire nursing consultation relationship if they fail to pay attention to the details of the gaining entry phase. The nurse consultant can jeopardize the consultation relationship by failing to clarify the consultee's concerns during environmental scanning activities. This failure can result in a contract that is meaningless. Ignoring the limitations of one's competence in relation to a problem issue will result in a contract that cannot be fulfilled. Promising too much and failing to be specific about what roles will be taken on are examples of nurse consultant oversights during contracting that can jeopardize a consultation relationship. Finally, failing to adapt to a client system's culture, concerns, and work processes may make it impossible for the nurse consultant to gain psychological entry into the client system. This will increase consultee resistance to change and set up the nursing consultation relationship for failure.

The consultee also has responsibilities during the gaining entry phase. Overlooking these responsibilities can put the entire nursing consultation process in jeopardy. Failure to clearly explain the consultation problem or verify a nurse consultant's skills can result in developing a contract that will fail to solve the problem issue. The consultee also needs to clarify specific expectations about the nurse consultant's roles and behaviors during the problem-solving process. Lastly, the consultee has the responsibility to be clear about any limitation of resources so that this is taken into consideration during development of a formal consultation contract.

Documenting the Activities of the Gaining Entry Phase

Just as nurses are accustomed to documenting their direct care interactions with patients, nurse consultants need to become accustomed to documenting their implementation of the nursing consultation process. A written record of a consultation relationship not only reminds the nurse consultant about what is occurring in a given consultation situation, it also serves as a learning device or record of what works and what doesn't work. A written record of a consultation relationship also serves as a means of demonstrating both fulfillment of the terms of the consultation contract and adherence to professional standards of practice. Documentation, therefore, can pro-

---

Box 8-7. Documentation Checklist: The Gaining Entry Phase

Documenting Initial Contact
☐ Date and time of contact
☐ Manner of contact—telephone call, letter, in person
☐ Contact person—name, title, position in the client system
☐ Referral source
☐ Stated consultation problem
☐ Stated desired consultation outcome
☐ Action taken and rationale

Documenting Environmental Scanning
☐ Date and time of scanning activity
☐ Activity undertaken—meeting, interview, reading, and so forth
☐ Information source (be exact)
☐ Information gained
☐ Implications of information for a consultation relationship
☐ Conclusions drawn
☐ Action taken and rationale

Documenting Contracting
☐ Preliminary discussions—date, persons present and their roles in the client system, content of discussion, decisions made
☐ Decisions about formal contract—format, who will develop, who will review, who will sign
☐ Keep a copy of signed contract

Documenting Effort to Gain Physical Entry
☐ Actions taken—date and time, by whom, members of the client system who were involved
☐ Follow-up—comments on effectiveness of actions
☐ Notes about what might have been more effective; possible next steps

Documenting Efforts to Initiate Psychological Entry
☐ Actions taken—date and time, rationale, parties involved and their response, personal feelings about the action's effectiveness
☐ Notes about possible next steps

---

vide legal protection to the nurse consultant. Box 8-7 provides a documentation checklist for the gaining entry phase of the nursing consultation process. Similar checklists will also be found in the next four chapters for the subsequent phases of the nursing consultation process.

Chapter Summary

The activities of the gaining entry phase of the nursing consultation process lay the foundation for the actual working phases of the consultation relationship. Environmental scanning is used to determine the fit between the nature of the nursing consultation request and the nurse consultant's interests and abilities. Activities undertaken in the process of gaining physical and initiating psychological entry into a client system establish the legitimacy of the nurse consultant's involvement and foster the nurse consultant's acceptance. Problems that occur during later phases of a nursing consultation relationship can often be traced to an unsuccessful or careless gaining entry phase. Specifically, failure to identify the real consultation issue, promising too much (especially with too few resources), failure to adequately specify roles and responsibilities, failure to recognize the limits of one's competence with respect to the identified problem, failure to acknowledge a "poor fit" with the problem situation, and failure to adapt to a client system's particular concerns and ways of working all reflect a lack of attention to the details of the gaining entry phase. This inattention can undermine the entire nursing consultation process.

Applying Chapter Content

Reflect on both a successful and unsuccessful consultation situation in which you have been involved. How did the entry phase seem to differ in these two situations? What would you have done differently in the unsuccessful scenario?

- What criteria would need to be met for you to consider a consultation opportunity a personal "good fit"? Consider your skills, values, and needs as you speculate on these criteria.

- Read the article by Badger (1988) that is listed as an additional reading. How was the entry phase of the nursing consultation process carried out in this consultation situation? What hidden agendas would you have looked for in this situation? Who was the client in this situation? What would you have done differently? How would you document what occurred?

- Read the article by Grabowski and Jens (1993) that is listed as an additional reading. In this article, the authors state, "... entry occurred when the nursing staff, nursing administration, and medical staff expressed concern to the CNSs about patient needs that were unidentified during hospitalization." What else would you do as an internal consultant to gain entry in this situation? How would you approach this situation differently as an external nurse consultant?

References

Dougherty, A. (1995). *Consultation: Practice and perspectives in school and community settings* (2nd ed.). Pacific Grove, CA: Brooks-Cole.

Kurpius, D., Fuqua, D., & Rozecki, T. (1993). The consulting process: A multidimensional approach. *Journal of Counseling & Development, 71*, 601-606.

Lippitt, G., & Lippitt, R. (1986). *The consulting process in action* (2nd ed.). San Diego: University Associates.

Metzger, R. (1993). *Developing a consulting practice*. Newbury Park, CA: Sage.

Monicken, D. (1995). Consultation in advanced practice nursing. In M. Snyder & M. Mirr (Eds.), *Advanced practice nursing: A guide to professional development* (pp. 183-195). New York: Springer Publishing.

Ross, G. (1993). Peter Block's *Flawless Consulting* and the Homunculus Theory: Within each person is a perfect consultant. *Journal of Counseling and Development, 71*, 639-641.

Schein, E. (1987). *Process consultation, volume II: Lessons for managers and consultants*. (2nd ed.) Reading, MA: Addison-Wesley.

Schein, E. (1988). *Process consultation, volume I: Its role in organization development*. (2nd ed.). Reading, MA: Addison-Wesley.

Ulschak, F., & SnowAntle, S. (1990). *Consultation skills for health care professionals*. San Francisco: Jossey-Bass.

Additional Readings

Badger, T. (1988). Mental health consultation with a surgical unit nursing staff. *Clinical Nurse Specialist, 2* (3), 144-148.
The author presents a case study that includes a description of gaining entry activities.

Dougherty, M. (1995). *Consultation: Practice and perspectives in school and community settings* (2nd ed.). Pacific Grove, CA: Brooks-Cole.
Chapter 3 of this text includes case studies about gaining entry in school and community consultation situations.

Grabowski, V., & Jens, G. (1993). The collaborative role of the CNS in support groups. *Clinical Nurse Specialist, 7* (2), 99-101.
This article presents an internal consultation scenario with a group consultee.

Kuh, G. (1993). Appraising the character of a college. *Journal of Counseling and Development, 71*, 661-667.
This article provides an excellent example of issues related to gaining entry to an academic institution. The content is readily transferable to the types of client systems with which nurse consultants are likely to work.

Metzger, R. (1993). *Developing a consultation practice*. Newbury Park, CA: Sage.
Chapter 5 discusses beginning a consultation relationship.

Ross, G. (1993). Peter Block's *Flawless Consulting* and the Homunculus Theory: Within each person is a perfect consultant. *Journal of Counseling and Development, 71*, 639-641.
The author presents a collaborative model of the gaining entry process. The development of a consultant-consultee team is emphasized.

Schein, E. (1987). *Process consultation, volume II: Lessons for manager and consultants*. Reading, MA: Addison-Wesley.
Chapter 7 includes an excellent discussion about determining who the client is in a consultation situation.

Problem Identification in Nursing Consultation

One needs to treat all data about the organization as valid and relevant. Also, one needs to remember that the presenting problem and the real problem are usually different. (Ross 1993)

Key terms: iterative, key informant, triangulation, diagnostic analysis

The problem identification phase of the nursing consultation process marks the beginning of the working relationship between the nurse consultant and consultee. The goal of the problem identification phase is to determine and then communicate the cause of the problems that prompted the request for nursing consultation.

The problem identification phase consists of three tasks: assessment, diagnostic analysis, and communication of assessment findings. The importance of each task to a successful nursing consultation outcome cannot be emphasized enough. The nurse consultant may solve the wrong problem—or solve the actual problem in an ineffective way—if incomplete or inaccurate information is collected or if conclusions about a problem's cause are inaccurate. A nursing consultation relationship is also likely to be unsuccessful if assessment findings and problem explanations are not effectively communicated to the client system or are not accepted by the client system. Box 9-1 reviews the purpose and focus of each task in the problem identification phase of the nursing consultation process.

The tasks of the problem identification phase are iterative in nature; that is, completing one task may require backtracking and refining what was done earlier. For example, if the consultee does not accept the nurse consultant's assessment findings and conclusions about the cause of the consultation problem, the nurse consultant will need to backtrack to the diagnostic analysis process. Likewise, the need to refine a problem diagnosis may require more information gathering. Figure 9-1 illustrates the iterative nature of the tasks of the problem identification phase.

This chapter explores each task of the problem identification phase: assessment, diagnostic analysis, and communication of assessment findings. Because an effective assessment is so important to the nursing consultation process, the chapter considers different purposes of assessment and different information-gathering strategies. Next, the implications of the theoretical perspective with which the nurse consultant approaches assessment and diagnostic analysis activities are illustrated. Finally, the chapter considers some of the difficulties that can arise during the problem identification phase of the nursing consultation process. As you read this chapter, think about the following questions:

- How does the purpose of a specific nursing consultation assessment affect information collection strategies, explanations about a problem's cause, and the problem solutions that will most likely be proposed?

Box 9-1. Tasks of the Problem Identification Phase
           in Nursing Consultation

Task #1: Assessment
Purpose: To identify factors in the nursing consultation problem situation that
    cause or contribute to the consultation problem.
Focus: Information-gathering activities

Task #2: Diagnostic Analysis
Purpose: To make a decision and reach a conclusion about the cause of the
    nursing consultation problem.
Focus: Analysis and interpretation of assessment findings

Task #3: Communication of Assessment Findings
and Diagnostic Conclusions
Purpose: To legitimize and create ownership of the problem's cause
Focus: Packaging and delivering information to different members of the
    client system

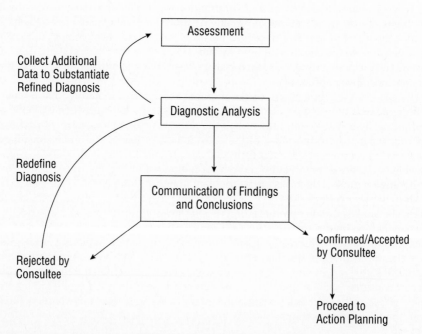

Figure 9-1. The Iterative Nature of the Problem Identification Phase
Performing one task may necessitate repeating what has already been done in a
previous task.

- How might a nurse consultant need to carry out the tasks of the problem identification phase differently for an individual versus group or organizational client?

- What specific skills does the nurse consultant need to effectively carry out this phase of the nursing consultation process? What nurse consultant roles predominate during this phase?

- What would be some advantages and disadvantages of carrying out problem identification activities as an internal and external nurse consultant?

Assessment: Gathering Information about the Nursing Consultation Problem

The first task in the problem identification phase of the nursing consultation process is assessment. The purpose of assessment is to determine the relationship between characteristics of the client system and problem setting and the nursing consultation problem. In a sense, assessment activities aim to identify the gaps between "what is" and "what ought to be" within the client system and problem setting. Thus the focus of assessment is information gathering. The information that the nurse consultant gathers provides data on which to base conclusions about a problem's cause. Because assessment uncovers strengths as well as weaknesses, it also provides a foundation on which to build problem-solving strategies.

The assessment activities that take place during the nursing consultation process are, in many ways, more complex than those that take place during traditional nurse-patient relationships. The increased complexity is due to the fact that the nurse consultant needs to cast a "wider net." A broader scope of assessment is needed because of the nature of the nursing consultation relationship: although a nurse consultant is interacting with a consultee, the ultimate goal of a nursing consultation relationship is enhanced client well-being. Therefore, assessment in nursing consultation must consider: (1) the client's response to a health care problem or health care delivery issue, (2) factors that contribute to the client's response, (3) the consultee's response to the client's problem, (4) factors that contribute to the consultee's response, and (5) the interaction between the consultee and client. These interactions and responses are possible causes of the nursing consultation problem and are also potential points for nursing consultation interventions. To detect these interactions and responses, the nurse consultant must clearly identify the purpose of the assessment (or answer the question, "What am I trying to find out?") and must select appropriate information-gathering strategies.

Identifying Assessment Purposes

Every nursing consultation assessment has one or more of the following purposes:

description
problem clarification
need assessment
desire analysis
resource identification
resource utilization
market analysis

Each assessment purpose reflects one or more key questions the nurse consultant hopes to answer about the problem situation. Identification of the purpose of an assessment is important because it influences the selection of information sources and information-gathering strategies. Clarity about the purpose of an assessment also helps the nurse consultant bring into focus details in the problem situation that might otherwise be overlooked or disregarded (Ridley & Mendoza 1993). Identifying the specific purpose of assessment activities and anticipating how the purpose is best addressed also increases the efficiency with which the assessment can be carried out.

Description The purpose of a descriptive assessment is to describe both factors in a problem situation that might be contributing to the consultation problem and resources that can be mobilized to solve the problem. A descriptive assessment, therefore, focuses on answering the question, "What is the history and context of this problem?" The information collected by a nurse consultant who is doing a descriptive assessment is primarily observational in nature. Put simply, a nurse consultant who is doing a descriptive assessment just "gets out and looks around" the problem setting. Occasionally, information gained by observation is supplemented by information from records and public documents.

A descriptive assessment is most useful for forming preliminary ideas about the possible causes of a nursing consultation problem. These preliminary ideas can then be used to formulate more comprehensive assessment activities. The following example illustrates this point. A nurse consultant is asked by representatives of a small rural community to help them determine reasons for their community's high incidence of cardiovascular disease so that preventive programs can be developed. The nurse consultant carries out a descriptive assessment and notes the following: the presence of a large number of fast-food restaurants within the community, a seemingly disproportionate number of obese individuals in the community, and evidence that it is only within the last five years that the community's rate of cardiovascular disease has exceeded that of surrounding communities. Based on this information, the nurse consultant's preliminary idea is that the consultation problem is linked in some way to residents' dietary habits.

The fact that a descriptive assessment provides only preliminary and not conclusive evidence about a problem's cause should be apparent from this example. Cardiovascular disease is a multifactorial problem and can have causes other than dietary habits; genetics, smoking, and exercise patterns are just three other possible explanations for this consultation problem. The descriptive assessment in this example merely provides the nurse consultant with some direction for a more focused assessment that considers, among other factors, whether or not residents actually eat at the fast-food restaurants and how their dietary habits have changed over the past five years.

Problem Clarification When the purpose of a nursing consultation assessment is problem clarification, assessment activities are designed to clarify the nature and magnitude of an identified problem and to identify factors that are associated with the problem. The key question in a problem clarification assessment is, "What factors are associated with this problem?"

A problem clarification assessment differs from a descriptive assessment in terms of the scope of information-gathering activities it entails. For example, when the purpose of an assessment is problem clarification, written surveys and interviews are often used to supplement observations. In addition, problem clarification may include comparing characteristics of members of the client system who are affected by the consultation problem with those who are not affected by the consultation problem.

A nursing consultation assessment can begin with the purpose of problem clarification. However, problem clarification assessment is often used to follow up on preliminary ideas about a problem's cause that have been developed as a result of a descriptive assessment. Consider how problem clarification could be used as a "phase two consultation purpose" in the preceding scenario. The nurse consultant suspects (because of findings from a descriptive assessment) that there is a link between the dietary habits of a community's residents and the community's high incidence of cardiovascular disease. To follow up on this preliminary idea about the problem's cause, the nurse consultant conducts a problem clarification assessment. Community residents are surveyed about their weight history and eating habits, particularly about eating fast food. Weight histories and eating habits are compared for residents with and without a known history of cardiovascular disease. To further clarify this problem, the relationship between residents' cardiovascular risk status (based on serum lipid levels), weight, and eating habits is explored. As this example illustrates, the scope and depth of a problem clarification assessment allow more confidence to be placed in a statement about a problem's cause.

Need Assessment A need assessment is the systematic and objective appraisal of the health-related service needs of a client system (Cook 1989). The purpose of a need assessment is to identify what type of program or service is needed to help a consultee achieve health-related client goals. A need assessment seeks to answer the question, "What is needed to have a healthier client system?" In order to answer this question, the nurse consultant may conduct interviews, administer surveys, review documents, and make observations.

In nursing consultation, a need assessment is indicated when a consultee needs help identifying and developing specific strategies to enhance client well-being. Need assessment is similar to a doctor-patient nursing consultation interaction pattern. Need assessment would be an appropriate assessment purpose if a nurse practitioner (the consultee) asked a nurse consultant to develop strategies in order to help a free clinic (the client) improve its financial well-being. Information collected during the need assessment might include supply use, staffing patterns, appointment scheduling, and donation patterns and sources. If assessment findings revealed that developing donation patterns and sources could solve the clinic's problem, the nurse consultant could work with the consultee to develop a fundraising program.

Desire Analysis When the purpose of a nursing consultation assessment is desire analysis, the nurse consultant focuses on identifying factors that will facilitate or hinder implementation of problem-solving activities, which have been specified by a consultee to achieve a specific goal. Thus the question that informs a desire analysis is, "How can we best implement this specific activity?" Nurse consultants gather information to answer this question by means of observations, interviews, surveys, and selected document review.

Desire analysis differs from a need assessment in that the consultee has already identified the specific problem to be addressed as well as how to address it, before seeking consultation. An assessment purpose of desire analysis, therefore, is consistent with a purchase-of-expertise nursing consultation interaction pattern.

Desire analysis would be the appropriate assessment purpose if, in the working example, the nurse practitioner had approached the nurse consultant with a request to develop and implement a fund-raising event to benefit the clinic. The nurse consultant's assessment would focus on identifying factors that could help or hinder implementation of this request.

Resource Identification When the purpose of a nursing consultation assessment is resource identification, assessment activities focus on enumerating and describing resources that are presently available to a consultee for dealing with a specific problem. The question that guides a resource identification assessment then, is, "What resources are available for dealing with this problem?" Resources of interest include existing programs, services, and work force. Observations, interviews, and surveys are the most frequently used information-gathering strategies in a resource identification assessment.

This type of assessment can help a nurse consultant and consultee decide if resources that already exist are adequate and can be mobilized to help solve a consultation problem, or if new programs or services need to be developed. A resource identification assessment helps avoid costly and unnecessary duplication of programs and services.

Resource identification would be an appropriate assessment purpose if a nurse consultant was asked by the director of a school of nursing to determine whether or not establishing a faculty practice clinic is the best way to help faculty meet clinical practice requirements for maintaining advanced licensure. By identifying currently available practice sites, the nurse consultant could help the nursing faculty meet their practice requirements more quickly and more cost-effectively, instead of having to develop a clinic from the ground up.

Resource Utilization The nurse consultant who is conducting a resource utilization assessment is trying to discover why currently available resources are not meeting a client's needs. The key question for this type of assessment is, "What factors are discouraging use of this resource?" Interviews and surveys are the predominant information-gathering strategies for this type of assessment.

Like a resource identification assessment, a resource utilization assessment can help a client system avoid unnecessary duplication of available resources. A resource utilization assessment, however, goes a step beyond resource identification: it considers the accessibility of resources, not just their existence.

Consider how a resource utilization assessment might be useful in the preceding scenario about the need for faculty practice opportunities. Perhaps a resource identification assessment reveals a number of clinical sites with opportunities for faculty practice. However, if the nurse consultant does not gather information about the *real* availability of practice opportunities at these sites, the school of nursing might mistakenly decide not to develop a faculty practice clinic. A resource utilization assessment could identify factors (such as hours of clinic operation that conflict with class commitments) that prevent these present sites from being used by faculty. This additional information offers the consultee more options for solving their problem: develop a new resource (the faculty practice clinic) or negotiate with existing resources to increase their actual availability.

Market Analysis When the purpose of a nursing consultation assessment is market analysis, assessment activities focus on identifying the fit between the service a consultee wants to offer and the needs of potential clients for that service. Market analysis is driven by the fundamental questions, "Would this service be used?" and "Would this service remain viable?" A nurse consultant gathers information by means of surveys, interviews, record review, and observation to answer these questions.

Consider how a nurse consultant could use a market analysis to help a nurse practitioner make a decision about opening an independent practice. The nurse consultant could collect information about the health status of the community's members, their patterns of health care utilization, how they pay for their health care, and health care providers or resources that could function as either supports or barriers to the proposed service. The findings of a market analysis can help a consultee package services so that the services meet the needs of both the intended client and the consultee. To

Box 9-2. Purposes of Nursing Consultation Assessment

Purpose	*Key Question*	*Focus*
Description	What is the history and context of this problem?	To discover factors that might contribute to a problem
Problem Clarification	What is causing this situation?	To clarify the nature and magnitude of an identified problem and to identify associated factors
Need Assessment	What is needed to have a healthier client system?	To appraise the service-related needs of a client system
Desire Analysis	How can we best implement this activity?	To identify factors that will facilitate or hinder desire fulfillment
Resource Identification	What resources do we have in place for dealing with this problem?	To identify resources that are currently available for solving a problem
Resource Utilization	What factors are discouraging use of this resource?	To determine why resources that are in place are not being used
Market Analysis	Would this proposed service be used? Would it remain viable?	To determine the fit between a consultee's proposed service and a target client's needs and desires

continue with the preceding example, a market analysis might help the nurse practitioner (consultee) decide to emphasize either acute and urgent care service or health maintenance and prevention services.

Box 9-2 summarizes the different purposes that can drive the assessment of a nursing consultation problem.

Selecting Information-Gathering Strategies

In addition to identifying the specific purpose of a nursing consultation assessment, the nurse consultant must determine the best way of collecting the needed information. While a nurse consultant's choice of information-gathering strategies should be based primarily on the purpose of the assessment, information-gathering decisions need to also take into account feasibility issues such as time, resources, and consultant and consultee abilities. The nurse consultant's goal should be to select strategies that will yield reliable, valid, and believable information as efficiently as possible.

Information-Gathering Options A variety of information sources and information-gathering strategies were mentioned in the preceding section about assessment purposes. This section highlights the strengths, limitations, and usefulness of the information-gathering strategies used most frequently by nurse consultants. In-depth discussions of these strategies can be found in any research methods textbook.

Surveys Surveys are a cost-effective means of collecting information about knowledge, perceptions, concerns, and attitudes from large groups. Surveys offer flexibility in terms of format (for example, they can use forced-choice as well as open-ended questions) and distribution options (such as mail or group administration). A major advantage of surveys is that they are unobtrusive and allow anonymous responses. As a result, individuals may be more likely to give accurate responses to somewhat sensitive questions such as attitudes about their work setting. The data generated by surveys tend to be quantitative in nature and lend themselves to high impact presentations such as tables, charts, and graphs.

A major disadvantage of surveys is the time required for their preparation. The format of a survey (such as Likert scale or checklist) needs to take into consideration both the types of information desired and the characteristics (such as reading level) of the survey's intended respondents. Careful wording to avoid cultural or gender bias, logical sequencing of questions, and attention to appearance are other details that the nurse consultant should attend to during the survey construction process. Another disadvantage of surveys is that they do not allow respondents to seek clarification to questions or elaborate on their responses. A final drawback is that the return rate for surveys tends to be fairly low. A low return rate can leave the nurse consultant wondering if the attitudes and perceptions of individuals who returned the surveys are different in any way from those who did not.

In nursing consultation assessments, surveys are useful for collecting information about personal characteristics that could be related to a problem's occurrence. Surveys are also useful for determining reasons why resources are not being used and for gathering opinions about how consultees would prefer to solve a specific problem.

Interviews Interviews allow a nurse consultant to collect more in-depth and detailed information than is generally possible with a survey. Interviews also allow the nurse consultant to probe and clarify responses.

A drawback of interviews is that they tend to be more costly to administer than are surveys, in terms of both time and human resources. As a result, interviews tend to be used selectively, that is, with carefully chosen key informants rather than large groups. Interviews also require a respondent to sacrifice anonymity; this may limit the content that individuals are willing to discuss in an interview. An additional drawback of interviews is that the data they yield tend to be more time-consuming to analyze than do survey data. In addition, because interview data tend to be narrative or qualitative in nature, the conclusions generated from interviews can be harder to sell to consultees who are accustomed to diagnosing problems and justifying change efforts with numbers.

Nurse consultants often use key informant interviews as a strategy for accessing expert or "insider" opinions and insights about a problem situation. For example, in a desire analysis assessment, a key informant interview might be a productive way of gathering information about factors in a client system that could facilitate or hinder a proposed problem solution.

Nurse consultants also use focus group interviews as a way of gathering information. A focus group format can be more efficient than multiple individual interviews and has the added advantage of enabling the nurse consultant to observe a group's communication and interpersonal processes. Thus a focus group interview can help a nurse consultant identify behaviors and group processes that could be contributing to the nursing consultation problem.

Observation Observation can be a relatively simple way of gathering information about a problem setting and how its members function on a day-to-day basis. A nurse consultant can use information obtained from observation to identify and clarify issues during subsequent surveys and interviews. Observations can also confirm information gained from other strategies.

A decision a nurse consultant must make before using observation as an information-gathering strategy is that of how much to tell the consultee (or other parties) about what is being observed. Observations that are made without awareness are more likely to capture "natural" behavior but raise ethical issues about informed consent and full disclosure. Also, the nurse consultant must carefully plan what to observe so that important details and behaviors aren't missed and so that observations are consistent and objective.

Reports and Records Nurse consultants can take advantage of a variety of existing reports and records that allow unobtrusive and relatively inexpensive information gathering. Records available from public health departments, for example, can help determine the severity of a nursing consultation problem (child abuse or teen pregnancy, for instance). A client system's financial records may help a nurse consultant identify the resources or lack of resources available for solving a consultation problem. Review of performance records over time (for example, records about medication errors) and changes in performance in response to events within the client system (such as downsizing) can help a nurse consultant detect possible causes of a problem. Finally, the nurse consultant can use reports and records to generate content for surveys and interviews as well as to confirm information obtained by other means.

Like other information-gathering options, reports and records are not without their limitations. The quality of information recorded can vary in terms of both content value and legibility. In addition, data from reports and records can be biased because of problems with selective recording, storage, and retrieval. That is, reports may provide information on only favorable or extreme (and not typical) cases, or records may be saved or retrieved for review only if they portray a problem setting favorably.

Box 9-3 summarizes the advantages and disadvantages of these different information-gathering options.

Triangulation The nurse consultant should incorporate triangulation into an assessment plan whenever possible. Triangulation refers to using multiple data sources and/or multiple data collection strategies to generate information. The purpose of triangulation is to "converge on the truth" about a consultation problem. Since each information-gathering option has its own limitations and each data source may have some inherent bias, it stands to reason that if a nurse consultant collects more than one type of data about a problem, the conclusions developed about a problem's cause are more likely to be accurate. The value of triangulation was illustrated earlier in this chapter: conclusions about the causes of cardiovascular disease in a community were more believable when they were based on both surveys and group comparison data rather than only observational data.

Box 9-3. Information-Gathering Options for Nursing Consultation

Option	Advantages	Disadvantages
Surveys	Cost-effective Can collect a variety of information Probably best option for collecting information from large groups Yield numerical data Offer anonymity	Require time to construct Low response rates
Interviews	Allow collection of in-depth and detailed information	Costly to administer Take more time to analyze No anonymity Narrative data may be less convincing than numbers to some groups
Observation	Can detect process and communication problems Inexpensive	May raise issues regarding disclosure and informed consent
Reports, Records	Inexpensive Generally easy to access	Problems with selective recording, storage, and retrieval

Diagnostic Analysis: Labeling the Cause of the Nursing Consultation Problem

The second task of the problem identification phase of the nursing consultation process is diagnostic analysis. Diagnostic analysis is the process of attaching meaning to the information obtained from the nursing consultation assessment. The purpose of diagnostic analysis is to draw conclusions about the cause of a nursing consultation problem. Diagnostic analysis also entails confirming or redefining the scope of a problem; that is, how much of the client system is affected by the problem, and how many different factors in the client system contribute to the problem.

Before conclusions can be made about the cause of a nursing consultation problem, the raw data from the assessment process need to be analyzed. While it is beyond the scope of this text to discuss data analysis procedures in detail, this section provides some simple and general guidelines.

When the assessment data that have been gathered are quantitative or numerical in nature, simple descriptive statistics are usually adequate for summarizing findings (that is, a tally of responses and calculation of the mean, median, and standard deviation). Sometimes it is meaningful to compare this information for different subgroups such as nursing staff on different shifts or before and after a key event such as downsizing.

Interviews and observations usually yield narrative data. The nurse consultant analyzes narrative data for recurring themes. The frequency with which the different themes occur can then be counted and compared for different subgroups or periods of time.

To a large extent, the success of a nursing consultation relationship is dependent on the ability of the nurse consultant to formulate causal statements with which the consultee agrees. Therefore, part of diagnostic analysis is getting consultees to both "buy into" a problem's cause and agree to assume their share of responsibility for its solution. One strategy the nurse consultant can use to create consultee buy-in to diagnostic statements is to involve the consultee in the actual analysis of the assessment data. For example, consultees can help tally numerical data and can also read narrative data to help identify relevant themes.

In addition to involving consultees in the diagnostic analysis process, it sometimes makes sense to also involve other members of the client system. For example, including administrators makes sense because they control the resources of the client system that will need to be accessed to solve the consultation problem. Involving other members of the client system in the diagnostic analysis process can also function as a form of "interpretive triangulation" and increase the accuracy of a diagnostic or causal statement because different perspectives are being brought into the interpretive process. This is important because a nurse consultant's unintentional misrepresentation of assessment findings and biased interpretation of information can be powerful barriers to the ultimate success of a consultation project.

A final strategy that a nurse consultant can use during the diagnostic analysis process is that of proposing several alternative causes for a consultation problem. This strategy is particularly useful for creating buy-in when consultees or other members of the client system have not been involved in diagnostic analysis activities. The nurse consultant can share these alternative causes with the consultee and allow the consultee to choose the problem cause to address during the subsequent phases of the nursing consultation process. Consultees may choose a problem cause on the basis of: (1) its reasonability or logic, (2) the feasibility of the problem solutions it implies, or (3) the consultees' motivation to respond to a particular causal issue (Dougherty 1995; Harrison 1994). Maslow's hierarchy of needs can also be used to help consultees prioritize and choose problem causes (Morgan, Burbank, & Godfrey 1993). This framework might lead a client system to address basic needs such as financial security before tackling higher-order needs such as job satisfaction.

Using a Theoretical Framework to Guide Assessment and Diagnostic Analysis

Theories identify linkages or relationships among the variables in a situation. For the purpose of assessment and diagnostic analysis activities, the theoretical framework a nurse consultant uses reflects a philosophy about linkages that are present among the various characteristics of a problem situation.

The advantage of using a theoretical framework to guide assessment and diagnostic analysis is that it helps to focus and bring order to what can otherwise seem like overwhelming tasks. In the problem identification process, a nurse consultant's theoretical perspective guides what kind of information is gathered during the course of assessment. The nurse consultant's theoretical perspective also influences how assessment findings are interpreted and the label or definition that is given to the problem cause. The definition of a problem's cause, in turn, influences its acceptability to the consultee. As mentioned earlier, if the problem is to be acted on, a consultee's acceptance of a problem cause is essential. These points are illustrated by the scenarios that occur throughout this section.

The theoretical frameworks discussed in this section are just a sampling of those that can be used to guide assessment and diagnostic analysis activities during the nursing consultation process. They have been chosen because they contrast sharply with one another and illustrate how the choice of a theoretical framework influences both data gathering and diagnostic analysis. Nurse consultants can use other nursing frameworks as well as frameworks from the social/behavioral sciences, business, management, and education as appropriate for both the consultation problem and the characteristics of the client system.

Neuman's Systems Theory

Betty Neuman, a nursing theorist, maintains that every system (individuals and their subsystems as well as groups and communities) is comprised of an inner core, a normal line of defense, a flexible line of defense, and lines of resistance. A system's normal line of defense represents its usual responses to its environment. An intact normal line of defense is associated with health or stability of a system's inner core. Flexible lines of defense reflect coping mechanisms that are activated when environmental stressors increase and a system's health or stability is threatened. Examples of flexible lines of defense include getting more rest with the onset of cold symptoms or seeking support from a colleague when things are not going well at work. Lines of resistance are coping mechanisms that are activated when the normal line of defense or usual level of health has been penetrated (because the flexible lines of defense have failed) and a system is experiencing symptoms of dysfunction. An individual's immune system is an example of a line of resistance (Anderson, McFarlane, & Helton 1991; Cross 1990). Neuman maintains that a system becomes dysfunctional when stressors overwhelm and penetrate the various lines of defense and resistance. Figure 9-2 is a schematic representation of Neuman's Systems Theory.

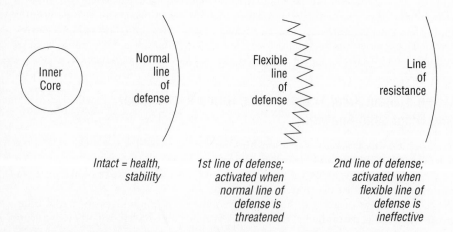

Figure 9-2. Schematic Representation of Neuman's Systems Theory
Neuman maintains that systems are comprised of layers of defense. A system is healthy when its normal line of defense is intact. A system's flexible line of defense and lines of resistance function to protect the system's inner core when it is threatened by environmental stressors.

Box 9-4. Assessing Low Morale Using Neuman's Systems Theory

A nurse consultant is asked to develop strategies to address the problem of low morale among nursing staff in a hospital that is undergoing work redesign. A problem clarification assessment, guided by Neuman's Systems Theory is carried out. Neuman's Systems Theory is chosen as the theoretical framework for the assessment because the nurse consultant believes that low morale occurs when stressors exceed a system's coping capacity. Thus to improve morale, stressors need to be reduced or coping strategies need to be improved. The consultee agrees with this perspective.

Assessment Questions:
What is the usual level of morale (normal line of defense)? How has this changed?
What stressors are being experienced by the nursing staff?
What are usual coping mechanisms (flexible lines of defense)? Are they being used? To what extent are they effective?
What new or emergency coping mechanisms (lines of resistance) are being used? To what extent are they effective?

Information-Gathering Strategies:
Survey staff perceptions of stressors and morale changes as well as identify coping strategies and their perceived effectiveness
Interview selected nurses to gather more in-depth information about perceptions to the low morale problem and possible contributing factors
Observe mood and interpersonal interactions for evidence of low morale

Findings:
Staff consensus that morale is lower than it was 12 months ago
Work redesign with associated downsizing and decrease in benefits seen as stressors
Usual coping mechanisms of teamwork and communication have been disrupted by staff changes and mistrust of management
"Emergency" coping mechanism such as complaining, calling in sick, and increased substance abuse tend to be ineffective

Diagnostic Analysis:
Low morale secondary to stressors that exceed coping abilities

Intervention Options:
Remove stressors (not feasible)
Enhance coping strategies—emphasize restoring flexible lines of defense or usual coping mechanisms so that lines of resistance don't need to be activated

A nurse consultant using Neuman's Systems Theory to guide an assessment would focus on identifying: (1) stressors, (2) whether present coping strategies represent flexible lines of defense or lines of resistance, and (3) the effectiveness of the coping strategies being used. What the nurse consultant wants to determine

---

Box 9-5. Assessing Low Morale Using the Health Belief Model

A nurse consultant is asked to address the problem of low morale among nursing staff in a hospital that is undergoing work redesign. The low morale is present despite opportunities for the nurses to be involved in planning and support groups. The nurse consultant carries out a problem clarification assessment that is guided by the Health Belief Model. This theoretical framework is chosen because the consultation contact person believes that more education about work redesign would help improve the nurses' morale.

Assessment Questions:
   How susceptible do nurses view themselves to be to adverse effects of work
      redesign? Do they perceive themselves to be at high or low risk?
   How seriously would nurses be affected on a personal level by the negative
      effects of work redesign?
   What benefits do nurses perceive in participating in the planning and
      support groups?
   What barriers do nurses perceive in participating in the planning and
      support groups?
   What cues to action are there regarding group participation?

Information-Gathering Strategies:
   Survey nurses about their perceptions of susceptibility and seriousness of the
      effects of work redesign and the perceived benefits and barriers to partici-
      pating in the planning and support groups
   Interviews not done because of concerns over the privacy of responses about
      a sensitive topic
   Observe for cues to action regarding group participation
   Review records of communication to nursing staff about the work redesign
      process

---

is which lines of resistance and defense are intact and which have been threatened or penetrated; these findings form the basis for a statement about the cause of the consultation problem. With this theoretical perspective, problems tend to be attributed to excess stressors and/or ineffective coping. Consultation interventions then, focus on removing stressors or bolstering coping strategies. Box 9-4 illustrates how a nurse consultant could use Neuman's Systems Theory to guide assessment of the problem of low staff morale after a hospital has undergone work redesign.

The Health Belief Model

The Health Belief Model (HBM) is frequently used to explain participation in disease-avoidance activities such as compliance with a treatment regimen. The HBM maintains that individuals' actions reflect their world view (Butterfield 1993). More specifically, behavior is determined by: (1) an individual's perceptions of personal susceptibility to a problem, (2) perceived seriousness of the problem if it occurs, (3) perceived benefits of engaging in a problem-avoidance activity, and (4) perceived barriers to participating in the problem-avoidance activity. These perceptions are modified by "cues to action"—environmental variables or events that encourage or

> **Box 9-5.** *(continued)*
>
> **Findings:**
> Nurses perceive themselves to be at "high risk" for layoffs, and so forth
> Many nurses are single parents and perceive being laid off as a very serious
>   problem
> No perceived benefits to participating in the planning and support groups—
>   "people just sit around and complain"
> Barriers to group participation include that group meetings do not occur dur-
>   ing regular work hours and there is no overtime pay for participating
> Cues to action—meetings are poorly attended, which tends to discourage
>   participation
>
> **Diagnostic Analysis:**
> *Low morale secondary to nurses' fear about the implications of work redesign; this is*
>   *aggravated by a perception of no benefits and the presence of barriers to participat-*
>   *ing in the planning and support groups*
>
> **Intervention Options:**
> Provide reliable information about the implications of work redesign
> Advertise the benefits of participating in the planning and support groups
> Emphasize nurses' professional responsibility to participate in the groups;
>   this is an attempt to induce guilt and override perceptions of barriers to
>   participation

discourage action. According to the HBM, a problem exists because of "errors" in an individual's perceptions; problems are solved then, by correcting these perceptual errors.

A nurse consultant using the HBM to guide assessment and diagnostic analysis activities would focus on identifying consultee attitudes, beliefs, and perceptions that could be the cause of the nursing consultation problem. Diagnostic analysis would identify an "error" in perception as the cause of the problem. Problem-solving interventions would consist of correcting the error in perception by reframing the meaning of the problem situation (making it seem more serious, for example) and increasing a consultee's knowledge or understanding of the situation. Box 9-5 illustrates how the consultation problem of low morale would be assessed if the nurse consultant used the HBM as the theoretical framework for assessment. Note that, in contrast to Neuman's Systems Theory, the HBM downplays environmental influences on problems and views the consultee as solely responsible for the problem situation.

Milio's "Upstream" Perspective

Nancy Milio's "upstream" perspective is presented as a third contrasting framework that a nurse consultant could use to guide assessment and diagnostic analysis activities. Again, the intent is to illustrate the implications of a nurse consultant's choice of framework for the tasks of the problem identification phase.

Milio's framework focuses on "upstream" or environmental factors that are precursors to "poor health" or dysfunction (Butterfield 1990, 1993: Milio 1976). Milio

---

Box 9-6. Assessing Low Morale Using Milio's "Upstream" Framework

A nurse consultant is asked to address the problem of low morale among nursing staff in a hospital that is undergoing work redesign. The hospital is attempting to address morale problems by offering nurses the opportunity to participate in planning and support groups. The nurse consultant decides to use Milio's "upstream" framework to guide a resource utilization assessment. The nurse consultant chooses this framework because it holds the hospital responsible for making the changes needed to solve the problem. The nurse consultant is able to convince the hospital administrator (consultation contact person) that this is an appropriate perspective for this problem situation.

Assessment Questions:
  Are nurses aware of the planning and support groups?
  Is group participation *really* feasible (easily accessible) for the nurses?

Information-Gathering Strategies:
  Survey nurses to gather information about awareness and accessibility of
    group opportunities
  Interview selected nurses and group facilitators in a focus interview format;
    the intent of the interview is to discover their points of agreement and dis-
    agreement about accessibility issues
  Review notices and communication about the planning and support groups
    in order to determine what messages are given about accessibility (group
    meeting times, and so forth)

Findings:
  Most nurses are unaware of the group opportunities
  Meetings are during the evening hours at the hospital
  No availability of the support group leader outside of group meeting times

Diagnostic Analysis:
  *Low morale secondary to no real opportunities to participate in planning and sup-
    port group activities*

Intervention Options:
  Increase publicity about meetings
  Offer meetings at multiple times
  Increase availability of support group's leader through regularly scheduled
    office hours

---

asserts that individuals will make healthy behavioral choices whenever such choices are the easiest ones to make. Milio maintains that poor health (or a nursing consultation problem) occurs when there is an imbalance between the conditions needed for health and the health-promoting conditions (choices) that are realistically available. Health is promoted then, by making healthy choices or conditions easily available. Milio's framework, therefore, emphasizes society's responsibility for the health of individuals. This contrasts with the HBM, which maintains that attitudes and perceptions cause an individual's health problems.

A nurse consultant using Milio's framework would focus assessment activities on identifying factors in the problem setting that are contributing to the consultation problem. Of particular interest would be the problem setting's policies and resources, the consultee's awareness of these resources, and resource accessibility. Box 9-6 illustrates how the consultation problem of low morale could be assessed using Milio's framework. Note that this framework assumes that health-promoting resources will be used if they are available. The "upstream" framework overlooks individual consultee factors such as values and perceptions that also influence behavior.

Choosing a Theoretical Framework

Because a single theoretical framework will not be equally suitable for all nursing consultation problems, nurse consultants need to be familiar with a variety of frameworks from nursing as well as from other disciplines. Ideally, the framework a nurse consultant selects to guide assessment activities will "fit" the nature of the consultation problem and will lead to meaningful, relevant, and acceptable problem solutions.

With experience, most nurse consultants come to favor certain theoretical frameworks over others. The nurse consultant needs to keep in mind, however, that consultees will only become involved in problem solving if they "buy into" explanations about the problem's cause. Because of this, the nurse consultant needs to make certain that the theoretical framework chosen in a given situation will explain problems in a way that is acceptable to the client system. Milio's "upstream" framework, for example, would only be effective if the client system accepted organizational (rather than individual) responsibility for problems and problem solving.

Involving Consultees in Assessment and Diagnostic Analysis Activities

The tasks of assessment and diagnostic analysis can be carried out by the nurse consultant alone or in a collaborative manner with the consultee. Both approaches have advantages and disadvantages. The approach that is used depends on the nature of the consultation problem (for example, its urgency) as well as the abilities and preferences of the consultee.

When consultees are involved directly in information-gathering and interpretation activities, they will often view conclusions about a problem's cause as more credible. This happens because consultees tend to see the information on a firsthand basis so they know it is valid. This can facilitate ownership of the problem and encourage buy-in or assuming responsibility for problem solutions.

Consultee involvement in information gathering has other benefits and can be especially helpful to external nurse consultants. Because consultees are the "insiders" to the problem situation, they can help an external nurse consultant locate and access needed information. They may also be more successful than the nurse consultant at retrieving certain types of data such as financial reports.

While a collaborative approach to assessment and diagnostic analysis has advantages, it also has disadvantages. Sometimes consultee involvement in information gathering and interpretation can cause other members of the client system to question the objectivity of the conclusions that are reached. For example, a consultee could be accused of interpreting data so that problem solutions will result in personal gain such as job protection. A collaborative approach to assessment and diagnostic analysis also takes more time than does a more consultant-directed approach. This is because consultees often need to be taught data collection, analysis, and interpretation skills.

Consequently, a collaborative approach is usually not feasible in urgent situations, such as a budget crisis or an infectious disease outbreak.

Communicating Assessment Findings

The third and final task of the problem identification phase of the nursing consultation process is communicating assessment findings and diagnostic conclusions to the consultee and other relevant members of the client system. The primary purpose of sharing findings with the consultee is to establish legitimacy and encourage ownership of the cause of the consultation problem. A second purpose of communicating assessment findings is to stimulate the consultee's thinking about how the problem might be solved. The communication process also gives the consultee the opportunity to give input and support or challenge the nurse consultant's conclusions about the problem's cause. This is important because, as emphasized earlier in this chapter, consultee acceptance of the problem cause is essential if the consultation process is to be successful.

The primary challenge for the nurse consultant in regard to communicating assessment findings is packaging the information effectively for different audiences. Often, nurse consultants need to share findings with such diverse groups as administrators, nursing staff, physicians, and community members or health care consumers. In most instances, language and style of presentation need to be altered in order to be responsive to the culture, knowledge level, and point of reference or vested interest of the particular audience. The two most common strategies for sharing consultation findings are written reports and formal presentations.

Written Reports

A written report of assessment findings and diagnostic conclusions should begin with an overview of the problem that triggered the request for nursing consultation. The overview should include the consultee's perspective of the problem (the symptoms and how they are problematic) as well as a history of the problem. The next section of the report should be a summary of how the assessment process was carried out (purpose, information-gathering strategies, and theoretical framework used), and how the information obtained was analyzed. Copies of any data collection tools (surveys and interview schedules, for instance) should be attached as appendices to the report.

The results section of a written report should be an objective reporting of the assessment findings. It is particularly effective to present information graphically (for example, with pie charts and bar graphs) and in tables rather than in a strictly narrative format. If narrative data have been collected, it is meaningful to include direct quotes, although care must be taken to protect the privacy of the individuals who are being quoted.

The final section of the report is the nurse consultant's interpretation of the assessment findings. This section is where the nurse consultant identifies the consultation problem's cause. Implications of the problem cause for possible problem-solving strategies are also addressed in this section.

It is important that a report is written in language that is appropriate for the intended audience. Nurse consultants need to be particularly careful about using technical jargon that may not be understood correctly by non-nurse consultees. Conclusions that are presented should be supported with specific facts and observations. Finally, individuals who provided specific information should not be named without their consent. Box 9-7 presents guidelines for preparing a written consultation report.

> ## Box 9-7. Preparing a Consultation Report
>
> Begin with an overview of the consultation problem—its history, the symptoms that prompted the consultation request, a description of the difficulties the problem is creating
>
> Summarize the assessment process—purpose, what kind of information was gathered, information-gathering strategies, information sources, who collected the information, theoretical framework used; state the rationale for these decisions
>
> Attach any information-gathering tools that were used
>
> Describe how the information was analyzed and who was involved in analysis activities
>
> Present results objectively—give specific examples, use quotes and graphs to enhance the discussion
>
> Protect the privacy of information sources
>
> Be sure that report is written in language that is appropriate for the audience

Formal Presentations

Many of the "ground rules" for preparing a written report can also be applied to formal presentations. Whenever possible, the nurse consultant should arrange for a personal meeting with the consultee or the consultation contact person before any formal group presentation of assessment findings and conclusions. This private meeting gives the consultee an opportunity to react to the findings. A private meeting avoids having the consultee become angry and defensive about any "negative" findings in a group setting. It also gives the consultee an opportunity to take part in planning the formal presentation.

The overall goals of a formal presentation about assessment findings and conclusions are to deliver the facts, facilitate discussion, have the consultee take responsibility for the problem situation, and plan the next steps for the nursing consultation relationship. Groups with whom it is appropriate to share assessment findings and conclusions are those who are being asked to take actions as well as those who might be affected by any action that is taken. A sample agenda that should accomplish these goals is presented in Box 9-8.

Communicating assessment findings and conclusions in a group setting can present a number of challenges to the nurse consultant. A particular concern of consultees is that the nurse consultant may catch them "off-guard" and that the nursing consultation assessment might have uncovered information that reveals problems that have been previously hidden (either intentionally or unintentionally). The nurse consultant needs to avoid becoming defensive and arguing with consultees when these reactions occur. Keeping a presentation objective and supporting conclusions with facts can often decrease consultee hostility. Another effective presentation strategy is to help the consultee realize that the problem is in the past and the focus is now on the future. In other words, a problem can be reframed as a goal to reach in the future (Kurpius, Fuqua, & Rozecki 1993).

Box 9-8. Sample Agenda for a Group Meeting about Assessment Findings

Introduction, review of the problem and reasons for nursing consultation *(The primary consultee or contact person should be encouraged to do this; this reinforces support of the nursing consultation process and the consultation relationship)*

Overview of the assessment and diagnostic analysis process

Presentation of assessment findings and their interpretation *(enhanced by graphics)*

Questions and comments from the audience

Validation of findings and conclusions with the audience

Recap—summarize what has been agreed upon as the next step

Potential Difficulties in the Problem Identification Phase

Both methodological and political difficulties can complicate the problem identification phase of the nursing consultation process. The nurse consultant who is aware of these possible problems will be more likely to recognize their occurrence and respond so that they are less likely to disrupt the tasks of the problem identification phase.

Methodological Difficulties

A methodological difficulty that can complicate the information-gathering process is reluctance of individuals being surveyed or interviewed to share unfavorable perceptions of a client system. Related to this difficulty is the issue of needing to sort out the meaning of conflicting ideas about the problem situation from different informants. These two dilemmas often represent opposing interests such as job security and fear of retaliation for revealing unfavorable information. The nurse consultant who encounters these difficulties needs to acknowledge the underlying concerns they represent. Additionally, the nurse consultant needs to reassure informants that the confidentiality of the information they share will be respected.

An additional methodological difficulty is constraints on information sources (people as well as documents) that can be accessed. Sometimes involving a consultee in information-gathering activities makes accessing these sources easier. Reassuring consultees about the confidentiality of information that is shared can also remove access barriers.

A final methodological difficulty that the nurse consultant may face during the problem identification phase is pressure to use quick and, perhaps, cursory and superficial information-gathering strategies. This pressure usually reflects consultee efforts to both save time and money as well as prevent discovery of additional problems within the client system. The nurse consultant can respond to this pressure by educating the consultee about the importance of a properly conducted problem identification phase for the ultimate success of the consultation process.

Political Dilemmas

A political dilemma the nurse consultant may face during the problem identification phase is that of being asked to share information obtained during assessment for purposes other than diagnosing a problem's cause. For example, a nurse consultant might be asked to provide input into personnel evaluations and decisions. The nurse consultant needs to respond to this pressure by emphasizing the confidentiality and purpose of the information that has been gathered. This dilemma can also be prevented (or at least protected against) by addressing the conditions under which assessment information will be shared in the nursing consultation contract.

Documenting the Activities of the Problem Identification Phase

Documenting the activities of the problem identification phase provides the nurse consultant with reminders of what has transpired during this phase of the nursing consultation process. Documentation also provides the nurse consultant with a learning tool about what works and what doesn't as a problem identification strategy. Finally, documentation is important because it provides evidence about appropriate fulfillment of the terms of the consultation contract. Thorough documentation can, therefore, provide the nurse consultant with legal protection against charges of inadequate assessment of the problem situation. Box 9-9 is a checklist that can be used for documenting the activities of the problem identification phase.

Box 9-9. Documentation Checklist: The Problem Identification Phase

Documenting Assessment Activities:
☐ Overall purpose of the assessment
☐ Theoretical framework that was used and why
☐ Date and time of each assessment activity
☐ Regarding each assessment activity—purpose, information-gathering strategy, information source, who collected the information; rationale for these decisions; attach any tools that were used
☐ Outcome of each assessment activity—information gathered; be objective and specific
☐ Difficulties encountered—how they were addressed, whether or not they were resolved
☐ Notes about possible next steps
☐ Impressions about the assessment process

Documenting Diagnostic Analysis Activities:
☐ Date and time of each activity
☐ Description and rationale for activity
☐ Identification of parties involved
☐ Difficulties encountered—how they were addressed, whether or not they were resolved
☐ Conclusion reached about the cause of the consultation problem
☐ Notes about possible next steps

Documenting the Presentation of Assessment Findings:
☐ Date and time of presentation
☐ Audience—be as specific as possible
☐ Format of presentation, rationale (attach copy of presentation or report)
☐ Difficulties encountered—how they were addressed, whether or not they were resolved
☐ Notes about possible next steps
☐ Overall (personal, subjective) impressions about how the presentation went

---

Chapter Summary

The problem identification phase is one of the most important phases of the nursing consultation process. The information gathered during this phase sets the stage for subsequent development of both problem-solving activities and the nursing consultation action plan. Clarity about the purpose of the assessment and selection of appropriate information-gathering strategies and theoretical framework helps to increase the meaningfulness and credibility of the findings and conclusions. Awareness on the part of the nurse consultant about the difficulties that might be encountered during the problem identification phase helps to insure that the tasks of the phase are accomplished as intended and achieve their purposes.

Applying Chapter Content

- Critique the problem identification activities carried out for the low morale problem presented in this chapter. Which of the frameworks do you think is most effective for this situation? Formulate an assessment for this same consultation problem using another theoretical perspective.

- Identify a nursing consultation problem in a health care setting with which you are familiar. Use two different theoretical frameworks to develop guidelines for implementing a nursing consultation assessment of this problem. Identify the implications of each assessment approach for possible explanations about the problem's cause as well as subsequent interventions. Which theoretical framework seems most appropriate for this problem? Why?

- Read the article by Grabowski and Jens (1993) that is listed as an additional reading. On page 100 of this article, the authors describe how they implemented the diagnostic phase of their consultation. Comment on the appropriateness of their assessment for the consultation problem. How would you carry out the problem identification phase for this consultation problem?

- Read the article by Kurlowicz (1991) that is listed as an additional reading. Look at the consultation requests listed in Tables 1 and 2 on page 126 of the article. Identify the nursing assessment purpose that would be most appropriate for each request. Explain your answers.

- Again, refer to the article by Kurlowicz (1991). Look at the first problem listed in Table 1 of this article. Speculate as to what explanations for this problem might be if (1) the Health Belief Model and (2) Milio's "upstream" perspective were used as the theoretical framework for problem identification.

References

Anderson, E., McFarlane, J., & Helton, A. (1991). Community as client: A model for practice. In K. Saucier, *Perspectives in family and community health* (pp. 59-65). St. Louis: Mosby.

Butterfield, P. (1990). Thinking upstream: Nurturing a conceptual understanding of the societal context of health behavior. *Advances in Nursing Science, 12* (2),1-8.

Butterfield, P. (1993). Thinking upstream: Conceptualizing health from a population perspective. In J. Swanson & M. Albrecht (Eds.), *Community health nursing: Promoting the health of aggregates* (pp. 80-108). Philadelphia: Saunders.

Cook, D. (1989). Systematic need assessment: A primer. *Journal of Counseling and Development, 67*, 462-464.

Cross, J. (1990). Betty Neuman. In J. George (Ed.), *Nursing theories: The base for professional practice* (3rd ed.) (pp. 259-278). Norwalk, CT: Appleton & Lange.

Dougherty, M. (1995). *Consultation: Practice and perspectives in school and community settings* (2nd ed.). Pacific Grove, CA: Brooks-Cole.

Harrison, M. (1994). *Diagnosing organizations: Methods, models, and processes* (2nd ed.). Thousand Oaks, CA: Sage.

Kurpius, D., Fuqua, D., & Rozecki, T. (1993). The consulting process: A multidimensional approach. *Journal of Counseling and Development, 71*, 601-606.

Milio, N. (1976). A framework for prevention: Changing health-damaging to health-generating life patterns. *American Journal of Public Health, 66* (5), 435-439.

Morgan, B., Burbank, P., & Godfrey, D. (1993). Health planning. In J. Swanson & M. Albrecht (Eds.), *Community health nursing: Promoting the health of aggregates* (pp. 109-127). Philadelphia: Saunders.

Ridley, C., & Mendoza, D. (1993). Putting organizational effectiveness into practice: The preeminent consultation task. *Journal of Counseling & Development, 72*, 168-177.

Ross, G. (1993). Peter Block's *Flawless Consulting* and the Homunculus Theory: Within each person is a perfect consultant. *Journal of Counseling and Development, 71*, 639-641.

Additional Readings

Badger, T. (1988). Mental health consultation with a surgical unit nursing staff. *Clinical Nurse Specialist, 2* (3), 144-148.
The author presents a case study of internal nursing consultation.

Barton, J., Smith, M., Brown, N., & Supples, J. (1993). Methodological issues in a team approach to community health needs assessment. *Nursing Outlook, 41*, 253-261.
The authors describe difficulties that can complicate a team approach to a needs assessment.

Beer, M., & Spector, B. (1993). Organizational diagnosis: Its role in organization learning. *Journal of Counseling and Development, 71*, 642-649.
The authors emphasize consultee involvement in problem identification activities. "Learning diagnosis" is presented as a means of increasing organizational effectiveness.

Berkey, K., & Hanson, S. (1991). *Pocket guide to family assessment and intervention.* St. Louis: Mosby.
Neuman's Systems Theory is applied to the concept of family assessment—a good example of how the theory can be extended to assessment situations other than those involving only individuals.

Butterfield, P. (1990). Thinking upstream: Nurturing a conceptual understanding of the societal context of health behavior. *Advances in Nursing Science, 12* (2), 1-8.
This article presents an overview of Milio's prevention framework and critical social theory, both of which are useful as approaches to nursing consultation assessment.

Dougherty, A. (1995). *Consultation: Practice and perspectives in school and community settings* (2nd ed.). Pacific Grove, CA: Brooks-Cole.
Chapter 4 of this text discusses the diagnostic stage of the consultation process which also includes assessment.

Finnegan, L., & Ervin, N. (1989). An epidemiological approach to community assessment. *Public Health Nursing, 6* (3), 147-151.
The authors describe the epidemiological approach to assessment and present ideas about how this approach can be applied to nursing consultation problem situations.

George, J. (Ed.). (1990). *Nursing theories: The base for professional practice* (3rd ed.). Norwalk, CT: Appleton & Lange.
This text is a basic reader on nursing theories; it includes case studies that illustrate how each theory can be applied.

Grabowski, V., & Jens, G. (1993). The collaborative role of the CNS in support groups. *Clinical Nurse Specialist, 7* (2), 99-101.
The authors present a case study of nurse consultants helping to develop a support group. The different phases of the nursing consultation process are illustrated.

Higgs, Z., & Gustafson, D. (1986). *Community as client: Assessment and diagnosis.* Philadelphia: F. A. Davis.
This classic text on community assessment includes examples of how nursing theory can be used to guide assessment activities. The ideas are directly transferable to nursing consultation situations.

Kurlowicz, L. (1991). Psychiatric consultation nursing interventions with nurses of hospitalized AIDS patients. *Clinical Nurse Specialist, 5* (2), 124-129.
The author describes activities of an internal nurse consultant.

Lippitt, G., & Lippitt, R. (1986). *The consulting process in action* (2nd ed.). San Diego: University Associates.
Chapter 7 of this text discusses diagnostic analysis.

Ross, G. (1993). Peter Block's *Flawless Consulting* and the Homunculus Theory: Within each person is a perfect consultant. *Journal of Counseling and Development, 71*, 639-641.
The author emphasizes the importance of a collaborative approach to consultation.

Schein, E. (1988). *Process consultation, volume I: Its role in organization development* (2nd ed.). Reading, MA: Addison-Wesley.
Chapter 12 frames the diagnostic process as a consultation intervention.

Stevens, P. (1989). A critical social reconceptualization of environment in nursing: Implications for methodology. *Advances in Nursing Science, 11* (4), 56-68.
The author presents a highly readable overview of critical social theory, a possible perspective for nursing consultation assessment.

Stevens, P., & Hall, J. (1992). Applying critical theories to nursing in communities. *Public Health Nursing, 9* (1), 2-9.
This article illustrates using critical social theory to guide assessment activities.

Ulschak, F., & SnowAntle, S. (1990). *Consultation skills for health care professionals.* San Francisco: Jossey-Bass.
Chapter 5 includes a thorough overview of information-gathering strategies for nursing consultation. Chapter 6 presents useful guidelines for presenting assessment findings.

~
10

Action Planning in Nursing Consultation

Whether consultees will accept an intervention appears to be a function of their perception of the fit between the problem and the intervention (for example, humaneness), the level of difficulty in implementing it, and the quality of the consultant-consultee relationship. (Dougherty 1995)

Key terms: goal, objective, Gantt chart, transition

Think of the last time you worked with a patient who was having some sort of pain. How did you decide what to do? Most likely, solving this problem involved setting goals (such as maximum pain relief with minimal side effects) and choosing an intervention on the basis of factors such as the nature of the problem (location and severity of pain) and the patient's characteristics (medication allergies, other health problems). The process of deciding on a problem solution is similar in nursing consultation. In nursing consultation, as in patient care situations, any presenting problem holds a variety of possible solutions. It is during the action planning phase of the nursing consultation process that the nurse consultant and consultee work together to decide how to specifically go about solving the consultation problem.

The action planning phase of the nursing consultation process consists of working with the consultee to accomplish the following four tasks:

setting goals
choosing a problem solution
developing an action plan
facilitating implementation of the action plan

These tasks occur in a fairly linear fashion despite differences in the nature of the nursing consultation problem, the problem setting, or the nursing consultation interaction pattern being used. Figure 10-1 depicts the tasks of the action planning phases as well as the various activities that occur as a part of each task.

The action planning and problem identification phases of the nursing consultation process are linked closely in a couple of ways. First, the theoretical framework that the nurse consultant selected to guide assessment and diagnostic analysis identifies possible points of intervention for responding to the problem. The selected framework also governs the range of interventions that are likely to be appropriate. Recall, for example, how problem causes and solutions differed in the low morale scenarios presented in Chapter 9 when the problem was approached from the perspective of Neuman's Systems Theory, the Health Belief Model, or Milio's "upstream" framework. The action planning phase is also linked to the problem identification phase because the basis for a solid action plan is thorough information gathering and solid data analysis. As noted in the last chapter, inadequate information can lead the consultant to attribute a problem to the wrong cause, which in turn, can lead to the development of inappropriate problem solutions. Furthermore, if information-gathering activities fail to detect barriers to potential problem solutions, the nurse consultant may propose a problem solution that the consultee cannot (or will not) implement.

The action planning phase of the nursing consultation process is important because it represents the first tangible action to resolve the problem that prompted the request for nursing consultation. The action planning phase is a bridge between the present state and the desired state of a client system. Therefore, the stakes are high in this phase for both the nurse consultant and the consultee. The goals that are set and the interventions that are chosen will determine not only whether the nursing consultation problem is resolved, they will also determine the side effects associated with solving the problem and whether the solution will produce long-lasting or only temporary results.

This chapter discusses each of the four tasks of the action planning phase. In the first section, strategies for working with consultees to set goals and establish priorities are considered. Next, the process of choosing a problem solution is discussed. The details of developing an action plan and strategies for facilitating implementation of the action plan are presented in the third and fourth sections of the chapter. The chapter concludes with a discussion of some of the difficulties that can arise during the action planning phase. As you read this chapter, consider the following questions:

- How might setting goals and developing problem solutions differ for internal and external nursing consultation situations?

- How might action planning differ with individual and consultees?

- What skills must a nurse consultant possess to be successful in the activities of the action planning phase? Which of these skills do you possess? Which do you need to aquire or further develop?

- What values and biases would you bring to the action planning phase? How might these affect your success as a nurse consultant?

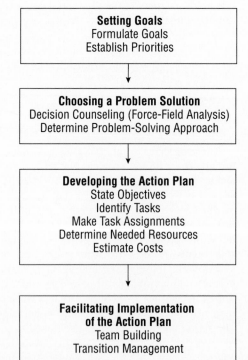

Figure 10-1. The Action Planning Phase of the Nursing Consultation Process
The tasks of the action planning phase occur in a fairly linear fashion despite differences in the nature of the nursing consultation problem, the problem situation, and the nursing consultation interaction pattern that is being used.

Setting Goals

Goals are statements about how the consultee wants things to be once the consultation problem has been resolved. Consultees often identify goals for the consultation relationship at the time of initial contact with the nurse consultant. These initial goals, however, are often vague or unrealistic ("We want to be more effective" or, "We want to decrease our medication error rate to zero within two weeks"). In most nursing consultation situations, new and more specific goals are identified once the consultation problem has been clarified and its cause has been determined. Once these new "working goals" have been identified, the nurse consultant and consultee work together to prioritize these goals.

The first task of the action planning phase in the nursing consultation process is to help a consultee set meaningful, acceptable, and realistic goals. In order to set goals, a consultee must have a clear picture about a *preferred* and *feasible* future. Developing meaningful, acceptable, and realistic goals is most likely to occur after two conditions are met. First, the tasks of the problem identification phase must be completed satisfactorily; that is, a thorough assessment must lead to an accurate problem diagnosis. Secondly, the consultee must be involved in the two activities of the goal-setting process: formulating goals and establishing priorities.

Formulating Goals

To formulate goals that are meaningful, it is often helpful to have the consultee consider exactly how the problem situation is problematic (that is, what "pains" are being experienced) as well as clarify what is *wanted* versus what is *needed* as a consultation outcome. Meaningful goals are value-driven because they reflect what the consultee would like to see happen in terms of problem resolution. Meaningful goals are also characterized by longevity; not only will they solve the immediate problem, they will also help a consultee respond to similar problems in the future.

Goals also need to be acceptable to the client system (that is, in keeping with the client system's culture and values) if they are to have longevity. Goal formulation, therefore, needs to consider the personal values of the consultee(s) and the culture of the client system, as well as how these factors might change in the future.

Organizational development consultants often have consultees explore the anticipated longevity of their goals by engaging in a process called "futurethink" (Chapter 18 discusses this process in greater depth). Consultees are asked to project an image of themselves and their organization five years into the future. In developing this image, consultees are asked to take into account trends in their own organization and work unit, as well as their personal ideas about what constitutes sound organizational practices. Nurse consultants can engage in a similar activity with both individual and group consultees during the goal-setting process. Family consultees, for example, might be asked to project the following: what their family will look like in five years (size, age distribution, geographic distance or proximity of members), what is going on within the family unit (aging, health issues, relationship changes, careers), and what is of value to them as a family unit (independence, togetherness, self-sufficiency). This exercise might help a family consultee develop more realistic and acceptable goals for the long-term problem of providing adequate care for a dependent family member with chronic health problems. By following a similar approach, a hospital unit consultee could develop meaningful goals about an optimum staffing mix by considering national trends in health care financing, occupancy trends in the institution, and personal as well as organizational values about what constitutes sound nursing care.

Box 10-1. Formulating Meaningful, Acceptable, and Realistic Goals

To establish meaningful goals:
Clarify what is problematic about the problem situation
Clarify what is *needed* versus what is *wanted* as a consultation outcome
Consider longevity of goals—"Will it still be meaningful in five years?"
Engage in "futurethink"

To establish acceptable goals:
Consider whether proposed goals are in keeping with personal and organizational culture and values
Consider longevity—"Will the goal still fit the organization's culture in five years?"

To establish realistic goals:
Identify resources needed for goal accomplishment
Review information from the nursing consultation assessment to identify resources available and resource-related barriers that are present
Conduct a resource identification or resource utilization assessment if necessary

---

In addition to being meaningful and acceptable, goals need to be realistic. Realistic goals can be achieved by the client system when its resources (for example, time, work force, financial resources, skill, and motivation) are taken into account. To formulate achievable or realistic goals, the consultant needs to help the consultee determine whether the resources needed to accomplish a goal are available. Reviewing information gathered during the nursing consultation assessment should provide information about resource availability. If not, the nurse consultant will need to conduct a new resource identification or resource utilization assessment. Appraising resources is important, as failure to identify resource-related barriers to goal accomplishment will leave the nursing consultation problem unresolved. In addition, new problems can be created if scarce resources are depleted or diverted from other needs in the client system. Box 10-1 summarizes strategies the nurse consultant can use to help a consultee formulate meaningful, acceptable, and realistic goals.

Establishing Priorities

The creative generation of goals for the nursing consultation relationship needs to be followed by a disciplined process of establishing priorities. The nurse consultant needs to help the consultee decide which goal to tackle first. Goals are often given top priority if they address an immediate and overriding problem. Using problem severity and impact as criteria for setting priorities makes sense because, as in patient care situations, goals such as self-care and learning new tasks are unrealistic until immediate problems such as pain, anxiety, and infection are addressed (this reflects Maslow's hierarchy of needs). In nursing consultation situations, consultee fear and anxiety are often immediate and overriding problems that need to be resolved before the real consultation problem can be addressed.

In other nursing consultation situations, it may make sense to identify some goals as high priority since their accomplishment will provide the consultee with knowledge or skills that will facilitate the accomplishment of other goals. For example, in a

---

Box 10-2. Establishing Priorities: Which Goal to Tackle First?

Goals that address immediate and overriding problems, including emotional
   reactions of consultees

Goals that will provide the consultee with knowledge or skills that will facilitate achievement of other goals

Goals that are easily attainable and will both increase consultees' perceptions of
   the credibility of the consultation relationship and build their confidence for
   proceeding with problem solving

---

work redesign project, it might make sense for initial goals to focus on learning skills
such as delegation and working as a mixed-skill team, because these skills are foundational to goals that address productivity and complication rates.

Finally, the nurse consultant might advise the consultee to give certain goals
higher priority because they are easily attainable. The accomplishment of these goals
can help demonstrate both the nurse consultant's credibility and the value of the
nursing consultation relationship. Accomplishing easily attainable goals can also
help the consultee build the confidence needed to pursue long-term and more ambi-
tious goals. Box 10-2 provides guidelines for prioritizing goals.

Choosing a Problem Solution

Goals and problem solutions are inextricably linked. The desire to achieve a specific
goal narrows the range of possible nursing consultation problem solutions. At the
same time, because most nursing consultation takes place in an open systems context
(see Chapter 5), there are multiple means to any end. Thus in any nursing consultation situation, the nurse consultant and consultee have a range of possible problem
solutions from which to choose. (Reviewing the scenarios presented in Chapter 9
might help to clarify this point.) Selecting the problem solution that is most likely to
be effective involves matching the problem's cause, the goals of the nursing consultation relationship, and the characteristics of the consultee (skills) and client system
(culture) to the appropriate problem solution. Two specific processes involved in the
task of choosing a problem solution are decision counseling and identifying the
appropriate problem-solving approach.

Decision Counseling

Decision counseling is the process of working with consultees to develop meaningful, acceptable, and realistic problem solutions (Dougherty 1995). Decision counseling is a give-and-take process between the nurse consultant and consultee and begins
with brainstorming about possible ways of attaining goals. Both parties assume
responsibility for identifying factors that make a particular problem solution more or
less acceptable and appropriate for a problem situation. Of particular interest in decision counseling is exploring both a proposed problem solution's side effects and situational variables which might act as driving or restraining forces to being able to
actually implement the problem solution.

Force-Field Analysis Force-field analysis is a useful exercise for identifying the driving and restraining forces related to a problem solution. Driving and restraining

---

Box 10-3. Variables to Consider as Possible Driving and Restraining Forces

The nurse consultant needs to consider the potential side effects of the problem-solving strategy on all levels of the client system—Desirable side effects should be considered a driving force, whereas undesirable side effects should be considered a restraining force.

Time and timing—how much is needed versus how much is available; if there is a "time crunch," a prescriptive approach to problem solving should be considered

Teamwork—how much is present versus how much is needed

Material resources—time, money, equipment

Human resources—availability, skills, willingness to participate

Trust—low trust can be a restraining force; try to increase trust with catalytic and confrontational interventions

Emotions—anxiety and fear are common restraining forces; try to resolve these with acceptant interventions

Culture and values

Power—consider who in the client system supports and does not support the problem solution

Historical considerations—Has this problem solution been used before? How did it work?

Politics—Who will the winners and losers be if this solution is implemented? What impact will this have?

---

forces are characteristics of a problem situation and client system that argue for or against a particular problem solution. Force-field analysis can help a nurse consultant and consultee gain perspective on a potential problem solution's possible pitfalls and strong points as they relate to the specific setting and situation within which the problem solution would take place. Variables that need to be considered as possible driving and restraining forces are identified in Box 10-3.

Once the driving and restraining forces related to a proposed problem solution are identified, the nurse consultant and consultee identify which driving forces can be strengthened and which restraining forces can be decreased. Next, they wieght each driving and restraining force (high, medium, and low) in terms of: (1) anticipated degree of impact, and (2) likelihood of occurrence. After the weighting process, driving and restraining forces are tallied separately. Problem solutions with restraining forces that outweigh driving forces are eliminated as viable problem-solving strategies. The force-field analysis process is summarized in Box 10-4.

Problem-Solving Approaches

Most problem solutions can be implemented in a number of ways. Once decision counseling has resulted in the identification of a problem solution, the nurse consultant needs to determine the most effective way to implement the problem solution. A "problem-solving approach" is the particular tactic or "manner" (the *how*) the nurse consultant uses to implement a problem solution (the *what*). Whereas decision counseling is a collaborative process between the nurse consultant and consultee, determining the problem-solving approach is generally the prerogative of the nurse consultant. The nurse consultant's decision about which problem-solv-

---

Box 10-4. The Force-Field Analysis Process

Step 1: Identify support for a solution
Identify the variables that are present that are supportive of a given problem solution. These are the driving forces for that solution.

Step 2: Identify barriers to a solution
Identify the variables that are barriers or restraining forces for a given problem solution. Take into consideration time, human and material resources, emotions, culture, and values.

Step 3: Identify possible consequences
Identify the possible consequences of the problem solution. Are side effects desirable, tolerable, or not acceptable? Are these consequences driving or restraining forces?

Step 4: Maximize supports and minimize restraining forces
Strategize ways in which driving forces can be maximized and restraining forces can be minimized.

Step 5: Weight factors
Weight each driving and restraining force (high, medium, and low) on the basis of its degree of impact and likelihood of occurring.

Step 6: Tally weighted factors
Tally the weight factors for both driving and restraining forces.

Step 7: Choose or reject the problem solution
If driving forces outweigh restraining forces, consider the solution useable. If restraining forces outweigh driving forces, eliminate the solution from further consideration.

---

ing approach to use to implement a problem solution will reflect the personal philosophy of the nurse consultant, but must also match characteristics of the consultee and client system.

Empirical-Rational Approaches   Empirical-rational approaches to problem solving are based on the assumption that individuals (consultees) are rational and, therefore, will change their behavior if they believe it is to their benefit to do so (Haffer 1986). When an empirical-rational approach is used, the nurse consultant focuses on providing consultees with the knowledge they need to change their patterns of behavior or thinking. Teaching, role-modeling, and demonstration are typical empirical-rational problem-solving strategies.

Theory-Principles Interventions   Theory-principles interventions (Blake & Mouton 1990) are a particular type of empirical-rational strategy that focus on helping consultees understand the cause and effect variables in a problem situation. The intended outcome of this type of intervention is that the consultee sees a problem situation more objectively, is able to think through both immediate and long-term implications of a problem solution, and curbs impulsive actions. Theory-principles interventions should increase a consultee's problem-solving skills because theories offer explanations for problems and provide problem solutions that can be generalized to similar future situations.

A nurse consultant using a theory-principles intervention would introduce a consultee to a relevant theory, help the consultee apply this theory to the current problem situation, and compare theory-based outcomes to those that might be attained otherwise. As an example, a nurse consultant might introduce a group of cardiac rehabilitation nurses to the Health Belief Model (this framework is described in Chapter 9). The nurses could be taught how to apply the model's concepts (a consultee's perceptions of seriousness, susceptibility, benefits, and barriers) to the nursing consultation problem of helping clients make permanent lifestyle changes. Client outcomes obtained when this model is applied would be compared to those outcomes obtained through other methods. This particular theory-principles application would be considered a success if the nurse consultees were convinced of the value of the model, began assessing and addressing client perceptions of lifestyle change requirements, and experienced a better success rate in achieving the desired outcomes of the rehabilitation program.

A limitation of theory-principles interventions and in fact, all empirical-rational problem-solving approaches, is that they tend to overlook the noncognitive issues in a problem situation. That is, empirical-rational approaches assume that knowledge is enough to inspire behavior change. Other issues that affect a consultee's willingness and ability to engage in problem solving (affective needs, time constraints, resources, and so forth) are also not addressed by empirical-rational approaches. As a result, empirical-rational approaches, when used alone, do not usually result in long-term problem solutions. Referring back to the preceding example, nurses' use of the Health Belief Model to guide their interactions with cardiac rehabilitation patients would most likely be short-term unless the client system also provided resources needed to incorporate the model into practice, such as rooms for conducting patient interviews and adequate staff. Nurses' needs for job satisfaction would also need to be met for the problem solution to be long-term.

Normative–Re-educative Approaches Normative-re-educative problem-solving approaches presume that people are guided in their actions by social norms, personal meanings, habits, and values. Changes in behavior occur then, only when a consultee's norms or values (or perceptions of these) change (Haffer 1986). The focus of normative-re-educative approaches to problem solving, therefore, is working with consultees to help them clarify and modify their attitudes and values. Teaching is probably the normative-re-educative strategy most frequently used by nurse consultants. Confrontation and catalytic interventions are other normative-re-educative problem-solving strategies.

Confrontation Confrontation is an appropriate type of intervention when there is a discrepancy between a consultee's professed values and actual behavior (Blake & Mouton 1990). A nurse consultant using confrontational tactics with a consultee would challenge the consultee to consider how the nursing consultation problem might be resolved if the consultee's existing behaviors or attitudes changed. Specific confrontational interventions the nurse consultant might use include asking questions such as "Why are things done this way?", pointing out discrepancies between a consultee's words and actions ("You say this, but your behavior implies..."), and playing devil's advocate. Examples of value/behavior discrepancies seen in nursing consultation include articulating a value of client autonomy but encouraging dependency and articulating a value of openness in communication but discouraging presentation of alternative viewpoints. Confrontation would be an appropriate intervention in either of these situations.

The major limitation of using confrontation as a normative-re-educative problem-solving approach is that it tends to trigger consultee defensiveness. Because of this risk, confrontation requires a fairly high level of trust between the nurse consultant and consultee.

Catalytic Interventions Catalytic interventions are another variation of a normative-re-educative approach to problem solving. Catalytic interventions are useful when the nurse consultant needs to both arouse a consultee's interest in being helped and create a willingness to participate in problem solving (Blake & Mouton 1990). Catalytic interventions are normative-re-educative in nature because they stimulate a dissatisfaction with the problem situation and sensitize a consultee to how the problem situation might be better if attitudes, norms, and habits are changed. Catalytic interventions that are frequently used by nurse consultants include involving consultees in setting goals, establishing priorities, and choosing problem solutions. Role-modeling behaviors and values so consultees can see their outcomes is another example of a catalytic intervention.

Prescriptive Approaches The basic premise of a prescriptive approach to solving nursing consultation problems is that the nurse consultant is the expert and authority and that the problem will be resolved if the consultee follows the consultant's recommendations. Thus prescriptive approaches involve delegating tasks to consultees and providing specific direction about actions that need to be taken. While this approach may sound counterproductive to the nursing consultation goal of consultees learning problem-solving skills, it is useful as an initial intervention when a consultee has "reached the end of their rope." It is also useful when a consultee has self-doubt and lacks the confidence to solve a problem alone (Blake & Mouton 1990). In these situations, a prescriptive approach can help a consultee realize an immediate result, which can help the consultee gain the confidence needed to become a more active participant in problem solving.

A prescriptive approach to problem solving is also indicated in problem situations where immediate action is needed (patient safety concerns or a severe budget crisis, for example) and there is not time for consultee involvement and deliberations about how to solve a problem. In these situations, a prescriptive approach can relieve pressure on the consultee to respond to the immediate crisis. Relieving this pressure helps the consultee gain the time and energy needed to be an active participant in formulating a long-term solution to the problem.

A third nursing consultation problem situation that may require a prescriptive approach is one in which there is consultee resistance to an imposed change such as work redesign (Haffer 1986). The nurse consultant's strategy in this situation is to "force" the change and make sure that those affected see or experience some immediate benefits associated with the change. Demonstrating these benefits should decrease further resistance and enable the consultant to continue problem solving with more participative approaches.

Acceptant Interventions Acceptant interventions are approaches to problem solving directed toward relieving emotional issues that can act as barriers to participation in problem solving (Blake & Mouton 1990). Active listening, acknowledgment, and expressing empathy are examples of acceptant interventions. In many nursing consultation situations, acceptant interventions need to be used before the real nursing consultation problem can be addressed; a parallel intervention in nursing would be taking care of a patient's fear or anxiety before trying to teach self-care. A danger with acceptant interventions is that a consultee may consider a problem resolved once the emotional issues are relieved. In a merger situation, for example, the danger of using

Table 10-1. Problem-Solving Approaches for Nursing Consultation Problems

Problem-Solving Approach	Assumptions	Possible Strategies
Empirical-Rational	Consultees will change their behavior if they think change will benefit them	Teaching (theory-principles, skills, knowledge) Role-modeling Demonstration
Normative-Re-educative	Attitudes, norms, and values must change before behavior will change	Confrontation Catalytic interventions Teaching (attitudes, values)
Prescriptive	Problems will be resolved if a consultee is told how to change	Delegation Direction
Acceptant	Emotional issues can act as barriers to problem solving	Active listening Empathy Acknowledgment

an acceptant intervention would be that consultees might feel better about their work (and even temporarily perform better) once they have had help dealing with their emotional responses to the consultation problem. However, this might not resolve the real problem of two groups of nurses who now need to merge different values and procedures to work as a single unit. Acceptant interventions are often followed by empirical-rational and normative-re-educative problem-solving strategies.

Table 10-1 summarizes the different problem-solving approaches for nursing consultation problems.

Developing the Action Plan

The action plan is a step by step blueprint of the work that is required to reach a goal. The action plan details how the problem solution that has been chosen by the nurse consultant and consultee will unfold. In a sense, an action plan is a contract of the activities that need to be completed in order for a goal to be reached. (The consultation contract is a more comprehensive document than the action plan because it addresses fees, confidentiality issues, and so forth. See Chapter 13 for a checklist of contract components.) In most cases, there are four standard parts to an action plan:

objectives
tasks
task assignments
resources needed, including estimated costs

A modified Gantt chart (see Figure 10-2) can be constructed to use as the basis from which to compile a narrative action plan, or can be used as the "working" action plan itself. A modified Gantt chart identifies objectives, tasks and their timeline, who is responsible for each task, and resources and costs associated with each task.

Stating Objectives

An action plan begins with a statement of the objective(s) of the nursing consultation relationship. An objective is a translation of the consultee's goal or desired end state, from a vague and abstract idea, into terms that are more concrete (Figure 10-2, A). For

NURSING CONSULTATION PROBLEM: Rural nurse practitioners need more opportunities to meet continuing education requirements

OBJECTIVE: Help a nurse practitioner group sponsor a 2-day conference in March that will attract 200 participants and provide 15 contact hours of continuing education

Task	Timeline/Person Responsible								Resources Needed	Estimated Cost
	Sept	Oct	Nov	Dec	Jan	Feb	March	April		
1. Survey members to identify conference topics	NNNN								Mailing list of members, paper, postage	Consultant time (4 hours), paper and postage for 500 surveys
2. Tally survey results		NN								Consultant time (4 hours)
3. Plan conference schedule, set date, identify speakers and location		NNNN CCCC								Consultant time (8 hours)
4. Contact and confirm speakers			CCC							Telephone calls
5. Develop conference brochure			NN CC							Printing costs for 1000 brochures
6. Mail brochures				CC					Mailing list	Postage for 1000 brochures
7. Obtain handouts from speakers					CCC					
8. Compile conference materials						NNN CCC				Paper and printing costs for 250 conference notebooks
9. Hold conference							NC		Site, audiovisual equipment	Consultant's time (16 hours), speaker fees, equipment rental fees, site fees, refreshments
10. Evaluate conference								NC		Consultant's time (8 hours)

Responsible party: NNN = Nurse consultant   CCC = Consultee

Figure 10-2. Modified Gantt Chart for a Nursing Consultation Action Plan

Refer to the letter keys in the text discussion for a complete explanation of the components of this chart.

example, the abstract goal of "provide better patient care" might be translated into the more concrete objective of "decrease medication errors by 80% within two months." Stating objectives in terms of a future condition that can be observed and measured builds in criteria for evaluating the success of the consultation project.

Identifying Tasks

The next component of the action plan is a list of the tasks that need to be completed in order to meet the specified objective (Figure 10-2, B). Particular attention needs to be given to sequencing and prioritizing these tasks. The nurse consultant and consultee collaborate to identify the tasks that need to be accomplished first in order to lay the foundation for later tasks. It is often helpful to list easier tasks early in the action plan because the successful completion of these tasks can build a consultee's confidence for tackling more difficult tasks. Moreover, placing simple tasks at the start of the plan gives the nurse consultant an opportunity to detect any unforeseen problems in the plan (for example, additional costs) as well as time to assess the consultees' skills and motivation to carry through with the plan. This strategy also gives the nurse consultant the opportunity to revise the plan if needed.

Making Task Assignments

An action plan must also identify who is responsible for each task and specify a timeline (start and end date) for when each task needs to occur (Figure 10-2, C). For the plan to have the best chance of succeeding, the nurse consultant should work with the consultee to identify who needs to be involved; a key to successful action planning is being clear about exactly where responsibility lies for the accomplishment of each task. Failure to specify responsibilities precisely can lead consultees to mistakenly assume that the nurse consultant is responsible for implementing the action plan (Ross 1993). Should this happen, the nurse consultant could be held wrongly accountable if the nursing consultation problem is not resolved.

Working with a Task Force   A specific task will sometimes need to be completed by a group of consultees and/or other members of the client system (a multidisciplinary "task force"). Task force members are usually selected on the basis of two considerations: the skills they can contribute and politics or the "clout" their involvement will carry.

When identifying task force members, the nurse consultant must be careful to avoid two common pitfalls. First, it is a mistake to assume that the people who have been chosen to work together are willing and able to do so. Thus consideration needs to be given to the compatibility of task force members and the time needed for team building (team building is discussed in a later section of this chapter). Secondly, it is easy for a task force to take on a life of its own and become alienated from the rest of the client system. An action plan should, therefore, incorporate strategies for regular communication between the task force and the rest of the client system.

Determining Needed Resources and Estimating Costs

Finally, an action plan should identify the human and material resources needed to carry out each task as well as the estimated cost of each task (Figure 10-2, D and E). Resources that need to be considered include personnel, time, office supplies, and information. Costs that need to be estimated include the consultant's fee, costs associated with consultee involvement in consultation activities (for example, paid time to attend meetings), travel expenses, and supplies. Identifying needed resources and costs up-front can help a client system avoid the pitfall of moving ahead with an action plan without having the material and financial resources needed to complete the plan.

Action Planning as Participative Learning

An action plan that is "owned" by the consultee has the greatest chance of being successful (Kurpius, Fuqua, & Rozecki 1993). Thus the nurse consultant needs to create opportunities for consultee "buy-in" to the action plan. Buy-in can be facilitated by involving consultees in the action planning process through participative learning strategies.

Participative learning—learning by doing—helps the nurse consultant achieve the tactical goal of developing a client system's own problem-solving skills. Using action planning as a learning opportunity also enhances consultees' capabilities and collaborative skills, encourages commitment and contributions to outcomes, raises consciousness about the dynamics of problem solving, and increases the likelihood of continuity of a problem's solution (Senge, Kleiner, Roberts, Ross, & Smith 1994).

Facilitating Implementation of the Action Plan

As discussed in the first chapter of this text, it is the nature of a nursing consultation relationship that responsibility for implementing the action plan rests with the consultee. Paradoxically, a nurse consultant's success as a consultant is judged, at least in part, by whether or not the consultee implements the action plan and whether the consultation problem is resolved. Nurse consultants then, have a vested interest in facilitating the implementation of action plans that they help to develop. Consequently, nurse consultants generally employ two strategies in their relationships with consultees that lay the groundwork for implementing the action plan: team building and transition management.

Team Building

"Team building" refers to interventions that are specifically designed to develop an effective consultant-consultee team (Dyer 1977). Adjectives that describe effective teams include "in harmony," supportive, motivated, committed, open, involved, interested, and productive. The goals of team building in terms of the action planning phase include active participation in problem-solving activities and ownership by all team members of the outcomes of the problem-solving process. Team building helps consultees see themselves as beneficiaries rather than as victims of the changes that accompany problem solving (Cohen & Murri 1995).

Team-building strategies focus on improving the "workings" of groups by enhancing relationships, problem-solving skills, and effectiveness. Thus team-building strategies focus on both the social and task-oriented processes (see Chapter 6) that occur within groups. Because team-building strategies decrease resistance and build understanding and support for change, they are an appropriate activity in all nursing consultation relationships.

The specific nature of team-building strategies is limited only by the creativity of the nurse consultant. Typically, team-building strategies incorporate catalytic, confrontational, and acceptant interventions. Team members are asked to engage in self and group review and analysis by reflecting on the group's image, processes, and values. One possible exercise is to have consultees first select a metaphor (animal, machine, kind of person) that describes their actual and preferred self and then explain the reason for their choice. This same exercise can also be used to generate perceptions of group behaviors and organizational processes. The point of this exercise is to promote discussion and increase consistency between values and actions. The exercise may also facilitate an appreciation and understanding of the diversity within a group.

Involving group members in problem identification activities and in planning problem solutions are additional team-building strategies. Providing continuous feedback to consultees about the value of their participation in these activities acts as a team-building strategy by maintaining the momentum of a group's problem-solving efforts. These activities enhance team members' capabilities, commitment, contributions, collaborative skills, and hence, the continuity of the problem solution (Senge et al. 1994).

Transition Management

Transition management strategies focus on the psychological processes that people go through as they come to terms with a new situation, such as adjusting to new behaviors that will need to be assumed in order to resolve a nursing consultation problem. These interventions acknowledge that "It isn't the changes that do you in, it's the transitions" (Bridges 1991). Including transition management strategies in the action planning phase can prevent consultee guilt, self-absorption, resentment, anxiety, and stress from interfering with developing and implementing a problem solution.

Transition consists of three phases: letting go, managing the neutral zone, and launching new beginnings. Nurse consultants can encourage problem solving by facilitating the passage through each phase. To help consultees let go of the past, the nurse consultant can use acceptant interventions such as identifying who is losing what and openly and sympathetically acknowledging the importance of these losses. Losses should be compensated for if possible. The nurse consultant should also clearly define what is over and what is not over and should treat the past with respect. In a merger situation, for example, nurses' loss of identity as members of one of the merging facilities could be compensated for by development of a new logo and name to which nurses from both facilities would have to adjust. The nurse consultant could acknowledge past successes of the individual merging facilities while emphasizing the importance of continuing quality care.

The core of the transition process and the focus of transition management interventions is the "neutral zone." The neutral zone is an "emotional wilderness" where old ways are gone but new ways don't yet feel comfortable (Bridges 1991).The middle of the neutral zone encompasses that period of time during which reorientation and role redefinition are taking place. A nurse consultant can facilitate passage through this transition phase by maintaining clear and consistent open lines of communication and by providing the training and education needed to make the change. Providing consultees with the opportunity to question usual ways of doing things and developing new and creative solutions to difficulties that arise during the transition also facilitate passage through the neutral zone. In a merger situation, for instance, some staff may need to learn to work with new equipment. Peer teaching sessions could be implemented to meet this need (and could simultaneously facilitate the development of teamwork).

Once a change has been implemented, there is an adjustment period during which consultees begin to incorporate the problem solution (new behavior, new attitudes, or new processes) into their usual way of work. The nurse consultant needs to help consultees accept the feelings of incompetence that often arise at this time. Strategies can be built into the action plan to lessen these feelings and let consultees "save face." These strategies will also help ensure that the action plan isn't abandoned because of

---

Box 10-5. Transition Management Strategies

To help consultees let go:
Identify who is losing what
Accept the reality and importance of subjective losses
Don't be surprised at "overreaction"
Acknowledge losses openly and sympathetically
Expect and accept the signs of grieving: anger, bargaining, anxiety, sadness,
    disorientation, and depression
Compensate for losses
Give people information … again and again
Mark the endings
Treat the past with respect
Let people take a piece of the old way with them
Show how endings ensure continuity of what really matters

To help consultees manage the neutral zone:
"Normalize" the neutral zone
Redefine and reframe the neutral zone; use metaphors such as "a bridge
    to be crossed"
Create temporary systems
Strengthen intragroup connections
Use a transition management team
Establish checkpoints
Use the neutral zone creatively: allow time for questions and innovation,
    provide training, encourage experimentation

To help consultees launch new beginnings:
Acknowledge ambivalence
Consider issues related to timing and allow time: explain the purpose of
    the change, paint a picture of how it will look and feel, give everyone a
    chance to participate and contribute
Reinforce new beginnings: give consistent messages, ensure quick successes,
    symbolize the new identity, celebrate successes

From Bridges, W. (1991). *Managing transitions: Making the most of change.* Reading, MA:
Addison-Wesley.

---

these feelings. An action plan, for example, might build in temporary lower expectations of quantity (reduced patient load) while still communicating expectations for quality. Box 10-5 summarizes transition management strategies.

Possible Difficulties in Action Planning

Conflict, ambivalence, and resistance are the dilemmas that are most likely to complicate the action planning phase of the nursing consultation process.

Conflict

Politics (competing needs and demands) are a frequent source of conflict during the action planning phase. One political conflict that a nurse consultant often faces is that of needing to decide whose needs to satisfy—the consultee's, the contact person's, the client's, or the consultant's. Sometimes a nurse consultant's own needs may override her/his judgment about what would be appropriate in a given situation. For example, a nurse consultant might want to use a process model of nursing consultation when the consultees have neither the time nor energy to do so.

Conflicts about goals or desired outcomes can also occur during the action planning phase. Consultees, contact persons, and the nurse consultant may disagree on what a desirable or feasible end state might be. As an example, the goal of "becoming more effective" can mean something different to each involved party.

Finally, methods conflicts can arise during action planning. Methods conflicts involve disagreements about both strategies and who should do what. There is a natural tendency for consultees to want a quick and easy problem solution. Consultees have often been living with the problem for some time, and once they decide to ask for help, they want it immediately (Kurpius et al. 1993). Nurse consultants can exacerbate methods conflicts by an inflexible insistence on using their favorite strategies to solve every kind of nursing consultation problem.

The nurse consultant is in a difficult position with all of these conflicts. Negotiation and the use of empirical-rational interventions can help resolve these conflicts.

Ambivalence

Ambivalence is a mix of positive and negative feelings about a situation. In the action planning phase, ambivalence is a natural reaction and usually reflects realistic concerns about how proposed interventions will affect a consultee on a personal level. While ambivalence should be legitimized as normal and expected (acceptant intervention), it also needs to be overcome so that consultees become committed to a problem-solving effort rather than merely compliant with it.

Nurse consultants can respond to ambivalence by using it as a resource (Lippitt & Lippitt 1986). Listening to and clarifying consultees' concerns often helps the nurse consultant identify important misinformation that needs to be corrected. Ambivalence can also be addressed by demonstrating the validity and feasibility of the action plan through role-modeling and rehearsal. Short-term demonstrable steps toward goal attainment can be developed, progress can be documented, and intermediate accomplishments can be celebrated and rewarded. In short, the nurse consultant can use ambivalence as an opportunity to involve consultees and enrich and revise the action plan so that it has a greater likelihood of success.

Resistance

Resistance to a specific proposed problem solution or to problem solving in general is a third dilemma that the nurse consultant often faces during the action planning phase. Cues that resistance might be building are highlighted in Box 10-6.

Sometimes, behavior that is labeled as resistance really is normal reality testing. The nurse consultant should respond to consultee comments such as, "I'm not sure we've thought this through" and, "I'm not sure this will work" by looking for possible holes in the action plan. When responding to these comments, it is important that the nurse consultant does not become defensive and try to change the consultee's attitudes. Rather, the nurse should use this as an opportunity for exploring the completeness and feasibility of the action plan.

Box 10-6. Is Resistance Building?

Possible cues ...
The action plan is attacked as impractical
Consultees act confused about what the problem is or what the goals of the
   plan are
Consultees intellectualize that the problem is really not a problem
The problem is labeled "no longer relevant"
Consultees moralize about "right" and "wrong" problem-solving strategies
More data and details are requested repeatedly
"No time" is used as an excuse for not accepting a specific solution or for not
   participating in the action planning process
There is pressure for an easy and quick solution
Passive-aggressive behaviors are present such as arriving late for meetings,
   leaving early, and acting bored

Resistance can also reflect a lack of understanding about the reason for a particular problem-solving strategy. When this is the case, the nurse consultant can use empirical-rational interventions to help a consultee gain knowledge and hopefully, understanding about the appropriateness of a particular intervention.

Documenting the Action Planning Phase

Documenting the activities of the action planning phase provides the nurse consultant with a track record of what has transpired during the nursing consultation relationship. Documentation can also serve as a learning tool and legal protection. The nurse consultant needs to document specific activities undertaken, parties involved, rationale for decisions, and outcomes of activities. In addition, many nurse consultants find it helpful to keep anecdotal notes about their impressions of how the consultation relationship is unfolding and ideas for next steps.

Box 10-7 provides a documentation checklist for the action planning phase of the nursing consultation process.

Chapter Summary

The activities of the action planning phase represent the first tangible "work" toward responding to the nursing consultation problem. Consequently, the action planning phase is a sensitive and somewhat risky phase of the nursing consulting process for both the nurse consultant and the client system. The consultant's reputation as an effective problem solver is on the line. At the same time, the client system is beginning to confront the transitions and losses that implementing the action plan (assuming it is accepted) may entail. Successful completion of the action planning phase can be determined only after the action plan has been carried out. However, matching goals and problem solutions to fit problem and client system characteristics, continually incorporating teamwork and transition management strategies, developing a sufficiently detailed plan of how an intervention should unfold, and being alert for

---

Box 10-7. Documentation Checklist: The Action Planning Phase

Documenting Goal Setting:

Identification of goal

How goal was determined: parties and process involved, rationale used

Conflicts about the goal: who, what, how it was resolved

Prioritization of goals: criteria used, who was involved in decision, conflicts
   (who, what, how resolved)

Documenting Intervention Selection:

Process used to select intervention: date and time, parties involved

Results of force-field analysis: driving and restraining forces identified, ideas
   about how to minimize and maximize these forces

Problem solution selected: criteria for decision

Conflicts about problem solution: who, what, how resolved

Resistance encountered: who, what, how resolved

Documenting the Action Plan:

Objectives and how determined

Sequenced list of tasks

Task assignments, rationale

Resources needed

Estimated costs

Attach Gantt chart if used

Documenting Implementation Facilitation:

Date and time of activity, parties involved

Description of activity (team building, transition management strategy),
   rationale

Results of activity

Ideas about possible next steps

---

and attending to possible dilemmas can facilitate development of an action plan that
is meaningful, acceptable, and feasible.

Applying Chapter Content

- Develop actions plans for the same nursing consultation problem using two different theoretical frameworks. State your rationale for the problem solutions and
  problem-solving approaches that you have chosen. Speculate as to what dilemmas
  you might encounter with each plan. Which plan do you think would have the
  greatest chance of success and why?

- Read the article by Huddleston (1992) that is listed as an additional reading. Critique the use of this problem-solving approach for this nursing consultation situation. How would you determine the appropriateness of this intervention for a
  particular family consultee? What difficulties do you think you might encounter

with this intervention? What transition issues would be faced in this situation? How would you deal with them?

- Analyze the effectiveness of a work team with which you are familiar. What team-building strategies would you use to enhance this team's effectiveness?

- Consider the following possible nursing consultation situations: (1) working with two clinics that are undergoing a merger, (2) opening a nurse practitioner clinic, and (3) working with a family to assume the long-term care needs of a handicapped child. What types of transition issues would be faced in each of these situations? How would you manage them?

References

Blake, R., & Mouton, J. (1990). *Consultation: A handbook for individual and organization development* (2nd ed.). Reading, MA: Addison-Wesley.

Bridges, W. (1991). *Managing transitions: Making the most of change.* Reading, MA: Addison-Wesley.

Cohen, W., & Murri, M. (1995). Managing the change process. *Journal of AHIMA, 66* (6), 40-47.

Dougherty, A. (1995). *Consultation: Practice and perspectives in school and community settings* (2nd ed.). Pacific Grove, CA: Brooks-Cole.

Dyer, W. (1977). *Team building: Issues and alternatives.* Reading, MA: Addison-Wesley.

Haffer, A. (1986). Facilitating change: Choosing the appropriate strategy. *Journal of Nursing Administration, 16* (4), 18-22.

Kurpius, D., Fuqua, D., & Rozecki, T. (1993). The consulting process: A multidimensional approach. *Journal of Counseling and Development, 71,* 601-606.

Lippitt, G., & Lippitt, R. (1986). *The consulting process in action* (2nd ed.). San Diego: University Associates.

Ross, G. (1993). Peter Block's *Flawless Consulting* and the Homunculus Theory: Within each person is a perfect consultant. *Journal of Counseling and Development, 71,* 639-641.

Senge, P., Kleiner, A., Roberts, C., Ross, R., & Smith, B. (1994). *The fifth discipline fieldbook.* New York: Currency-Doubleday.

Additional Readings

Albee, G., & Ryan-Finn, K. (1993). An overview of primary prevention. *Journal of Counseling and Development, 72,* 115-123.
  The author describes a proactive approach to consultation.

Blake, R., & Mouton, J. (1990). *Consultation: A handbook for individual and organization development* (2nd ed.). Reading, MA: Addison-Wesley.
  This classic text provides a thorough discussion of problem-solving approaches.

Bridges, W. (1991). *Managing transitions: Making the most of change.* Reading, MA: Addison-Wesley.
  This text emphasizes and provides strategies for managing the psychological dimension of change.

Dyer, W. (1977). *Team building: Issues and alternatives.* Reading, MA: Addison-Wesley.
  This classic text is a wealth of team-building principles and strategies.

Fuqua, D., & Kurpius, D. (1993). Conceptual models in organizational consultation. *Journal of Counseling and Development, 71,* 607-618.
  The authors provide an excellent overview of different approaches to problem solving.

Haffer, A. (1986). Facilitating change: Choosing the appropriate strategy. *Journal of Nursing Administration, 16* (4), 18-22.
The author applies Hersey and Blanchard's situational leadership model to choosing problem-solving strategies.

Harrison, M. (1994). *Diagnosing organizations: Methods, models, and processes* (2nd ed.). Thousand Oaks, CA: Sage.
Chapter 2 of this text discusses using an open systems perspective to determine problem solutions.

Huddleston, J. (1992). Family and group psychoeducational approaches in the management of schizophrenia. *Clinical Nurse Specialist, 6* (2), 118-121.
The author provides a case study of a consultation intervention.

Lippitt, G., & Lippitt, R. (1986). *The consulting process in action* (2nd ed.). San Diego: University Associates.
Chapter 6 discusses designing participative learning. Chapter 8 includes examples of consultation in action.

Schein, E. (1987). *Process consultation, volume II: Lessons for managers and consultants.* Reading, MA: Addison-Wesley.
Chapter 10 describes different problem-solving approaches.

Schein, E. (1988). *Process consultation, volume I: Its role in organization development* (2nd ed.). Reading, MA: Addison-Wesley.
Chapter 5 discusses group problem solving and decision making. Chapter 13 talks about confrontational interventions.

Senge, P., Kleiner, A., Roberts, C., Ross, R., & Smith, B. (1994). *The fifth discipline handbook.* New York: Currency-Doubleday.
This text is a compendium of strategies for creating a "learning organization."

Ulschak, F., & SnowAntle, S. (1990). *Consultation skills for health care professionals.* San Francisco: Jossey-Bass.
Chapter 7 discusses taking action in internal consultation situations.

Evaluating Nursing Consultation Efforts

*Despite the fact that virtually every kind of business,
government, and service organization has been involved
in consultation to some extent, only a limited amount of
research exists on evaluating the consultation process.*
(Lippitt & Lippitt 1986)

Key terms: formative evaluation, summative evaluation,
effectiveness criteria, performance standard, impact evaluation

Gaining entry, problem identification, action planning, evaluation, and disengagement—these phases of the nursing consultation process represent distinct sets of activities that occur in a predictable sequence. Recall from earlier discussion, however, that the activities of adjacent phases may actually overlap (see Figure 2-1), and that there can be a certain amount of back-and-forth movement between phases. Thus the nursing consultation process is an iterative process; what occurs in one phase provides feedback about the previous phase and may necessitate backtracking and repeating tasks. For example, the inability to agree on goals during the action planning phase may signal a need to revisit the results of the diagnostic analysis that occurred as part of the problem identification phase. Another characteristic of the nursing consultation process is that some activities occur on a more or less continual basis throughout the process. To a certain extent, the nurse consultant is always assessing, diagnosing, planning interventions, and evaluating (Dougherty 1995).

In nursing consultation, evaluation involves systematically collecting data and making and communicating judgments about both the activities and outcomes of the nursing consultation relationship. Because a consultee may not actually implement a proposed action plan, the evaluation of a nursing consultation relationship does not always focus on determining the success of a particular problem solution or intervention. Instead, the "intervention" that the nurse consultant evaluates is the entire nursing consultation relationship. The evaluation process in nursing consultation consists of the following three tasks:

planning evaluation activities
conducting the evaluation
giving evaluation feedback

Much of the first task—planning—takes place during the action planning phase of the nursing consultation process. The second and third tasks—conducting the evaluation and giving evaluation feedback—occur on two levels. First, these tasks occur as distinct phases of the consultation process and are carried out in order to draw conclusions about the nursing consultation relationship (summative evaluation). Secondly, these tasks occur on a more or less continual basis and provide the nurse consultant with information for revising the nursing consultation process while it is still underway (formative evaluation). Thus evaluation in nursing consultation can be thought of as a feedback mechanism that provides ongoing as well as summative information to both the nurse consultant and consultee about their success in meeting the goals of the nursing consultation relationship.

This chapter begins with a discussion of how evaluation fits into the nursing consultation process. Next, the specific tasks associated with evaluation—planning evaluation, conducting the evaluation, and giving evaluation feedback—are discussed. The chapter concludes by considering some of the difficulties associated with implementing evaluation activities in the nursing consultation process. While the content in this chapter focuses primarily on summative evaluation as a distinct phase of the nursing consultation process, much of the content applies to the ongoing or formative evaluation activities that take place throughout the entire consultation relationship. As you read this chapter, think about the following questions:

- How are assessment and evaluation activities which both occur continuously throughout the nursing consultation process distinct from one another?

- How might the evaluation phase of the nursing consultation process be different when the consultee is an individual and when the consultee is a group?

- How might the evaluation phase vary with purchase-of-expertise, doctor-patient, and process consultation interaction patterns?

- What types of difficulties might internal and external nurse consultants encounter during the evaluation phase?

Evaluation and the Nursing Consultation Process

Evaluation is one of the more complex sets of activities undertaken by a nurse consultant because, in addition to being a distinct phase in the nursing consultation process, evaluation occurs on a more or less continual basis. Evaluation is more likely to be carried out effectively if both the nurse consultant and consultee understand the difference between formative and summative evaluation, appreciate the purposes of evaluation, and understand how evaluation links to and affects other phases of the nursing consultation process.

Formative and Summative Evaluation

As indicated, evaluation is both an ongoing activity and a distinct phase in the nursing consultation process. Formative evaluation is the evaluation activities that occur on an ongoing basis throughout the nursing consultation process. The purpose of formative evaluation is to provide the nurse consultant and the consultee with a steady stream of information about how the nursing consultation relationship is progressing. Formative evaluation provides the nurse consultant with an answer to the question, "Are we on the right track?" Formative evaluation is a decision-making tool that helps the nurse consultant determine: (1) the consultation relationship is progressing effectively and should be continued as planned, or (2) the consultation relationship is not progressing effectively and earlier phases of the nursing consultation process need to be revisited.

Formative evaluation is often conducted in an informal manner. That is, formative evaluation can be accomplished by simply questioning consultees about their perceptions of how the consultation relationship is progressing. Formative evaluation should

---

Box 11-1. Questions Addressed by Formative and Summative Evaluation of a Nursing Consultation Relationship

Formative Evaluation

What are the objectives at this point in time and have we accomplished these objectives?

Are we proceeding on our timeline?

What stumbling blocks are we encountering? How are we dealing with these?

Are any new problems arising?

Do we need to make any changes in the way this project is being carried out?

What about the clients' openness versus resistance to consultation? Is this changing? If so, in what direction?

Are needs and issues being met or unmet?

Summative Evaluation

Was the action plan carried out? If not, why not?

Were revisions in the plan needed? Why?

Have the interventions achieved their desired purpose?

Were there any unanticipated effects?

What factors facilitated success?

What factors subtracted from success?

What factors contributed to effectiveness and efficiency?

What factors subtracted from effectiveness and efficiency?

Were the terms of the contract met?

Did investments of time, money, and effort pay off?

Was the consultant helpful?

Did we "pass" or not?

Would the consultant be recommended or contacted again?

---

also entail checking the progress of the nursing consultation relationship against the proposed project timeline and anticipated costs.

Summative evaluation describes those evaluation activities that comprise the fourth phase of the nursing consultation process. Summative evaluation activities predominate as the nursing consultation relationship is winding down. The purpose of summative evaluation is to provide the nurse consultant and consultee with answers to the questions, "Have we been successful?" and, "Did we do what we planned to do in an efficient and effective manner?"

Like formative evaluation, summative evaluation is a decision-making tool. Information obtained from summative evaluation helps the nurse consultant decide whether: (1) the consultation relationship has been successful and can be terminated, (2) the relationship has been partially successful but additional problem-solving efforts are needed and earlier phases of the nursing consultation process need to be revisited, or (3) the relationship has not been a success but should go no further and an "autopsy" should be done (Ulschak & SnowAntle 1990). Box 11-1 compares the specific questions addressed by formative and summative evaluation of a nursing consultation relationship.

Other Purposes of Evaluation

Evaluation has other purposes in the nursing consultation process besides that of being a decision-making tool. Evaluation can serve as a quality control and accountability device, legal protection, a learning device, and a marketing tool. Evaluation, therefore, is beneficial in a number of ways for both the nurse consultant and the consultee.

As a quality control device, evaluation provides the nurse consultant and the consultee with information about the validity of the problem definition that was generated from earlier assessment and diagnostic analysis activities. In other words, if problem-solving efforts are unsuccessful, it may be because the wrong problem cause was identified. Evaluation also provides information about the quality of decision making that went into goal setting and action planning. For example, were feasibility issues related to proposed problem solutions considered?

Evaluation promotes accountability in both the nurse consultant and consultee by verifying whether and to what extent they have met the terms of the nursing consultation contract. In this way, evaluation also offers both the nurse consultant and the consultee legal protection because it helps to identify whether failing to meet agreed upon and contracted responsibilities are to blame for an unsuccessful nursing consultation relationship.

The information obtained from evaluating a nursing consultation relationship can also serve as a learning device. Evaluation can help a consultee recognize additional needs or areas and skills that need more work if problem solutions are to be long-lasting. Evaluation can also help a consultee identify problem-solving skills and interventions that could be useful in similar problem situations that might occur in the future.

Evaluation information may also serve as a learning tool for the nurse consultant. Evaluation feedback such as consultee satisfaction or perceptions of effectiveness can help a nurse consultant identify the need for improvement in particular skills or services. In addition, feedback from many consultation relationships, over time, can help the nurse consultant understand how different consultation approaches and problem-solving strategies are more or less effective for different consultation situations (Kurpius, Fuqua, & Rozecki 1993).

A final purpose or benefit of evaluation is that both the nurse consultant and the consultee can use information obtained from evaluation as a marketing tool. Consultees can use evidence of improved performance as a tool for attracting future clients. Favorable satisfaction and effectiveness ratings can promote positive public relations for both internal and external nurse consultants. Since as much as 75% of a consultant's activity is from consultee referrals and repeat business (Cosier & Dalton 1993), this benefit or side effect of evaluation cannot be overlooked.

Linkages between Evaluation and Other Phases of the Nursing Consultation Process

Formative evaluation, evaluating the nursing consultation relationship as it is unfolding, is one way in which evaluation-related activities permeate the entire nursing consultation process. Evaluation is linked to other phases of the nursing consultation process in another way as well; activities that take place during earlier phases of the consultation process lay the foundation for the summative evaluation activities that comprise the fourth phase of the nursing consultation process.

During the gaining entry phase, the nurse consultant needs to communicate to the consultee or contact person that evaluation is both an expectation of the nursing consultation relationship as well as crucial to its success. To reinforce this expectation, it is important that the nursing consultation contract includes an explicit agreement that evaluation will occur. The contract should also specify any limitations (such as time,

Table 11-1. Evaluation and the Nursing Consultation Process

Phase of Nursing Consultation Process	Evaluation-Related Activity	
Gaining Entry	Communicate evaluation and feedback as important components of the nursing consultation relationship Establish expectations that evaluation will occur	Formative Evaluation
Contracting	Agree to evaluation Identify limits to evaluation activities	
Problem Identification	Plan to evaluate the nursing consultation relationship: Identify data sources for post-consultation comparison	
Action Planning	Plan to evaluate specific interventions and problem solutions: Establish effectiveness criteria Identify performance standards Determine data sources and data collection strategies	
Evaluation	Conduct the evaluation: Gather evaluation information Determine whether standards have been met Share evaluation feedback Utilize evaluation findings 1. Goals met → disengage 2. Goals not met → disengage, do autopsy 3. Problem still exists → recycle to earlier phase 4. Unanticipated results → implement secondary interventions	Summative Evaluation

budget, or access to information) that may restrict how evaluation activities are implemented in the consultation relationship.

Throughout the problem identification phase of the nursing consultation process, the nurse consultant should attempt to identify possible sources of evaluation data. The nurse consultant should also be alert for information that it might be meaningful to compare on a before and after basis as a way of determining the effectiveness of the consultation relationship. Take, for example, a consultation project that is addressing the problem of nurses not adequately meeting the psychosocial needs of patients with HIV/AIDS. During the problem identification phase of the consultation process, the nurse consultant might collect information on nursing staff attitudes toward caring for patients with HIV/AIDS. As this information is being collected, the nurse consultant should make at least a mental note to reassess these attitudes as a way of determining the effectiveness of the consultation relationship.

During the action planning phase, the nurse consultant and consultee lay an additional foundation for summative evaluation by collaborating to determine how to evaluate specific problem solutions and interventions. To do this, the nurse consultant and consultee develop effectiveness criteria and performance standards for each intervention. In addition, they outline in advance the specific strategies for measuring the objectives of the action plan in order to ensure that the objectives are realistic. If the objectives of the nursing consultation relationship cannot be measured, the nurse consultant and consultee cannot know whether they have attained the objectives or if the objectives are even attainable. Table 11-1 summarizes the evaluation-related activities that occur during each phase of the nursing consultation process.

Because assessment and evaluation both involve data gathering and interpretation and both occur on an ongoing basis throughout the nursing consultation process, the two sets of activities are sometimes confused with each other. As Figure 11-1 illustrates, assessment and evaluation differ in terms of their orientation and utilization as

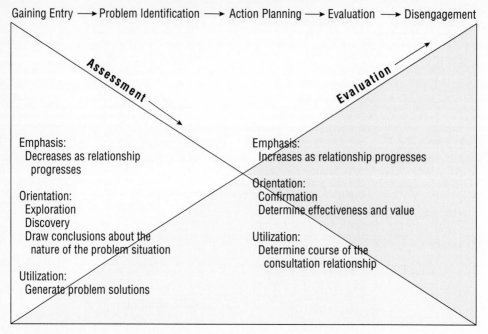

Figure 11-1. Assessment and Evaluation in the Nursing Consultation Process
Assessment and evaluation both occur continuously throughout the nursing consultation process. Assessment activities predominate in the earlier phases of the process and decrease as the consultation relationship progresses; the opposite occurs with evaluation activities. Assessment and evaluation also have different foci and their findings are used for different purposes.

well as in the relative emphasis assumed during the course of the nursing consultation process.

Assessment activities predominate during the initial phases of the nursing consultation process and taper off as the consultation relationship progresses; the opposite progression occurs with evaluation activities. Assessment activities focus on discovering new information about the problem situation and using this information for shaping problem solutions. In contrast, the focus of evaluation is gathering information for determining whether the nursing consultation relationship is on track or needs midcourse correction.

Planning Evaluation Activities

Even though evaluation is not emphasized until the fourth phase of the nursing consultation process, as the preceding discussion implies, much of the groundwork for these evaluation activities takes place prior to the evaluation phase itself. In fact, much of the summative evaluation plan is developed during the action planning phase. The evaluation plan reflects decisions about the content of evaluation (what to evaluate), effectiveness criteria, performance standards, appropriate data sources, and data collection strategies. A carefully constructed evaluation plan helps prevent evaluation from being burdensome to implement and yielding data that are meaningless or ignored.

Identifying Evaluation Content

The first step in planning evaluation is identifying evaluation content. Because nursing consultation consists of a product (the problem solution) as well as a process, evaluation activities need to consider both the services provided by the nurse consultant and how well the nurse consultant provided the services. More specifically, evaluation should focus on the following three focal areas: (1) consultee progress toward goal attainment, (2) specific events in the nursing consultation relationship, and (3) the working relationship between the nurse consultant and the consultee (Lippitt & Lippitt 1986).

Each focal area that is evaluated in nursing consultation also needs to be considered in terms of three potential impact levels. Nursing consultation relationships can affect individuals, groups, and the total client system (Lippitt & Lippitt 1986). At the individual level, nursing consultation affects the consultees with whom the nurse consultant is interacting as well as the clients on whose behalf consultation was sought. Groups that can be affected by a nursing consultation relationship include work units, families of clients, and aggregates of patients. Nursing consultation can also have far-reaching effects on the client system as a whole. The content that needs to be considered in the evaluation of a nursing consultation relationship then, can be pictured as a "Focal Area vs. Impact Level Matrix." This matrix and sample issues it might address are illustrated in Box 11-2.

Focal Area #1: Goal Progress   This focal area centers around progress towards or accomplishment of the agreed upon goals of the nursing consultation relationship. If the action plan is sufficiently detailed and has clearly stated objectives and a timeline, goal progress evaluation should be straightforward. The nurse consultant can simply collect information about whether or not tasks are being carried out and whether or not this is occurring on schedule.

Individual level impacts of goal progress that might be considered include changes in consultee behavior and changes in client well-being. Group level impacts of goal progress include changes in work group productivity. At the total client system level, effects of goal progress on profit margin and market share might be evaluated.

Goal evaluation provides the nurse consultant with valuable information about the quality of both the problem identification and action planning phases of the nursing consultation process. For example, goal evaluation can provide feedback to the nurse consultant about the feasibility of both goals and the timeline of the action plan.

Focal Area #2: Event Evaluation   Event evaluation focuses on specific events that have occurred during the course of the nursing consultation relationship. Examples of specific events a nurse consultant might want to evaluate are education or training sessions, feedback meetings, and specific data gathering events such as interviews and surveys. Event evaluation considers reactions to and perceived value of the specific event.

At the individual level, evaluation of a training session would include participants' comments about the teaching methods used and usefulness of content. Group level impacts of the same training session that could be evaluated include how much the session disrupted the work unit's productivity. A total client system impact of a training system to consider would be the cost/benefit ratio; that is, did expenses for the session pay off?

Event evaluation provides the nurse consultant with information that can be used to improve similar future events that are scheduled to occur during a particular consultation relationship. It also provides information that the nurse consultant can use when designing future consultation projects with other client systems.

Box 11-2. Focal Area vs. Impact Level Matrix for Evaluating
the Nursing Consultation Process

Evaluation Area	Individual Impact Level	Group Impact Level	Total Client System Impact Level
Goal Progress	Have there been changes in consultee behavior, skills, or attitudes? How has goal progress affected consultee workload? Has there been an improvement in client well-being? What side effects have been experienced by the client?	How has care delivery changed for the client group? How has goal progress affected the client's family? What impact has goal progress had on morale and productivity of the work unit?	Has there been any change in market share of business from the client group? What has been the cost/benefit ratio of goal accomplishment?
Specific Events	What was the perceived effectiveness of teaching sessions? How did consultees react to involvement in problem identification and action planning activities?	Was the event disrupting to the work flow of the unit? Were all work groups able to participate in the event?	How much time and productivity was lost because of participation in the event?
Nurse Consultant-Consultee Relationship	Have there been any changes in consultee insight and problem-solving skills?	How did the relationship with the consultant affect teamwork, collaborative skills, and productivity?	Has the consultant-consultee relationship had any impact on public relations?

Focal Area #3: Relationship Evaluation   One of the most significant predictors of successful consulting is the relationship the nurse consultant is able to establish with the consultee and other members of the client system (Ross 1993). For this reason, the nurse consultant needs to be continuously gathering information and informally monitoring how individuals, groups, and the total client system are reacting to him/her as a consultant. In many ways, relationship evaluation assesses the extent to which the nurse consultant has been able to gain psychological entry into the client system. Thus relationship evaluation considers the nurse consultant's abilities to establish rapport and credibility and communicate effectively. These abilities reflect an awareness of the culture of the client system and an ability to accommodate interactions and interventions to the system's culture. Relationship evaluation also focuses on the consultee's perceptions of the nurse consultant's fulfillment of the consultation contract and technical skills as a consultant.

Individual level impacts of the nursing consultation relationship that could be considered include individual consultees' development of insight and problem-solving skills. Group level relationship impacts could include increased teamwork and collaborative skills. A possible systems level relationship impact could be an enhanced public image secondary to engaging in the consultation relationship. Feedback about perceptions of the nurse consultant/consultee relationship can help the nurse consultant identify areas for personal and professional development.

Selecting Effectiveness Criteria

The second decision made in relationship to the evaluation plan is selecting the criteria that will be used to determine the effectiveness or success of the nursing consultation relationship. Selecting effectiveness criteria can be one of the more difficult tasks in developing an evaluation plan. It is also one of the most important tasks, because if effectiveness criteria fail to pass the tests of meaningfulness and relevance, it may prove difficult to persuade the consultee that undertaking evaluation is worthwhile. Even if evaluation is undertaken, if effectiveness criteria are perceived by the consultee as being irrelevant or meaningless, it is unlikely that the evaluation results will be used.

Effectiveness criteria should be selected by both the nurse consultant and consultee. Occasionally, clients and other members of the client system may also be involved in developing criteria. For example, administrators (who are paying the nurse consultant's fee) may want to have some say about what constitutes effectiveness in an organization-wide consultation project in which the entire organization is the client. Questions that can be used to help select meaningful and relevant effectiveness criteria are, "What needs to happen for this relationship to be considered a success?" and, "What would success look like in this situation?" Five categories of effectiveness criteria should be considered for evaluating any nursing consultation relationship.

Cost benefit ratio This criterion considers the net "payoff" of the nursing consultation relationship: did what was gained from the relationship outweigh costs (time, money, stress, and so forth)?

Behavior or performance change This criterion considers whether behavior changes among consultees occurred as planned and contributed to the problem solution.

Cognitive or knowledge change Some nursing consultation relationships are considered effective if consultees' knowledge changed in such a way as to contribute to the problem solution.

Affective or attitude change If this criterion is used, a nursing consultation relationship is considered effective if consultees' attitudes changed in such a way as to contribute to the problem solution.

Reactions This effectiveness criterion considers consultees' satisfaction with the nursing consultation relationship and perceptions of the relationship's effectiveness.

Which of these criteria are meaningful and relevant will depend on the nature of the nursing consultation problem, the goals of the consultation relationship, and the identity of the client. Not all criteria are appropriate in every nursing consultation situation. What is more, different effectiveness criteria might be appropriate for different impact levels of a nursing consultation relationship. For example, a change in knowledge might indicate effectiveness of the nursing consultation relationship at the individual impact level, while work group efficiency might be a more valid effectiveness criterion at the group impact level. At the total client system impact level, cost/benefit information might be considered the most meaningful and relevant indicator of effectiveness. The scenario presented in Box 11-3 illustrates determining effectiveness criteria.

Box 11-3. Determining Effectiveness Criteria:
         A Nursing Consultation Scenario

The Consultation Problem:
A physician group asks a nurse consultant to help increase the group's caseload
   of pediatric patients.

Parties Involved:
Consultee = physicians in the group
Client = the group practice
Stakeholders = pediatric patients and their parents, other physicians in the area

Possible Effectiveness Criteria:
Cost/Benefit Ratio: Has the change in caseload of pediatric patients been
   enough to offset the costs associated with the nursing consultation relationship?
Behavior/Performance Change: Have the consultees' behaviors changed in a
   way that will attract more pediatric patients on a continual basis?
Cognitive or Knowledge Change: Have the consultees gained knowledge that
   will enable them to attract and maintain more pediatric patients?
Affective or Attitude Change: Have the consultees' attitudes changed in such a
   way as to continue to attract more pediatric patients to the practice?
Reactions: How did the physicians rate their satisfaction with the consultant
   and the consultation relationship?

It is important to recognize that effectiveness evaluation is different from impact
evaluation. Effectiveness evaluation focuses on goal accomplishment. In contrast,
impact evaluation considers the effects of the nursing consultation relationship, and
effectiveness is only one possible effect. Referring to the scenario in Box 11-3, note that
effectiveness evaluation is concerned with determining the extent to which outcomes
and reactions associated with the nursing consultation process resulted in achieving
the goal of increasing the physician group's goal of an increased caseload of pediatric
patients. Impact evaluation would consider other possible effects of the nursing consultation relationship and its outcomes, for example, healthier children, better access to
care, increased waiting time for an appointment, increase in practice revenue, increased
expenses incurred by the physician group as a result of seeing more pediatric patients,
changes in physician work time, and so forth. In summary, while there can be many
favorable outcomes at different impact levels for any nursing consultation relationship,
effectiveness evaluation focuses only on goal accomplishment and, therefore, the effect
of the relationship on client well-being. In our working scenario, this would translate
into increased financial well-being of the physician group practice.

Specifying Performance Standards

The third decision that the nurse consultant needs to make in developing the nursing
consultation evaluation plan is that of performance standards. A performance standard is a reference point against which specific consultation outcomes are compared
in order to make a judgment of success or failure. A nursing consultation relationship
is successful when its outcomes match or exceed agreed upon performance standards.

Common performance standards include the following: operating more effectively than before the nursing consultation relationship, meeting minimal accepted standards such as those established by an accrediting agency, and meeting ideal standards established by oneself or some group (Harrison 1994).

What constitutes an appropriate performance standard is determined by the nature of the nursing consultation problem and the consultee's goals. For example, in the scenario about the nurse consultant working with the physician group, performance standards that could be used to determine the success of the nursing consultation relationship include the following:

the group's caseload of pediatric patients doubles in volume as compared to its pre-consultation level

the group's pediatric caseload accounts for 50% of daily office visits

the group's pediatric caseload accounts for 35% of the practice's revenue

Identifying Data Sources

The fourth decision that needs to be made when formulating an evaluation plan for a nursing consultation relationship involves selecting sources of evaluation data. Data sources that should be considered include consultees, clients, and other members of the client system (for example, the consultation contact person, fee payers, or family of an affected patient group). Recall that one of the distinguishing characteristics of nursing consultation is that patients always stand to be affected by the consultation relationship, either directly as clients or indirectly as stakeholders. With this in mind, the nurse consultant should always make an effort to gather evaluation information from patients, regardless of their role in the nursing consultation relationship.

Evaluation data from clients and stakeholders who are patients can target current performance, perceptions, and reactions to the consultation relationship as well as expectations about future performance. Again, using the scenario of the nurse consultant working with the physician group, current evaluation data from the parents of pediatric patients might focus on satisfaction with the care provided on a single occasion. Future-oriented evaluation data might focus on the likelihood that parents will use the physician group for their child's future health care needs. Future-oriented evaluation data can provide the nurse consultant and consultee with information about both the longevity of their problem solution and the need to conduct additional problem-solving interventions on an ongoing basis.

An additional source of evaluation information in a consultation relationship is oneself as the consultant. One's own perceptions about how things went and what worked (as well as what didn't and why) provide valuable information for structuring subsequent consultation relationships and increasing one's effectiveness as a nurse consultant. Essentially, what the nurse consultant needs to ask is, "If I had to do it over, what would I do the same and what would I do differently?" The nurse consultant should also evaluate any reactions (such as satisfaction) to the consultation relationship and personal cost/benefit ratio. This self-evaluation can provide the nurse consultant with information about what types of problem situations are a good fit for her/his skills and about how to formulate future consultation contracts.

Determining Data Collection Strategies

The final decision that needs to be made by the nurse consultant and consultee about the consultation evaluation plan is how to collect the evaluation data, including data collection techniques, the timing of data collection, and collecting comparison data. Ideally, individuals who are affected by the consultation relationship should be involved in making the decisions about how evaluation data will be collected. In addition, involving consultees in collecting and analyzing evaluation data increases the credibility of the findings and the likelihood that the information will be used.

Data Collection Techniques Observations, interviews, surveys, and document review can all be used to gather evaluation data about the nursing consultation relationship. The usefulness and limitations of each of these techniques were discussed in Chapter 9. The nature of the information desired, who the data sources are, and feasibility issues all influence decisions about how specific evaluation information would be best obtained.

One specific technique for generating evaluation data involves compiling a case study by the nurse consultant about the client system. A case study is an in-depth narrative report that includes detailed descriptions of observations of changes in the consultee, the client, and the total client system that occur as a particular consultation relationship unfolds. Case studies have the advantage of generating rich qualitative data on an ongoing basis. These data can contribute to a nurse consultant's own learning and can be shared with a consultee to provide positive feedback and increased insight into how the consultee's behavior and values influenced the consultation outcome. Case study data alone, however, may be less convincing than quantitative data to administrators, payers, and other stakeholders in a consultation relationship. Case study data are also inherently subjective and, therefore, prone to consultant bias. A nurse consultant, for example, may "see" hoped-for improvements in staff morale that cannot be confirmed objectively.

The Timing of Data Collection Deciding how to best time the collection of data in order to get a reliable indication of effectiveness requires consideration of a different set of issues. Evaluation data from surveys and consultee interviews might produce overly positive results due to a "novelty" effect if collected too soon after a problem has been resolved. That is, the evaluation results might appear positive only because the intervention or change is new and different and its side effects have not had a chance to develop. On the other hand, data collected too soon could reveal largely negative results if consultees are reacting to the discomfort of being in an adjustment period. Finally, if evaluation data are collected too late, changes that occurred may have become accepted as the status quo and thought of as "how things have always been." In these situations, effectiveness or success might be underestimated. Timing dilemmas are often handled best by collecting both immediate and delayed evaluation data.

Collecting Comparison Data Decisions about data collection strategies also involve consideration about what kinds of comparisons need to be made in order to demonstrate effectiveness of the nursing consultation relationship. Comparisons can be made over time as well as between groups.

Pre- and Post-Comparisons Comparisons of relevant pre- and post-consultation data from any source can provide objective and quantitative data about changes in attitudes or the frequency of undesirable behaviors or events. A pre- and post-consultation review of the frequency of abnormal blood glucose readings, for example, would provide a nurse practitioner with one piece of information about the effectiveness of consultation efforts about diet and exercise recommendations with the family of a newly diagnosed juvenile diabetic. The drawback of pre- and post-consultation data is that they require obtaining the same information from the same source at two points in time. If the data source is records, changes in documentation practices may have occurred between the pre- and post-data collection points. If before and after attitudes are being compared, testing effects (such as recall of previous responses) and attrition

---

Box 11-4. Strategies for Collecting Comparison Data
for Nursing Consultation Evaluation

Pre- and Post-Consultation Comparisons:
What it involves: Collecting the same information from the same sources
  before and after the nursing consultation relationship
Advantages: Since information is gathered from the same source, changes in
  performance are easy to see and interpret
Disadvantages:
  Can be cumbersome
  Practices of recording the data to be compared (for example, in medical
    records) may have changed between the two data collection periods
  Testing effects—individuals may recall their previous responses and
    respond in the same way
  Low response rates may bias post-consultation results

Longitudinal Comparisons:
What it involves: Collecting outcome data at multiple points in time
Advantages: Probably the best way of identifying the effects of the consultation
  relationship on variables that have fluctuating values; also the best way to
  determine long-term effects of a problem solution
Disadvantages:
  Takes time
  Is costly to implement
  Delays achieving closure of the nursing consultation relationship

Comparison Groups:
What it involves: Collecting information on the same variable from individuals
  who were participants in the nursing consultation relationship and those
  who were not
Advantages: No need to worry about testing effects
Disadvantages:
  Need to find a valid comparison group
  Pre-existing group differences may explain differences in performance
  "Contamination" of nonparticipants by participants in the consultation
    relationship

---

or "dropout" of some group members may bias findings and affect their meaningfulness and accuracy.

Longitudinal Comparisons When the purpose of a nursing consultation relationship is to effect change in a variable that has fluctuating values (such as sick days), it is often appropriate to track indicators of effectiveness over a longer period of time. In a longitudinal comparison, it is desirable to see a general trend of improvement that overrides any natural transient or situational variations. A nurse consultant working with a unit to improve staff morale might look for a general trend in decreased absenteeism over time despite occasional and expected increases that could be explained

---

Box 11-5. Planning Summative Evaluation: Essential Decisions

Decision #1: Evaluation Content
Focal Areas: goal progress, specific
  events, the nurse consultant-consultee relationship
Impact levels: individual, group, total
  client system

Decision #2: Effectiveness Criteria
Cost/benefit ratio
Behavior change
Knowledge change
Attitude change
Reactions

Decision #3: Performance Standards
Before and after changes
Compare to other groups
Compare to minimum standards
Compare to an ideal

Decision #4: Data Sources
Consultee
Client
Other members of the client system
Patients
Nurse consultant

Decision #5: Data Collection Strategies
Techniques:
Surveys
Interviews
Observations
Case study
Timing:
Immediate
Delayed
Comparisons:
Pre- and post-consultation
Longitudinal
Comparison group

---

by the flu season or holidays. Time and cost factors are the primary barriers to collecting longitudinal data about the effectiveness of nursing consultation interventions. Longitudinal evaluations can also delay bringing closure to a nursing consultation relationship.

Using a Comparison Group Comparisons between groups that were exposed to the nursing consultation relationship and those that were not can also be a means of generating effectiveness information. One difficulty of using this type of comparison, however, is the possibility of pre-existing differences between the groups. For instance, different styles of leadership on two nursing units, only one of which participated in the nursing consultation intervention, might be the real explanation of any post-consultation differences that are detected between the two units. A second drawback of using comparison groups is the possibility of "contamination effects." Staff on the unit involved in the consultation relationship might share what they learned with staff on the comparison unit and cause changes in their behavior. Box 11-4 summarizes the advantages and disadvantages of these different strategies for collecting comparison data.

The importance of triangulation was emphasized as a strategy for providing a check against bias during the problem identification phase of the nursing consultation process; it is also a recommended strategy for evaluating nursing consultation efforts. Combining reports of improved morale with time-series data about lower staff attrition and work-related injury rates, for example, would provide a more convincing picture of a nurse consultant's effectiveness than would either piece of information alone.

Box 11-5 summarizes the decisions the nurse consultant needs to make when planning the summative evaluation of a nursing consultation relationship.

Conducting the Evaluation

Evaluation can be conducted in either a consultant-directed or a collaborative manner. An evaluation that is carried out solely by the nurse consultant can often be completed in a more timely manner than can a collaborative evaluation. A consultant-directed evaluation allows the nurse consultant to work quickly and not have to rely on consultee cooperation or teach the consultee evaluation-related skills. Consultant-directed evaluation is most appropriate when the nurse consultant is under pressure to wrap up the consultation relationship in a hurry and when the inability to conduct evaluation in a timely manner might mean that evaluation would not be conducted at all. It is also appropriate when consultees are focused on implementing the action plan and dealing with the psychological transitions that accompany problem solving to the exclusion of actively contributing to the evaluation process. A disadvantage of consultant-directed evaluation is that its findings may be perceived as biased by the consultees and other members of the client system. For example, the nurse consultant might conclude that the consultation relationship has been successful, but the consultees might perceive otherwise since they have not had firsthand experience "seeing" and "hearing" the evaluation data.

Conclusions that are derived from an evaluation that has been conducted in a collaborative manner are often more believable to consultees and other members of the client system. This is because consultees have an opportunity to see and hear the evaluation data as the data come in. Consultees who are involved in the evaluation process also see how effectiveness and impact evaluation can offer different perspectives on the success of the consultation relationship. Another advantage of involving consultees in evaluation activities is that it gives them the opportunity to develop skills that will enable them to conduct their own evaluations in the future. Finally, consultees who are involved in evaluation have the opportunity to see the importance of evaluation as a feedback mechanism and learning device; this increases the likelihood that they will incorporate evaluation activities into their own work setting.

Giving Evaluation Feedback

Evaluation is useless unless the information that has been gathered is acted on and used to either make midcourse corrections in the nursing consultation relationship or reinforce positive changes that have occurred in the problem situation. Sharing evaluation findings with consultees and other members of the client system is the first step in using the findings to shape the subsequent course of the nursing consultation relationship.

Feedback helps evaluation serve its purposes. If consultees are not aware of evaluation findings, they will be unable to use the information as a decision-making, learning, or marketing device. Giving evaluation feedback then, functions as a catalytic intervention (see Chapter 10) because it increases awareness of how the nursing consultation relationship is progressing. Feedback can also serve as reinforcement for continuing the nursing consultation relationship and problem-solving efforts. Sharing evaluation findings also helps to bring closure to the nursing consultation relationship.

Strategies for Giving Effective Feedback

For evaluation feedback to be effective, the nurse consultant must make decisions about who needs to hear what information and how this information can be "packaged" so that it is accepted and used. In a consultation situation where a clinical nurse specialist is providing internal consultation to a staff nurse about a patient management issue, the nurse consultant would want to provide detailed ongoing (formative) evaluation feedback to the staff nurse consultee. Most likely, this feedback would be shared informally and verbally. Depending on the situation, it might also be important to share evaluation information with the patient, other nursing staff, the patient's physician, various levels of hospital administration, and other departments within the hospital such as the pharmacy. The content and format of an evaluation report would most likely vary, however, for each of these audiences.

If evaluation findings are to be shared in a public forum such as with all nursing staff, it is wise to first present the findings privately to the primary consultee or contact person. This provides an opportunity for the nurse consultant to preview possible reactions to and enlist support for the evaluation findings as well as involve the consultee or contact person in the group presentation. This involvement is perceived by the audience as a sanctioning of the evaluation findings and increases the likelihood that they will be used.

Because evaluation includes a component of judgment, sharing evaluation findings is different from sharing other kinds of information such as problem assessment findings. Before a client will hear judgmental news, the nurse consultant must be perceived as both credible and trustworthy. There also needs to be "readiness to hear" or agreement that feedback is a legitimate activity to engage in at this point in time.

The difficulty involved in giving needed negative feedback about consultation effectiveness can tempt a nurse consultant to withhold negative information in order to save face and avoid consultee reactions such as defensiveness. However, negative evaluation findings are at least as important as favorable findings in terms of being a learning device. Sometimes negative findings can be neutralized by being paired with positive findings. For example, a nurse consultant might be able to neutralize negative evaluation findings about the cost/benefit ratio of a consultation relationship by pairing them with favorable reports of staff and patient satisfaction. Negative findings can also be reframed as opportunities for further growth.

Throughout the feedback process, the nurse consultant needs to be mindful of the feelings that may be triggered by evaluative feedback and alert for possible signals of poor timing or violation of cultural norms. Both defensiveness and a too eager acceptance of feedback can signal recognition as well as denial of the validity of the evaluation findings. Premature closure of a feedback session often indicates confirmation of, but lack of support for, evaluation findings. A nurse consultant can deal with these reactions by acknowledging the validity of the feelings that most likely underlie the reaction (frustration or embarrassment, for example), making an effort to share favorable findings and strengths, and trying to reframe evaluation findings. For example, an immediate post-consultation finding of ineffectiveness in terms of cost/benefit ratio could be reframed as poorly timed evaluation and an indication for additional follow-up. Other strategies for effectively communicating findings from the evaluation of a nursing consultation effort are highlighted in Box 11-6.

Evaluation can be a painful and anxiety provoking process for all involved. Because evaluating nursing consultation efforts entails gathering data about the nurse consultant's own effectiveness as well as about goal attainment by the client system, the nurse consultant, too, can react to evaluation findings with defensiveness and denial. Many of the tips in Box 11-6 for effectively sharing feedback can be reinterpreted and used by the nurse consultant as strategies for interpreting personal evaluation findings. For example, the nurse consultant needs to consider how timing can affect personal receptivity to evaluation findings (bad news is always worse when one is tired!). The nurse consultant should also look for specific examples to support general statements about personal effectiveness and avoid putting too much stock in

---

Box 11-6. Giving Effective Evaluation Feedback

Keep the feedback objective and nonjudgmental

Keep feedback pertinent to the focal issues (that is, the nursing consultation experience and its effectiveness); remember relevance and meaningfulness

Support conclusions with specific examples; avoid broad generalities

Share strengths as well as weaknesses —what was accomplished or effective as well as what was not

Consider timing issues

Consider cultural norms

Recognize the need of all parties to "save face"

Share formative evaluation findings with clients on an ongoing basis

Keep individual evaluation responses confidential

Give verbal feedback before written feedback

Share findings privately with key players in the problem situation before "going public"

Try to demystify evaluation and reframe negative findings

Consider that sharing evaluation findings can function as both a catalytic and confrontational intervention

---

broad generalities. Finally, just as consultees are expected to accept only meaningful and relevant evaluation information, the nurse consultant should only attend to evaluation comments that address effectiveness in the present consultant role, not other roles (such as expert clinician or supervisor) in which the nurse consultant may also be familiar to the consultee.

Possible Difficulties in Evaluating Nursing Consultation Efforts

Many of the difficulties related to evaluating nursing consultation efforts such as timing, effectiveness issues, and the emotional responses to evaluation have been mentioned in earlier sections of this chapter. In this section, the focus is on three specific sets of potential difficulties: political dilemmas, hidden agendas, and barriers to implementing evaluation.

Political Dilemmas

A political reality of working with groups is the tension between securing private (individual level) and public (group or total client system level) benefits. Because repeat business is such a large part of any consultant's "portfolio," there is a myopic temptation to share only good news with a client system. While buying into the motto "the customer is always right" and sharing only favorable evidence of effectiveness may help all parties initially save face, it can be disastrous for both the nurse consultant and the client system in the long run, especially if interventions produce only short-term change or result in unanticipated side effects or costs. A response to this difficulty is learning to package unfavorable findings so they are more acceptable to the consultee and client system.

Hidden Agendas

One of the nurse consultant's tasks during the gaining entry phase of the nursing consultation process is to determine what, if any, hidden agendas might be prompting the consultation request. During the evaluation phase, a consultee's hidden agendas may place limits on what can be evaluated, what data can be accessed, and what findings are appropriate to share with which parties in the client system. Among the hidden agendas that can become apparent during the evaluation phase is the tendency to use findings to either protect an ineffective but popular individual or program or get rid of an effective but unpopular individual or program. For instance, the nurse consultant may be asked to reframe negative findings about a hospital's inability or unwillingness to provide the resources to implement a change in patient care strategies as staff inability or unwillingness to meet patient care needs within the existing structure of care delivery. The potential difficulty of hidden agendas can be addressed proactively when the nurse consultant and consultee establish parameters for reporting evaluation information in the nursing consultation contract and the evaluation plan.

Nurse consultants can also have hidden agendas that compromise the integrity of the evaluation phase of the nursing consultation process. Because favorable evaluations are effective consultation marketing tools, the temptation exists for evaluation activities to be structured and findings to be used strictly to serve marketing purposes. The danger, of course, with following this agenda is that the nurse consultant's needs, and not those of the consultee, are served by the evaluation. For example, a clinical nurse specialist can use a log that documents consultation activities to justify a continuing position within an organization. Failing to gather or report data about the impact of interventions, however, might hide the fact that many repeat requests for consultation reflect an inability to help clients solve certain types of problems on the first attempt. The nurse consultant needs to recognize that this shortsighted response to negative evaluation findings is unlikely to protect his/her reputation on a long-term basis. Instead, negative evaluation findings need to be used as guidelines for further professional development.

Barriers to Implementing Evaluation

Because evaluation can be an uncomfortable process, both consultees and consultants tend to come up with excuses for not including it as part of the consultation process. Evaluation is often perceived as an activity that only adds more time and expense to a consultation relationship. Evaluation also is often viewed as self-serving for the nurse consultant but of little value to the consultee or client system. In today's health care environment of cost-containment, these arguments are understandable but also somewhat misguided. Monitoring, documenting, and ensuring the quality of changes in health care practices that have resulted from consultant recommendations is vital for protecting and promoting the practice of nursing and nursing consultation as well as for ensuring that patient care and its outcomes are not compromised. Nurse consultants need to actively educate consultees about the purposes and benefits of evaluation.

The barriers that are most difficult to overcome in evaluating nursing consultation efforts are determining what constitutes meaningful, relevant, and feasible effectiveness criteria and valid performance standards. Few effectiveness criteria will suit the interest of all participants and stakeholders in the consultation process equally; this dilemma can result in avoidance of the entire evaluation phase. One response to the effectiveness dilemma is developing an evaluation plan that incorporates multiple focal areas and impact levels. Also, incorporating the concept of triangulation into data collection strategies can give a more convincing and accurate picture of effectiveness.

Documenting Evaluation Activities in Nursing Consultation

Documenting the evaluation activities that occur during a nursing consultation relationship serves many of the same purposes as evaluation itself. More specifically, documenting evaluation activities provides visual feedback and reminders to the nurse consultant about how to proceed with the nursing consultation relationship as well as serves as a learning tool in terms of providing information about interactions and interventions that were more and less successful. Documenting evaluation activities can also provide protection against possible legal charges of not adapting the consultation process to the evolving needs of a particular nurse consultant-consultee relationship. Box 11-7 provides a checklist for documenting the evaluation activities that take place during the nursing consultation process.

Chapter Summary

The benefits of evaluating nursing consultation relationships—for both nurse consultants and their consultees—underscores the importance of ensuring that the difficulties inherent in evaluation don't cause evaluation to be avoided as a part of nursing consultation. Systematically planning and implementing evaluation activities increases the likelihood that evaluation is feasible and yields information that is meaningful and relevant. Evaluation is more likely to be perceived as a worthwhile activity if it is kept simple and evaluation findings are actually used to enhance the effectiveness of the nursing consultation process.

Applying Chapter Content

For each of the following scenarios, describe how you would evaluate the effectiveness of your consultation efforts. Specifically address the following issues:

    areas to evaluate (including focal areas and impact levels)
    effectiveness criteria
    performance standards
    sources of data
    methods of data collection (including timing and comparisons)
    reporting strategies
    dilemmas or difficulties you might encounter and how you would
        respond to them

Scenario #1
You are a nurse-educator who has been providing consultation to a department of nursing as they formulate their self-study report in preparation for an accreditation site visit. Your primary interventions have been meeting with the faculty and sharing with them your impressions of their program and areas that might be problematic in the report. You also read the final self-study report before it is submitted to the accrediting agency.

Scenario #2
You are a nurse practitioner who has been providing consultation to a family. The issue that prompted consultation was perceptions of "acting out" behaviors by the family's adolescent son. Your interventions have included education about adolescent developmental issues, evaluation of family dynamics and communication patterns, and suggestions about setting limits and communication strategies.

Box 11-7. Documentation Checklist: Evaluation Activities

Documenting Formative Evaluation
☐ Consultee and nurse consultant perceptions of task accomplishment
☐ Consultee perceptions of key events and cost/benefit ratio
☐ Consultee perceptions of nurse consultant effectiveness
☐ Nurse consultant's impressions about the effectiveness of the nursing consultation relationship to date
☐ Adherence to timeline for tasks (if no, give rationale)
☐ Adherence to budget (if no, give rationale)
☐ Unanticipated side effects and how they are being responded to
☐ Date and time of each evaluation activity
☐ Source and method of data collection for each evaluation parameter
☐ Parties with whom formative evaluation findings were shared and reactions of these parties
☐ Actions taken as a result of evaluation findings

Documenting Summative Evaluation
☐ Goal accomplishment (give evidence)
☐ Consultee and nurse consultant evaluation of key events
☐ Consultee and nurse consultant evaluation of the nurse consultant-consultee relationship
☐ Other effects of the consultation relationship—describe, provide specific examples, identify as positive or negative
☐ Adherence to timeline (if no, give rationale)
☐ Adherence to project budget (if no, give rationale)
☐ Consultee satisfaction with the consultation relationship
☐ Nurse consultant satisfaction with the consultation relationship
☐ Cost/benefit ratio of the consultation relationship
☐ Date and time of each evaluation activity
☐ Data sources for each evaluation parameter
☐ Data collection strategy (timing, method, who implemented) for each evaluation parameter (attach tools)
☐ Effectiveness criteria and performance standards used for each evaluation parameter
☐ Difficulties encountered during summative evaluation—how they were handled, whether or not they were resolved
☐ Parties with whom evaluation findings were shared—format, their reactions
☐ Actions taken as a result of summative evaluation findings

Scenario #3

You are a nurse-manager who is working as an internal consultant with a unit that has recently undergone work redesign. The issues that prompted the consultation request were perceptions of low morale on the unit and patient care concerns. Specifically, ratings on patient satisfaction surveys have dropped and there has been an increase in incident reports. Your interventions have included listening to staff complaints, explaining the rationale behind redesign, and providing in-service education on communication and delegation skills.

Scenario #4

You are a clinical nurse specialist on an oncology unit. A nurse colleague asks you for help dealing with a patient who seems to be in denial about his poor prognosis and is refusing pain medication. Your interventions with the nurse can be characterized as being acceptant and confrontational in nature. You also make some specific suggestions for intervening with this patient.

References

Cosier, R., & Dalton, D. (1993). Management consulting: Planning, entry, performance. *Journal of Counseling and Development, 72,* 191-196.

Dougherty, A. (1995). *Consultation: Practice and perspectives in school and community settings.* Pacific Grove, CA: Brooks-Cole.

Harrison, M. (1994). *Diagnosing organizations: Methods, models, and processes* (2nd ed.). Thousand Oaks, CA: Sage.

Kurpius, D., Fuqua, D., & Rozecki, T. (1993). The consulting process: A multidimensional approach. *Journal of Counseling and Development, 71,* 601-606.

Lippitt, G., & Lippitt, R. (1986). *The consulting process in action* (2nd ed.). San Diego: University Associates.

Ross, G. (1993). Peter Block's *Flawless Consulting* and the Homunculus Theory: Within each person is a perfect consultant. *Journal of Counseling and Development, 71,* 639-641.

Ulschak, F., & SnowAntle, S. (1990). *Consultation skills for health care professionals.* San Francisco: Jossey-Bass.

Additional Readings

Alvarez, C. (1992). Are consultation notes always necessary? *Clinical Nurse Specialist, 6* (4), 214.
The author addresses the issues related to demonstrating the effectiveness of consultation efforts through ongoing evaluation and documentation.

Badger, T. (1988). Mental health consultation with a surgical unit nursing staff. *Clinical Nurse Specialist, 2* (3), 144-148.
This article provides a useful case study of the consultation process and includes evaluation activities.

Baird, S., & Prouty, M. (1989). Administratively enhancing CNS contributions. In A. Hamric & J. Spross (Eds.), *The clinical nurse specialist in theory and practice* (pp. 261-283). Philadelphia: Lippincott.
This chapter includes a discussion of the need to evaluate the multiple role components that comprise the clinical nurse specialist role.

Dougherty, A. (1995). *Consultation: Practice and perspectives in school and community settings.* Pacific Grove, CA: Brooks-Cole.
Chapter 5 of this text is a discussion of the evaluation phase of the consultation process.

Harrison, M. (1994). *Diagnosing organizations: Methods, models, and processes* (2nd ed.). Thousand Oaks, CA: Sage.
Chapter 3 of this text includes a thorough discussion of different ways in which effectiveness can be demonstrated.

Lippitt, G., & Lippitt, R. (1986). *The consulting process in action* (2nd ed.). San Diego: University Associates.
Chapter 17 presents the authors' model for evaluating the consultation process.
Ridley, C., & Mendoza, D. (1993). Putting organizational effectiveness into practice: The preeminent consultation task. *Journal of Counseling and Development, 72,* 168-177.
The authors present a model for defining organizational effectiveness.
Ulschak, F., & SnowAntle, S. (1990). *Consultation skills for health care professionals.* San Francisco: Jossey-Bass.
Chapter 7 discusses how to evaluate internal consultation efforts, including how to develop an evaluation design.

12

Disengagement in Nursing Consultation

If the entry stage is characterized by the question,
"Hello, what can I do for you?" then the disengagement
phase is characterized by the question, "What do we
need to take care of before I say good-bye?"
(Dougherty 1995)

Key terms: readiness, dependency, psychodynamics

Typically, traditional nurse-patient relationships "just end." In the traditional nursing process, a patient's discharge may be anticipated or even planned, but, as desirable as it may be, there is seldom an opportunity for a systematic and planned relationship closure process. In the nursing consultation process, however, there is a formal disengagement phase. Disengagement is the strategically planned and mutually agreed upon series of activities that ultimately results in the termination of the nurse consultant-consultee relationship. Disengagement then, is a process rather than a single abrupt event.

This chapter begins with an overview of the disengagement phase—its purposes, its importance, and its relationship to the other phases in the nursing consultation process. Next, the nurse consultant's tasks in the disengagement phase are discussed. The chapter closes by considering some of the difficulties that the nurse consultant may encounter when implementing the disengagement phase. As you read this chapter, think about the following questions:

- How might implementation of the disengagement phase differ for internal and external nurse consultants?

- How can disengagement be carried out by a nurse practitioner who has been providing consultation to a family or peer consultee?

- What facilitates and impedes successful implementation of the disengagement phase?

- How would you approach disengagement if you were "fired" as a nurse consultant?

An Overview of Disengagement

The themes of the disengagement phase are "letting go" and "securing the future." The theme of "letting go" applies to both the nurse consultant and the consultee. What is "let go," however, is only the problem-solving relationship between the nurse consultant and consultee. Disengagement does not necessarily mean that all personal or professional contact with a consultee ends. For example, in an internal consulting situation, the nurse consultant remains a part of the client system and most likely interacts with the consultee (and perhaps, the client) after the nursing consultation or problem-solving relationship has ended.

The second theme of the disengagement phase is "securing the future." Disengagement is an opportunity for both the nurse consultant and consultee to link the past with the future. That is, the activities of the disengagement phase provide an opportunity for the nurse consultant and consultee to review what has happened during the nursing consultation process and to ensure a secure future for the problem solution and resulting changes in the consultee and client system.

The Purposes of Disengagement

Although "letting go" and "securing the future" describe the overall focus of the disengagement phase, the more immediate goal of disengagement is to ensure that any problems that have been solved as a result of the nursing consultation relationship remain solved. Thus the primary purpose of disengagement is to facilitate "refreezing," that is, fostering the consultee's incorporation of a new point of view and new behaviors into everyday working relationships (Schein 1987).

A second purpose of disengagement is to encourage consultee self-reliance and prevent dependency on others for problem solving. This purpose supports the overall goal of nursing consultation to provide a consultee with problem-solving skills that can be transferred to future problem situations. This purpose of disengagement is also in line with the professional responsibility of nurse consultants to become progressively unnecessary to a consultee and client system (Lippitt & Lippitt 1986). The disengagement phase in the nursing consultation process helps prevent continuing a consulting relationship when it would only serve to meet the needs of the nurse consultant.

The Importance of Disengagement

How many times have you been involved in a consultation situation, either as a nurse consultant or as a consultee, in which the changes that had resulted from the consultation relationship evaporated as soon as the consulting relationship ended? On occasion, consultation efforts result in only short-term change and consultees regress to old ways of interacting with a client. In other situations, change is so fragile that counter-reactions arise and must be dealt with quickly in order to protect the problem solving that has occurred (Lippitt & Lippitt 1986). A strategically planned disengagement phase is important as a strategy for fostering the continuance of the outcomes of the nursing consultation relationship.

The disengagement phase is an opportunity to acknowledge the relationship that has developed between the nurse consultant and consultee. Very often, nursing consultation occurs because of a difficult and complex problem situation. As the nurse consultant and consultee work together to solve problems, a valued, trust-based, interpersonal relationship develops. Disengagement is an opportunity for the nurse consultant to recognize and validate the importance of this dimension of the nursing consultation relationship (Barron 1989). This validation is important for establishing a basis for future personal and professional contact between the nurse consultant and consultee.

Keep in mind that disengagement culminates in the termination of the nurse consultant-consultee relationship only in regard to a particular problem-solving activity. When disengagement activities have been successful, termination should be accompanied by a mutual sense of satisfaction about both the consultation relationship and what has been accomplished. If the problem-solving relationship between the nurse consultant and consultee has been mutually satisfying, the door is always open for reinvolvement or additional work at the consultee's request.

Linkage to Other Phases in the Nursing Consultation Process

While disengagement is a distinct phase in the nursing consultation process, much of the groundwork for successful disengagement is laid in earlier phases. During the gaining entry phase of the nursing consultation process, the nurse consultant needs to clearly establish the temporary, problem-focused nature of the consultation relationship. The nurse consultant needs to make sure that the consultee understands that the focus of the nursing consultation relationship is solving a particular problem and learning problem-solving skills for future use. The nursing consultation contract should clearly identify the criteria that will be used to set the activities of the disengagement phase into motion.

During the action planning phase of the nursing consultation process, the nurse consultant and consultee decide together how the nurse consultant will transfer responsibility for maintaining change to the consultee and the time frame for this transfer. In particular, the nature of the supports and resources that will be developed and installed into the client system in order to facilitate permanence of the problem solution need to be identified (Lippitt & Lippitt 1986). The action plan should be clear in terms of who is responsible (the nurse consultant, the consultee, or someone else in the client system) for developing and securing these supports.

The disengagement phase is linked most clearly to the evaluation activities that occur during the nursing consultation process. Ongoing formative evaluation may provide the nurse consultant and consultee with feedback that success is unlikely in a particular problem-solving relationship. For example, formative evaluation information may reveal a lack of resources or consultee motivation for continuing the nursing consultation relationship in any kind of an effective manner. If this is the case, the nurse consultant and consultee should proceed with disengagement activities (Kurpius, Fuqua, & Rozecki 1993).

In many nursing consultation situations, disengagement begins with the onset of summative evaluation activities. Collecting "end-point" evaluation information (on satisfaction or perceptions of success, for example) often serves as a "natural" signal to consultees that the nursing consultation relationship is winding down. In other cases, disengagement doesn't begin until after findings of summative evaluation provide the nurse consultant and consultee with the information needed to decide whether or not the goals of the nursing consultation relationship have been accomplished. If the nursing consultation problem has been resolved or the consultee has accepted the nurse consultant's recommendations, the nurse consultant and consultee can proceed with the previously planned disengagement activities. If, on the other hand, evaluation findings indicate that the nursing consultation problem remains unresolved, the nurse consultant and consultee have three options available to them: continue with current problem-solving efforts, revisit an earlier phase of the nursing consultation process (such as problem identification or action planning), or proceed to the disengagement phase because success seems unlikely (Ross 1993). (Recall that in some cases, evaluation findings will indicate a need to implement secondary or supplemental interventions in response to new problems or side effects to problem solving that have occurred.) Figure 12-1 illustrates how the disengagement phase is linked to other phases in the nursing consultation process.

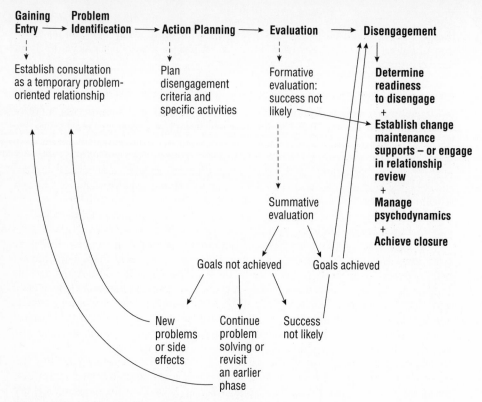

Figure 12-1. Disengagement in Nursing Consultation

While disengagement is a distinct phase in the nursing consultation process, the foundation for successful disengagement is laid during the gaining entry and action planning phases of the nursing consultation process. Information from both formative and summative evaluation activities helps the nurse consultant and consultee decide whether to proceed with disengagement activities or revisit an earlier phase in the nursing consultation process.

Nurse Consultant Tasks in Disengagement

Nursing consultation is characterized by a peer relationship between the nurse consultant and consultee. That is, the nurse consultant and consultee share responsibility for completing the tasks of each of the phases of the nursing consultation process. The situation is somewhat different in the disengagement phase, in which the nurse consultant assumes primary responsibility for successful task completion. This makes sense, because disengagement occurs at a point in the nursing consultation relationship when the consultee needs to concentrate on new ways of thinking and new behaviors that will ensure that the nursing consultation problem remains resolved after the nurse consultant leaves the client setting. To accomplish the goals of the disengagement phase (and of the entire nursing consultation process), the nurse consultant must successfully complete four tasks: (1) accurately determine the consultee's readiness to disengage, (2) put supports in place to maintain the changes that have occurred as a result of the consultation relationship, (3) manage the psychodynamics that accompany disengagement, and (4) achieve closure or terminate the nursing consultation relationship.

Determining Readiness to Disengage

The activities of the disengagement phase of the nursing consultation process should not begin until both the nurse consultant and consultee agree that the consultation relationship should be terminated. Ideally, this occurs because the goals of the nursing consultation relationship have been achieved and the nurse consultant is no longer of value to the client system. However, this sometimes occurs because it has become clear that a successful outcome to the nursing consultation relationship is unlikely. In either case, the nurse consultant should be alert for cues or indications that it is time to wind down the consultation relationship.

Information from the summative evaluation of the nursing consultation relationship should provide the nurse consultant with evidence (in terms of consultee behavior and characteristics of the nursing consultation relationship) that it is appropriate to proceed with the tasks of disengagement. Attainment of project goals or acceptance of the nursing consultation action plan is one piece of evidence that suggests it is appropriate to proceed with disengagement. Another cue of readiness to disengage would be consultee statements about readiness and self-confidence to continue without the nurse consultant (such as, "I think I've got it now"). Evidence that refreezing has occurred and that new behaviors, attitudes, and problem-solving skills have become the norm for the consultee and client system also supports disengagement. The best evidence that it is appropriate to proceed with disengagement is when the nurse consultant hears mutually developed recommendations and conclusions about a problem's cause being verbalized and owned by the consultee (Monicken 1995). An undesirable but nonetheless important indicator of readiness to begin disengagement is evidence that the consultee is growing more dependent on the consultation relationship in spite of new problem-solving abilities and goal achievement. Increased dependence is suggested by consultee passivity and withdrawal from problem-solving activities and by "stall tactics" such as the reappearance of previously resolved resistance to the problem solution and the changes it implies.

As an example of how readiness to disengage might present itself, consider the scenario of a psychiatric nurse practitioner (PNP) who has been providing consultation to a family nurse practitioner (FNP) colleague about the management of a patient with depression. One indicator of readiness to disengage could be evidence from the patient's record that indicates the FNP's competence in managing the patient. Another cue could be the FNP's expressions of increased comfort and confidence in managing the patient. In contrast, increased or continuing reliance on the PNP for management advice despite stabilization or improvement in the patient's condition could indicate dependency and a need to begin disengagement activities as a strategy to promote the FNP's autonomy and future problem-solving skills. In this case, however, a lack of knowledge and skill or increased acuity of the patient's condition would need to be ruled out as explanations for what appears to be dependency.

Sometimes, the disengagement phase needs to begin because there is evidence that success is unlikely in a particular nursing consultation relationship. This conclusion may result from either formative or summative evaluation findings. Evidence that success is unlikely in a nursing consultation relationship includes the consultee's withdrawal from problem-solving activities, unfulfilled promises of client system support for problem-solving activities, and verbalization by the consultee (or other influential parties in the client system) that the nursing consultation problem no

---

Box 12-1. When to Disengage

A nurse consultant's sense of timing is a key factor in successful disengagement. The nurse consultant needs to be alert for the following cues that indicate it is appropriate to proceed with the disengagement phase of the nursing consultation process:

Attainment of the goals of the nursing consultation relationship
Refreezing has occurred; new behaviors and problem-solving skills have become the norm for the consultee and client system
Consultee dependency
Success in the consultation relationship is unlikely even with recycling to an earlier phase
The nurse consultant is becoming enmeshed with the consultee and client system and is losing objectivity

---

longer exists. Continuing a nursing consultation relationship under these circumstances only serves to meet the needs of the nurse consultant.

The preceding point is especially important, for the nurse consultant needs to be alert for indications of becoming too enmeshed in the client system. The danger of prolonging the nursing consultation relationship in this situation is that the nurse consultant loses objectivity and, consequently, becomes less helpful in problem solving. When a nurse consultant trades empathy for emotional enmeshment with a consultee, problem solutions that are developed are less likely to take into account the needs of the client system and more likely to be developed to meet needs of the nurse consultant. Nurses who are providing consultation in emotionally charged problem situations that are similar to situations they have lived through (for example, downsizing and work redesign) are particularly at risk for becoming enmeshed with a consultee and losing their objectivity. Again, this is an indication to initiate disengagement activities and, possibly, turn the situation over to another nurse consultant.

Box 12-1 summarizes indicators of readiness to disengage.

Maintaining Change

The nurse consultant's second task in the disengagement phase is to develop strategies that will enable the client system to maintain the changes that have occurred as a result of the nursing consultation relationship. Reduced involvement, intermittent follow-up, and the development of "continuity supports" are typical change maintenance strategies that are used by nurse consultants (Lippitt & Lippitt 1986).

Reduced Involvement   Reducing involvement with the client system forces the consultee to take on more responsibility for ongoing problem solving. The nurse consultant's contact with the client system should not abruptly drop to zero, but should decrease gradually and strategically as the consultee demonstrates more skill and self-confidence. For example, a clinical nurse specialist (CNS) who has been providing consultation to a group of staff nurses might first decrease full-time involvement and presence on the nursing unit to daily "drop-in" contact. The next step might be to only attend staff meetings rather than have a predictable presence on the unit. The nurse consultant needs to keep in mind that decreasing involvement means reducing regular presence within a client system but not eliminating availability to deal with problems that may arise during the disengagement phase.

Intermittent Follow-up While disengagement requires the nurse consultant to reduce contact with a client system, this phase also involves planned intermittent follow-up or checking back with the consultee and client system. Intermittent follow-up that is initiated by the nurse consultant facilitates early discovery of possible difficulties with the problem solution that is being implemented. Intermittent follow-up, therefore, provides the nurse consultant and consultee with opportunities to salvage an action plan that is not as effective as had been anticipated. Follow-up also demonstrates the nurse consultant's continued availability for assistance with problem solving and provides the opportunity to give positive feedback. Finally, follow-up that is initiated by the nurse consultant enables a consultee to "save face" by not needing to ask for help at a time when increased capability at problem solving is supposed to be demonstrated.

Continuity Supports "Continuity supports" are situation-specific mechanisms developed and put into place to help ensure that the consultee and other members of the client system don't regress to old patterns of thinking and behaving once the nursing consultation relationship has ended. Continuity supports also help prevent the development of counter-reactions to the changes in the client system that have occurred as a result of the nursing consultation process.

Training the consultee or another influential member of the client system to be an internal consultant or "change maintainer" is one continuity support strategy. As an example of this strategy, an external nurse consultant who has been working with the nursing staff of two rival home health care agencies as they merge their services could train one or two of the nurses in group facilitation and mediation skills. This particular type of continuity support might be appropriate because communication problems, value conflicts, and power struggles are most likely to be the issues that will compromise the ability of these two former competitors to work together.

Another strategy that can be used as a continuity support is a "minimum periodic maintenance plan." A minimum periodic maintenance plan is a regular schedule of self-evaluation that is undertaken by the consultee to make sure that the performance objectives established during the nursing consultation action plan continue to be met. This continuity support strategy might be used by a CNS who has been providing consultation to a nursing unit as the unit implements critical pathways. Members of the nursing unit could be assisted to develop a chart audit process for periodically gathering, analyzing, and responding to data on effectiveness indicators such as patient lengths of stay, cost of care, and complication and readmission rates.

Yet a third continuity support strategy that can be put into place by a nurse consultant is referral of the consultee to a formal support program. This strategy is appropriate when change maintenance is likely to require ongoing external support that it is unrealistic for the nurse consultant to provide. This strategy might be used by a nurse practitioner who has been providing consultation to the spouse of a recent myocardial infarction (MI) patient in regard to facilitating lifestyle changes (such as diet, exercise, and stress reduction) that have been prescribed for the MI patient. In this case, the nurse practitioner might use referral to a cardiac rehabilitation program as a strategy for continuity support.

Managing the Psychodynamics of Disengagement

Disengagement can trigger a variety of emotions in consultees. Most commonly, disengagement triggers feelings of inadequacy and abandonment. These emotions can result in dependency behaviors, withdrawal, passivity, or increased conflict within the client system. The emotions triggered by disengagement activities and consultees' reactions to these emotions are referred to as the "psychodynamics of disengagement." The nurse consultant's third task in the disengagement phase is to manage these psychodynamics so that the consultee isn't overpowered by them to the extent that there is regression to old habits and former patterns of behavior.

The nurse consultant should inform a consultee about the anticipated timeline for disengagement. By doing so, the nurse consultant may prevent or allay some of the consultee's feelings of abandonment. A "weaning period" of gradually reduced frequency and intensity of contact between the nurse consultant and consultee can also ease these feelings. The nurse consultant can also attempt to decrease the stress of disengagement by leaving the door open for future consultation with the consultee.

The nurse consultant can respond to the feelings of inadequacy that arise in the consultees as the disengagement process gets underway by providing reassurance and evidence to consultees about their readiness to disengage. The nurse consultant can also remind consultees that proceeding with disengagement is actually a vote of confidence about their abilities to maintain the changes that have been put in place during the nursing consultation relationship.

Continuity supports that have been developed as change maintenance strategies can also be used to respond to the psychodynamics of the disengagement phase. Consider how the continuity supports described in the previous nursing consultation scenarios might also be used to help manage the psychodynamics of the disengagement phase.

In the first scenario, the nurse consultant working with the merging home health care agencies might anticipate increased inter-staff conflict once termination of the nursing consultation relationship becomes apparent. With the nurse consultant present less frequently, the competing staffs might each believe that now is their last chance for hanging on to their former ways of doing things. Staff members who have been trained in mediation skills could help the nurses respond to these reactions.

The second scenario was about a nursing unit working with an internal (CNS) nurse consultant to implement critical pathways. This client system might respond to disengagement with passive resistance and might perceive decreased contact with the nurse consultant as an opportunity to regress to the former way of delivering care on the nursing unit. Periodic self-evaluation and feedback in the form of chart audits, however, could serve to hold the nurses accountable for the patient care outcomes intended by the critical pathways.

The spouse of the MI patient in the last scenario could be expected to feel overwhelmed and abandoned as termination of the consultation relationship with the nurse practitioner becomes apparent. The nurse practitioner could manage these emotional reactions by acknowledging their validity. In addition, providing evidence of goal accomplishment (for example, weight loss or lowered blood pressure in the patient) could help to replace feelings of inadequacy with feelings of accomplishment and self-confidence.

Achieving Closure

The nurse consultant's final task in the disengagement phase is to achieve closure of the nursing consultation relationship. Achieving closure acknowledges both the problem solving that has occurred and the interpersonal relationships that have developed during the course of the consultation process. Closure activities require a degree of intentionality so that both the nurse consultant and the consultee have a sense of satisfaction and pride about what they have accomplished and how it has taken place. Numerous strategies and rituals can be used to facilitate closure, the scope of these activities being limited only by the creativity of the nurse consultant. Closure activities must also be sensitive to the culture of the client system.

The final consultation report is one strategy that can be used to formally signal the transfer of responsibility for maintaining change and ongoing problem solving to the

> ## Box 12-2. Strategies for Successful Disengagement
>
> Know when it is time to leave
>
> Provide warning that termination is forthcoming; be specific about when, why, and how it will be done
>
> Explain what has happened as a result of the nursing consultation relationship; consider goals that have been met as well as other changes in the culture and climate of the client system that have occurred
>
> Recognize members and processes of the client system that have been especially helpful; be generous with thank-yous
>
> Share recommendations for reinforcing the changes that have occurred
>
> Celebrate successes
>
> Always leave the door open for future contact

consultee. A final report generally includes an overview of what has occurred and been accomplished during the consultation process, acknowledgment of persons and processes that have contributed to success, and the nurse consultant's thoughts about what the future holds and issues that need ongoing attention. A final "closure report" typically ends with a thank-you for the consultation opportunity and an offer to be of future assistance. In nurse practitioner consultation relationships, the final report is often shared only verbally with the consultee. In other consultation situations, a written final report is provided to the consultee and other appropriate members of the client system.

Other termination strategies can be more symbolic indicators of the completion of a change process—a celebration, a mock funeral, ceremonially discarding of old equipment, and so forth. Consider how these types of closure strategies might be incorporated into the disengagement phase of the nursing consultation scenarios used earlier in this chapter.

In the home health care agency merger scenario, closure could involve an open house of the facility, introduction of a new logo, and new equipment bags for staff, as well as a final report.

The CNS who has worked with the nursing unit to implement critical pathways could stage a closure celebration that includes shredding old chart forms and opening packages of new forms.

The nurse practitioner who has been providing consultation to the spouse of the MI patient could present the consultee with a "graduation" certificate to the cardiac rehabilitation program.

Strategies for successful disengagement are summarized in Box 12-2.

Possible Difficulties in Disengagement

As is the case with the other phases of the nursing consultation process, difficulties can arise during disengagement. These difficulties, if not resolved, can undermine successful disengagement. Timing issues and role-related dilemmas are two potential threats to successful disengagement. Another difficulty the nurse consultant may need to face is that of completing the disengagement phase when the nursing consultation relationship has been unsuccessful.

Timing

Even the most carefully planned disengagement phase can end up being ineffective if it is carried out too soon or not soon enough. All too often, disengagement activities are premature. Ending a nursing consultation relationship is sometimes seen by either the nurse consultant or consultee as the best or easiest way out of a consultation relationship or project that is not progressing as anticipated. In other situations, starting disengagement too soon reflects a desire by either the nurse consultant or the consultee to "bail out" when the going is getting rough and the consultation relationship is becoming characterized by conflict and confrontation. Nurse consultants who are working with consultees about process issues (communication patterns, power, values, interpersonal dynamics, and so forth) are at particular risk for beginning disengagement activities too soon or carrying them out over too short a period of time. At the same time, consultees in these situations can pressure a nurse consultant to disengage before readiness is actually present.

Terminating a nursing consultation relationship too soon can have negative consequences for both the nurse consultant and the consultee. When disengagement occurs too soon or is rushed, the consultee is at risk for regressing to old patterns of behavior. When this occurs, everything that has been accomplished during the nursing consultation relationship can become undone. Once the nurse consultant leaves the client system, it is easy for the consultee to blame the nurse consultant for this "failure." When a consultee returns to business as usual with a current consultation problem unresolved, more problems are likely to follow because the consultee has probably not incorporated problem-solving skills into daily behavior patterns (Kurpius et al. 1993).

Sometimes, disengagement does not begin soon enough or is stretched out over too long a period of time. Dependency needs on the part of either the nurse consultant or consultee are usually the forces behind this situation. For the nurse consultant, there is somewhat of a conflict of interest in disengagement because ending a consultation relationship means ending any consultation-related fees or benefits. Delaying disengagement then, can reflect financial as well as psychological dependency needs. A nurse who is working as an internal consultant might be tempted to delay disengagement in order to prolong possible benefits such as better work hours, prestige, and avoidance of regular work responsibilities.

A key question to ask in regard to the timing of disengagement is whose and what needs are being met by the push to disengage or delay disengagement. In other words, is the timing of disengagement activities optimum for ultimate success of the nursing consultation relationship or does it reflect other issues and other needs?

Role-Related Dilemmas

Some difficulties that arise during the disengagement phase reflect the uniqueness of each nursing consultation situation as well as how a nurse has been enacting the consultant role.

For an external nurse consultant, disengagement and termination might be misinterpreted by the consultee as meaning that the nurse consultant is no longer available to provide help with problems. Unless this is the message the nurse consultant intends, care must be taken that this is not the message that is inadvertently conveyed. Another difficulty frequently faced by external nurse consultants is a lack of any opportunity to see the long-term consequences of their efforts. To some extent, this is simply inherent in the nature of any consultation relationship. However, formal post-termination follow-up can be built into both evaluation and disengagement plans. Also, less formal follow-up opportunities are generally present through networking, mutual acquaintances, and professional activities.

Box 12-3. Relationship Review: The Disengagement Phase in Unsuccessful Nursing Consultation Relationships

The focus of a relationship review is figuring out the reason for the unsuccessful consultation relationship by systematically reviewing what happened during each phase of the nursing consultation process. The following questions should be asked:

Were the right conditions in place for the nursing consultation interaction pattern that was used?

Were the implicit expectations of the nursing consultation relationship made explicit in the contract?

Were the tasks of each phase in the nursing consultation process carried out completely?

Was there an effective working relationship between the nurse consultant, the consultee, and other members of the client system? That is, had the nurse consultant achieved psychological entry into the client system?

Were there quality data on which to base both conclusions about a problem's cause and feasible solutions?

Was the problem definition accurate and owned by the consultee?

How ready and willing was the consultee and client system to problem solve and change?

Were the system supports needed for change in place?

Were the consultation goals and action plan jointly developed by the nurse consultant and consultee? Were the goals and action plan owned by the consultee? Were proposed goals meaningful and feasible for the client system?

Did evaluation occur on an ongoing basis? Were the results used?

The nurse who has been functioning as an internal consultant generally has the opportunity to observe the outcomes of the nursing consultation relationship; the tradeoff is that there is no real opportunity (other than quitting!) to exit the client system. This can create the dilemma of being perceived as continuously available for troubleshooting, problem solving, and giving advice. Initially, this may be somewhat flattering. Constant availability for problem solving, though, can foster dependency in both the nurse consultant and the client system. It can also create role conflicts and place substantial and generally uncompensated demands on the nurse consultant's time if it goes unchecked. Parameters of post-consultation availability need to be made explicit in the nursing consultation contract.

Nurse practitioners who provide consultation to patient groups or families need to be aware that disengagement and termination can be perceived as abandonment by the consultee and client. While disengagement activities should always be mutually planned and agreed on, it is especially critical that nurse practitioners communicate to their consultees and clients that it is only a specific problem-solving relationship, not the entire practitioner-patient or care-provider relationship, that is the focus of disengagement. Completely terminating a care-provider relationship with a patient involves its own specific and legally prescribed set of disengagement activities.

Box 12-4. Documentation Checklist: The Disengagement Phase

Evidence of readiness to disengage—about identity specific indicators, as well
    as who initiated disengagement
Anticipated timeline for the disengagement phase
Pattern of reduced involvement—describe, give rationale, document consultee
    reaction to this decision as well as reactions to subsequent interactions
Intermittent follow-up activities—date, purpose, who initiated, what occurred
Continuity supports—describe, give rationale
Psychodynamics that occurred during disengagement—how they were
    responded to, results of nurse consultant's response
Closure activities—date, describe activity and response, attach copy of final
    consultation report
Difficulties encountered—how they were addressed, whether they were resolved

---

Disengagement in Unsuccessful Nursing Consultation Relationships

Unfortunately, not all nursing consultation relationships are successful in terms of
resolving the consultee's presenting problem. A disengagement phase still needs to
occur in unsuccessful situations, but the disengagement task of "maintaining change"
is replaced by the task of "relationship review." In other words, the focus of disengagement in an unsuccessful nursing consultation relationship is determining what
went wrong in the relationship.

To accomplish a relationship review, the nurse consultant and consultee should
together review what happened during each phase of the nursing consultation
process. Sometimes what is discovered is that elements from each phase of the consultation process contributed to the "failure" by having an additive effect. It is more
likely, though, that some of the foundational conditions for a successful consultation
relationship were missing. Box 12-3 presents questions the nurse consultant can use to
guide the disengagement phase in an unsuccessful nursing consultation relationship.

There is a tendency by both the nurse consultant and consultee to want to rush disengagement activities when the nursing consultation relationship has been unsuccessful. This reflects a cultural tendency to overvalue success and undervalue failure.
Rushing through the disengagement phase of an unsuccessful nursing consultation
relationship ignores that learning can occur in both positive and negative situations.
What is learned from an unsuccessful consultation relationship can be used by the
nurse consultant to increase the likelihood of success in future relationships.

Documenting the Disengagement Phase

Because the nursing consultation relationship essentially ends once the tasks of the
disengagement phase have been completed, it is tempting to overlook documentation
responsibilities for this phase of the consultation process. However, documentation is
as important in the disengagement phase as it is in earlier phases of the nursing consultation process, for what it can provide the nurse consultant in terms of reminders
(what has been done and what needs to be done next) and a learning device (what
works and what doesn't). In addition, documentation can provide the nurse consul-

tant with evidence to counter possible charges of premature or delayed closure of the consultation relationship or charges of abandonment. Box 12-4 is a checklist for documenting the disengagement phase of the nursing consultation process.

Chapter Summary

The disengagement phase of the nursing consultation process is a time of letting go and an opportunity for both the nurse consultant and consultee to celebrate success, acknowledge the problem-solving skills and relationships that have developed, secure the future, and learn from mistakes.

While the onset of the activities of the disengagement phase usually coincides with the presentation of findings from the summative evaluation of the nursing consultation process, the groundwork for disengagement is laid much earlier. The specific tasks of the disengagement phase—identifying readiness to disengage, developing strategies to maintain change, managing the psychodynamics of disengagement, and achieving closure—are intended to prevent dependency and ensure the continuity of changes and problem solving that have occurred. In an unsuccessful nursing consultation relationship, completion of the disengagement phase can provide the nurse consultant and the consultee with insight about what needed conditions of a successful consulting relationship were lacking. When disengagement is thoughtfully planned and carefully implemented, both the nurse consultant and consultee should leave the consultation relationship with a sense of satisfaction about what has been accomplished.

Applying Chapter Content

Refer to the article by Badger (1988) that is listed as an additional reading. How was disengagement carried out in this case study? How would you have done it differently?

Develop a checklist of skills and outcome criteria needed for successful disengagement for a consultation scenario that is typical of those in which you are most likely to be involved. Compare your list to those developed by students in other practice roles. Which skills and effectiveness criteria seem to be universal and which seem to be role specific? How can you explain these differences?

References

Barron, A. (1989). The CNS as consultant. In A. Hamric & J. Spross (Eds.), *The clinical nurse specialist in theory and practice* (2nd ed., pp. 125-146). Philadelphia: Saunders.

Kurpius, D., Fuqua, D., & Rozecki, T. (1993). The consulting process: A multidimensional approach. *Journal of Counseling and Development, 71*, 601-606.

Lippitt, G., & Lippitt, R. (1986). *The consulting process in action* (2nd ed.). San Diego: University Associates.

Monicken, D. (1995). Consultation in advanced practice nursing. In M. Snyder & M. Mirr (Eds.), *Advanced practice nursing: A guide to professional development* (pp. 183-195). New York: Springer Publishing.

Ross, G. (1993). Peter Block's *Flawless Consulting* and the Homunculus Theory: Within each person is a perfect consultant. *Journal of Counseling & Development, 71,* 639-641.

Schein, E. (1987). *Process consultation, volume II: Lessons for managers and consultants.* Reading, MA: Addison-Wesley.

Additional Readings

Badger, T. (1988). Mental health consultation with a surgical unit nursing staff. *Clinical Nurse Specialist, 2* (3), 144-148.
  The author illustrates the nursing consultation process through an internal consultation scenario.
 Dougherty, A. (1995). *Consultation: Practice and perspectives in school and community settings.* Pacific Grove, CA: Brooks-Cole.
  Chapter 6 of this text discusses activities that take place during the disengagement phase.
Schein, E. (1988). *Process consultation, volume I: Its role in organization development* (2nd ed.). Reading, MA: Addison-Wesley.
  Chapter 16 reviews disengagement strategies.
Ulschak, F., & SnowAntle, S. (1990). *Consultation skills for health care professionals.* San Francisco: Jossey-Bass.
  In Chapter 3 of this text, the authors discuss disengagement in internal consultation situations.

Market Segmentation and Analysis

Market segmentation is the process of dividing the market (all potential consultees) into groups or "niches" with shared characteristics (Lachmann 1996). For example, the potential market of all primary care providers might be segmented as follows: solo practices, group practices, urban versus rural practices, practices that offer versus those that do not offer obstetrical care, and so on. These groups are then analyzed in terms of their current and future needs. The following are questions a nurse consultant can use to direct the market segmentation and analysis process.

- Who are my intended consultees? What group am I most interested in working with?

- What needs does this group have or are they likely to have?

- What does this group buy (for example, education, support services, trouble-shooting)?

- When do they buy? That is, are they reactive or proactive? (Franck 1991)

This list of groups and their needs is then compared to the nurse consultant's proposed services. If a nurse consultant's proposed services are a good fit with the market niche of interest, there is an increased likelihood of service and business viability. On the other hand, if there is a poor fit between proposed services and preferred market niche, the nurse consultant can either change "product" characteristics to better meet the needs of the preferred market niche or target a different market niche whose needs are more compatible with the proposed services. Market segmentation and analysis, therefore, helps a nurse consultant identify to whom to promote proposed consultation services. Examples of niche marketing by nurse consultants include offering team-building services to organizations that are undergoing restructuring, providing medication and symptom management consultation services to families of individuals with schizophrenia, and providing research development consultation services to primary care providers.

Product Promotion

The third principle of the marketing process is product promotion. In nursing consultation, product promotion includes all of the activities the nurse consultant undertakes to inform the target market or niche about the availability of services (Longworth & DiNardo 1995). Product promotion includes personal selling, advertising, and all types of publicity. The goal of a nurse consultant's promotional activities is gaining recognition and having an image and reputation that attracts referrals and is known for producing results (Lachmann 1996). Promotion strategies can be either direct or indirect.

Direct Promotion Strategies Direct promotion is analogous to advertising. Nurse consultants engage in direct promotion when they directly approach a potential consultee and inform them about one's consultation services. Direct promotion can involve face to face appointments ("cold calls"), telephone solicitation, and mailings. Occasionally, a consultant will host an informational meeting (usually with a meal) for a group of consultees (Lippitt & Lippitt 1986; Metzger 1993). However, because the time involved in hosting meetings is not income-generating and because relatively few potential consultees can be reached at any one meeting, most consultants use *targeted* mailings as their primary direct promotion strategy. Mass mailings are generally avoided because of their low cost/benefit ratio; a mass mailing to 10,000 potential consultees will most likely yield only 200 inquiries and only one contract

(Lewin 1995). Consultants tend to rely on the following four types of printed materials for direct promotion: announcements of services, brochures, a consulting vita, and capability statements.

An announcement of services (Figure 13-1) is generally sent to potential consultees at the time the nurse consultant first establishes services, moves services from one location to another, or changes the focus of offered services. The announcement is in the form of a letter that defines the nurse consultant's overall objective and describes typical situations for which the consultant's services are appropriate. The announcement should be printed on good quality letterhead stationery, addressed to the specific potential consultee, and personally signed by the nurse consultant. The nurse consultant should enclose a professionally produced business card or telephone index card with the announcement of services. Art departments of local colleges are often a good source of reasonably priced help for designing a letterhead and logo.

An announcement of services is frequently accompanied by a brochure, consulting vita, or capability statement. A brochure (Figure 13-2) should include a brief statement about the nature of the consultation services being offered, the consultant's background and experience, and a description of how assignments are conducted (Lewin 1995). An effective brochure is characterized by a professional layout and attention to readability. A brochure needs to make a potential consultee aware of the services being offered in 3 seconds of reading time or less if it is to be given any attention (Lewin 1995).

A consulting vita (Figure 13-3) highlights the nurse consultant's experiences and qualifications that directly support or demonstrate the ability to offer the advertised consultation services. The goal of a consulting vita is to concisely convey a nurse consultant's credibility (Metzger 1993). Most consulting vitae also list a "few other interesting things" (hobbies, for instance) about the nurse consultant in an attempt to demonstrate balance and establish identity with potential consultees (Lewin 1995).

A capability statement (Figure 13-4) is the fourth type of promotional material that nurse consultants find useful. A capability statement lists the specific skills and abilities that undergird or are a part of a nurse consultant's services. The intent of a capability statement is to give potential consultees ideas about the specific tasks and types of problem solutions the nurse consultant is capable of implementing.

Announcements of services and capability statements can be adapted into advertisements for placement in business and professional journals or for publication in telephone directories. The intent of all these direct promotion activities is to create a "mental hook" so that when a potential consultee has a need for specific services, an immediate picture is formed of who should be contacted to provide those services.

Indirect Promotion Strategies   The focus of indirect promotion is to gain the recognition of those who are in a position to help one's career as a nurse consultant. Indirect promotion activities increase one's visibility and educate specific as well as more general audiences about one's nursing consultation services. Speaking engagements, publishing, professional memberships, and volunteerism are common indirect promotion activities.

Public speaking offers nurse consultants an opportunity to get their name and face and credentials in front of a lot of potential consultees in a short period of time. Whether the investment of the time spent in public speaking has a long-term payoff, however, depends on who is in the audience (administrators or staff nurses, for example). A nurse consultant can also gain visibility by becoming a spokesperson about topics within their own area of expertise for local radio and television stations.

Publishing gives a nurse consultant an opportunity to build a reputation and establish credentials as an expert. Publishing establishes name recognition and can bolster

Perinatal Solutions, Inc.
Nursing Consultation Services
Partners for promoting healthy mothers, babies,
families, and communities

Leslie Norton, RNC, MSN
12703 125th Avenue, SE
Bellevue, WA 98772

Phone: (208) 546-9808
FAX: (208) 546-9888
email: peri.1342.aol.com

Dr. Sandra Davison
Director of Obstetrical Services
Mercy Medical Center
1720 NW Mountain Blvd.
Bellevue, WA 98605

January 15, 1999

Dear Dr. Davison,

I have recently established a consulting practice to share my twenty years of experience in obstetrical nursing and ambulatory health care. My primary objective is to help care providers meet the challenge of providing safe and cost-effective family-centered obstetrical care in today's health care environment of managed care, higher risk clients, and increasing malpractice costs. The strength of my practice is the breadth and depth of my experience, my extensive knowledge of both obstetrics and health care systems, as well as my creativity and passion for my work. Below are a few of the situations in which my services are most likely to be useful.

• Facility design or redesign (inpatient or outpatient) to enhance productivity while maintaining safe, family-centered care

• Developing perinatal and obstetrical care programs (protocols, fees schedules, and so forth) for non-obstetrical providers such as family practice physicians, home health care agencies, and community-based clinics

• Staff development—inpatient cross-training, perinatal home care services

• Market research regarding the need for services or satisfaction with services

• Development of documentation and evaluation systems

• Expert testimony

Should you learn of or encounter any situations in which my services may be of help, please call. All consultations are strictly confidential and a preliminary meeting is free of charge or further obligation. I have enclosed a telephone index card for your convenience.

Sincerely,

Leslie Norton

Leslie Norton, RNC, MSN

Figure 13-1. Sample Announcement of Nursing Consultation Services
An announcement of services is used to notify potential consultees of new, relocated, or revised consultation services.

WHAT WE DO...

We sit down and work with you to clearly envision your future.

We gather information on what changes you would like to see take place. We work with you to identify causes of current problems or reasons for making a proactive change in services. We also identify your internal resources, the harnessing of which will reduce your costs and enable you to maintain any implemented changes.

We include you in the problem-solving process.

We recognize that *you* are the expert about what will and will not work in your system. We rely on your input and insight to help us develop problem solutions that will be meaningful, feasible, culturally sensitive, and long-lasting.

We do the legwork and negotiation.

Often, change and problem solving involves negotiating and working with other parties such as insurance providers, other care provider systems, equipment vendors, and the legislative/political system. We will contact these people on your behalf and introduce you to key players. We want to facilitate change for you and enable you to maintain the change on a long-term basis.

We empower you!

Our role is to facilitate change and ensure that change is long-lasting. We recognize that change will be long-lasting only when you can maintain it after we leave. To this end, we provide you with the training and support needed to manage change on an ongoing basis. We will also work with you to develop system supports such as policies, protocols, and reward (salary and benefit) structures.

We won't leave you high and dry.

Too often, consultants end up abandoning consultees at the end of a contract. We are always available for follow-up, support, and troubleshooting.

WHO WE ARE...

Perinatal Solutions, Inc. was founded to help health care providers meet the challenges of providing safe and cost-effective family-centered obstetrical care in today's rapidly changing— and challenging — health care environment. Our goal is to promote the health of mothers, babies, families, communities, and society. We are a group of expert perinatal nurses who have combined our extensive and varied experiences into a system that helps providers solve a range of problems and plan for the future as an obstetrical care provider. Our services include the following:

- Inpatient or outpatient facility design or redesign
- Program development, including perinatal curriculum for educational systems
- Staff development
- Market research
- Development of quality assurance programs
- Expert testimony

Perinatal Solutions, Inc. was founded by Leslie Norton, RNC, MSN. Ms. Norton has more than 10 years experience as a consultant and over 20 years experience in perinatal nursing. She is also a Women's Health Care Nurse Practitioner. Ms. Norton holds courtesy faculty appointments in both the School of Business and the College of Health Professions at Northwest Washington University.

Ms. Norton is a member of a variety of professional and civic organizations and is certified by the Association of Health Care Consultants and the American Nurses' Credentialing Center. In her spare time, she designs quilts and raises Labrador retrievers.

Perinatal Solutions, Inc.
Nursing Consultation Services
Partners for promoting healthy mothers, babies, families, and communities

12703 125th Avenue, SE
Bellevue, WA 98772

Phone: (208) 546-9808
Fax: (208) 546-9888
email: peri.1342.aol.com

Figure 13-2. Sample Brochure for Nursing Consultation Services
A brochure needs to be professional and readable. It needs to make a potential consultee aware of the sevices being offered within 3 seconds of reading.

Leslie Norton, RNC, MSN
Founder and President
Perinatal Solutions, Inc.

Leslie Norton is founder and President of Perinatal Solutions, Inc., a local consulting firm that has served the health care industry throughout the Northwest for more than 10 years. Ms. Norton has worked with hospitals, HMOs, home health care agencies, and private care providers to develop creative ways of delivering perinatal services in today's changing health care environment.

Ms. Norton is a member of the faculty of Northwest Washington University where she holds courtesy appointments in the School of Business and the College of Health Professions. She teaches courses in nursing consultation, marketing, health care policy, and evaluation research.

Ms. Norton began her career in health care as a registered nurse working in the labor and delivery unity of a Level 3 medical center. Her area of study for her MSN was Parent-Child Nursing. She has also worked in home health care and is a women's health care nurse practitioner. She regularly conducts research in health promotion during high risk pregnancies.

Ms. Norton is a member of the National Academy of Nurse Consultants, the Association of Home Health Care Nurses, and the Association of Perinatal and Women's Health Care Nurse Practitioners. She holds specialty certifications from the Association of Health Care Consultants and the American Nurses' Credentialing Center.

Perinatal Solutions, Inc.
Nursing Consultation Services
Partners for promoting healthy mothers, babies,
families, and communities

12703 125th Avenue, SE
Bellevue, WA 98772

Phone: (208) 546-9808
Fax: (208) 546-9888
email: peri.1342.aol.com

Figure 13-3. Sample Consulting Vita
In contrast to a traditional academic curriculum vita, the consulting vita focuses only on experiences and qualifications that directly support the consultation services that are being promoted.

Capabilities of Leslie Norton, RNC, MSN, Founder and President of Perinatal Solutions, Inc. as a nurse consultant for high-risk obstetrics home health care services

- Conduct community assessments to determine the need for and feasibility of services

- Develop a marketing plan, including promotional brochures for services; this plan can be targeted to specific market segments such as physicians, hospitals, or consumers

- Develop protocols and standards of care for common high risk obstetrical conditions

- Provide staff training and competency validation in regard to nursing knowledge and skills needed for effective delivery of high risk obstetrical home health care services; this can be delivered in traditional or self-study formats

- Develop billing guidelines for services

- Identify equipment needs and purchasing options

- Assist with recruiting and interviewing for staff positions for high risk obstetrical home health care services

- Develop risk management programs

- Work with staff to develop and implement an ongoing quality assurance program

- Conduct program evaluations, including cost-effectiveness and satisfaction

- Serve as a clinical consultant to nursing staff and physicians in regard to problematic cases

Perinatal Solutions, Inc.
Nursing Consultation Services

Partners for promoting healthy mothers, babies,
families, and communities

12703 125th Avenue, SE
Bellevue, WA 98772

Phone: (208) 546-9808
Fax: (208) 546-9888
email: peri.1342.aol.com

Figure 13-4. Sample Capability Statement

A capability statement is a task-oriented listing of skills that informs a potential consultee about the nature of problem solutions a nurse consultant is qualified to implement.

market clout, generate consultation inquiries, and prompt invitations to speak at meeting and conferences. In addition to seeking publication opportunities in professional journals, a nurse consultant might also explore publishing in the lay press or writing a regular newspaper column.

Attending professional meetings gives a nurse consultant the opportunity to network with colleagues. Volunteering, serving on community boards, and sponsoring selected community activities are other strategies a nurse consultant might use to gain name recognition. Finally, nurse consultants need to keep in mind that attention to personal presentation, maintaining professionalism in dealing with others, and the quality of their business cards, brochures, and stationery are ways of creating a professional image and enhancing one's reputation.

To a certain extent, the amount of time a nurse consultant spends on promotional activities limits the amount of time that is available to carry out income-generating consultation activities. A challenge for nurse consultants, then, is to maintain a balance between conducting business and creating new business opportunities. A one-to-four or two-to-three rule is used by many consultants to maintain this balance. More specifically, one or two days are spent on promotional activities for every three or four days of billable work (Lewin 1995; Metzger 1993).

Promotion Strategies for Internal Nurse Consultants Nurses who work as internal consultants also need to engage in activities that will enhance their visibility and credibility as a nurse consultant. This is particularly important when the nurse consultant or consultant role is new to the client system.

Internal nurse consultants can begin the marketing process by meeting with the key people in the client system (for example, nursing staff and administrators in a hospital) to identify their service needs. These meetings also give the nurse consultant an opportunity to describe and garner support for the consulting role. These activities can help prevent two common causes of failure of the internal nurse consultant role: unrealistic expectations of staff or a distorted view of consultation (Barron 1989).

Members of a client system can also be educated about the nurse consultant role through brochures and announcements like those an external nurse consultant would use. Consultation referral forms and telephone index cards are additional strategies an internal nurse consultant can use to increase name and service recognition.

Money Issues in Nursing Consultation

Typically, nurses have not been paid fees that are linked directly to the services they provide and are unaccustomed to charging others for their acquired skills, time, and talent. As a result, nurses who are establishing themselves as nurse consultants frequently find establishing and collecting fees to be a difficult task. However, the fees a nurse establishes for consulting services can have implications for the marketability of these services; fees that are too low unintentionally discredit oneself and one's services, whereas fees that are too high can price oneself out of business. In addition, as discussed in Chapter 14, issues related to fees and their collection can be a cause of legal action against a nurse consultant. The challenge of establishing and collecting fees for nursing consultation services, therefore, is to balance self-interest, guilt, and other factors with consultee and client needs for one's services (Lanza 1996).

Setting Fees: Guidelines and Options

The true value of one's work as a nurse consultant reflects both beliefs about the worth of one's time and skills and what the market will bear (Metzger 1993). A reasonable starting place for establishing fees is to find out the going rate. This information can be obtained from other consultants, individuals or organizations that have recently used consultation services, and employment advertisements. If employment ads are used as a source of information, the fees or salary they quote needs to be adjusted (if one is practicing as an independent nurse consultant) to account for the costs of overhead and benefits (Finnigan 1996). Typically, hourly fees or salaries cited for employment by a consulting agency are lower than what an independent nurse consultant would charge because benefits (insurance, vacation, and so forth) are also received as part of an employment package.

Fees also need to take into consideration the actual cost of offering one's services, needed or desired income, and hours available for generating that income. Finally, the fees one can realistically establish for nursing consultation services are affected by the laws of supply and demand. That is, the value of one's nursing consultation services will decrease if the same service is also being offered by others (Finnigan 1996). Consequently, nurse consultants must carefully differentiate their services and be aware of their competition as well as what the market will bear. Box 13-1 presents several common formulas for establishing consultation fees.

Many nurse consultants will vary their fees according to the nature of a consultation contract (for example, whether the contract is for a few hours, a day, or an extended period of time). It is often helpful to get some sense of the nature and scope of a nursing consultation project before citing a definite fee. If a nurse consultant is pressed for a fee at the initial meeting with a consultee, it is often best to quote a range of fees with the explanation that actual fees depend on the circumstances. Other consultants suggest quoting a flat daily rate that can then be broken down by the hour (Schein 1987). Most consultants identify a minimum billing time and bill in increments of an hour (for example, "Fees are calculated in 15 minute increments; minimum billing time is 4 hours"). Some consultants also state a project maximum (for example, "Fees will be calculated at the rate of $150 per hour, not to exceed $7500 for the project").

In general, consultants bill for all preparation time as well as actual contact time with a consultee. Travel within a reasonable distance to a consultation workplace is usually not billed. Some consultants will charge more for making a presentation (such as an in-service education offering) than they will for activities such as reviewing documents and attending meetings to help a consultee with process and communication issues (Schein 1987).

As discussed in Chapter 8 ("The Gaining Entry Phase"), consultants differ in terms of whether or not they charge for an exploratory meeting with a consultee or organization contact person. Some consultants advocate treating an initial meeting as a marketing strategy and a cost of doing business (Frings 1991). Other consultants routinely charge for an initial meeting because they have found that often enough advice is shared with a consultee during an initial meeting so that no further intervention is needed (Schein 1987). If a nurse consultant decides to charge for an initial meeting, the amount needs to be agreed upon in advance rather than arbitrarily decided on by the nurse consultant after the meeting has taken place.

Just as nurse consultants may vary their fees with the nature of the nursing consultation contract, they may also vary them for different consultees. Nurse consultants must keep in mind, however, that discounting their work without valid reason in a manner that is inconsistent from consultee to consultee demeans their work (Frings 1991). In the case of a truly needy consultee who cannot afford the nurse consultant's usual fees, nurse consultants will often accept or offer a contract for intangible payoffs such as the opportunity to gain or practice skills, work with a certain individual or

Box 13-1. Establishing Fees for Nursing Consultation Services

Several simple formulas exist for helping nurse consultants (and other entrepreneurs) establish fees for their services.

Option #1:
1. Identify base salary desired
2. Divide this by 2000 hours to get hourly rate
3. To this number add 100% for overhead* and 100% of salary rate for profit ("take home" pay)

Option #2:
1. Look at the fixed plus variable expenses in your business plan
2. Add profit desired ("take home" pay)
3. Divide by expected billable time** to get service price

Option #3:
1. Establish income goal
2. Add what is needed (by you personally) for benefits (includes vacation, sick leave, insurance, and so forth)
3. Add overhead* from business plan
4. Add desired percent for profit
5. Divide by billable hours**

Option #4:
1. Calculate days or hours available for consulting per year—Full-time = 22 working days per month x 8 hours/day = 176 billable hours per month
2. Subtract ⅓ of these hours (176 x .33 = 58) for new business development plus 1 day per week for administrative time (32 hours per month)
3. Adjusted billable hours per month = 176-58-32 = 86
4. Divide #3 into income desired from consultation hours = hourly fee
5. To this add 40% to cover operating expenses

* Most experts say "double the overhead." That is, in calculations for overhead enter double what was already calculated in your business plan.
** Billable hours = hours available for consultation activities

References: Finnigan, S. (1996). Getting started in business: From fantasy to reality. *Advanced Practice Nursing Quarterly, 2* (1), 1-8; Lewin, M. (1995). *The overnight consultant.* New York: John Wiley & Sons; and Metzger, R. (1993). *Developing a consulting practice.* Newbury Park: Sage.

group, or get a foot in the door for other possible paying opportunities. Some nurse consultants will reduce their fees for a needy consultee in exchange for having the client system be responsible for completion of specific tasks such as taking notes of meetings and making logistical arrangements for training sessions. Nurse consultants need to remember, however, that in the eyes of many potential consultees, a nurse consultant's worth is determined by cost (Frings 1991). While a modest amount of discounted or free work can bring excellent results, too much can drive a nurse consultant out of business (Franck 1995).

Because nurses who are working as internal consultants are usually engaged in consultation projects during their regular work hours, they are usually more time- than money-conscious. For internal nurse consultants, involvement in a consultation project typically occurs in lieu of other work tasks. Internal nurse consultants do, however, need to be clear about the resources (time, personnel, equipment, and so forth) they will need in order to complete a project. If time in addition to regular work hours will be needed for a project, the nurse consultant should arrange for compensatory time or for these additional hours to be paid at their regular rate of pay or as overtime.

Collection Issues

The use of inappropriate methods to collect fees is a frequent reason for legal action against consultants (this is discussed in Chapter 14). Regardless of how a nurse consultant decides to handle fees and billing and collection procedures, expectations should be discussed in advance with the consultee or contact person. Fees and collection issues must also be spelled out in the nursing consultation contract.

Most consultants bill a consultee as soon as the contracted service has been completed (Finnigan 1996; Metzger 1993). The bill should restate the fees and payment terms that were agreed to in the nursing consultation contract (for example, "Terms: net 30 days"). Receiving payment for nursing consultation services is facilitated by getting to know the client system's payment processes such as the need for a purchase order, payment cycle, and who is responsible for paying the bills. Detailing exactly what is being billed (time, travel, other reimbursable expenses) tends to prevent the client system's questioning of the charges (Box 13-2 identifies expenses that are usually billed to consultees). Many consultants find that their bill is less likely to be challenged if they present it in person and accompany it with a progress report (Lewin 1995).

A nurse consultant who is going to be working with a consultee over a prolonged period of time may want to get the consultee to agree to a monthly itemized bill for "progress payments" (Metzger 1993). A bill for a progress payment usually incorporates charges for supplies as well as the nurse consultant's time. Nurse consultants who are working with a particular consultee or client system for the first time will sometimes ask for start-up supply costs as well as a down payment ($\frac{1}{3}$ to $\frac{1}{2}$ of the estimated total) on the actual nursing consultation fees as evidence of "good faith" (Metzger 1993; Tepper 1985).

Contracts for Nursing Consultation Services

The process of contracting in nursing consultation is discussed in Chapter 8. The focus of the discussion in this section is the components of formal contracts and the ways in which consultation contracts can be structured.

From a legal perspective, a contract is formed every time two parties come together and enter into an arrangement that involves (1) an offer (that is, for a specific consultation service), (2) acceptance of the offer, and (3) consideration (Remley 1993). "Consideration" refers to something of value that is given in exchange for service. In external nursing consultation situations, consideration is usually money, but can also be intangibles such as access to information or people. In internal nursing consultation situations, consideration is more likely to consist of intangibles such as release from usual duties, an office, travel, and so forth. Without consideration, or the exchange of something of value, a contract does not exist. However, nurse consultants need to realize that they have a legal contractual obligation even in many circumstances in which they are not being paid. In nursing consultation, a contract can be offered by either the nurse consultant or the consultee.

Box 13-2. Charging for Expenses

Expenses that are incurred while completing a consultation project are generally charged back to the consultee or client system. The following expenses should be itemized on the billing statement:

- Long-distance telephone calls to or on behalf of the consultee
- Printing and copying costs
- Overnight mail (not ordinary postage) charges
- Materials—binders, folders, and so forth (but not paper as this is covered in copying costs)
- Parking
- Airplane or public transportation costs
- Hotel and meal expenses
- Travel—50% of hourly rate plus mileage at current rates (local travel is generally not billed)
- Books, software, and so forth; purchased for the consultee or as needed to complete the project, as preapproved
- Training needed to complete an assignment, as preapproved. If training is one-time and essential for a project, the consultee is usually charged 100% of incurred costs. If training can be applied to future consultation situations, the consultee is usually charged 50%

Reference: Lewin, M. (1995). *The overnight consultant*. New York: John Wiley & Sons.

Contracts do not necessarily have to be in writing. In most cases, any time a verbal offer is made and accepted and consideration exists, there is a legal contract. In some states, common law requires that contracts that transfer property (money) must be in writing (Remley 1993). Nurse consultants will want to check their state statutes regarding contract issues.

Nurses who are working as internal consultants should be aware that a legally enforceable contract *does not* exist when an individual in an organization agrees to provide nursing consultation services to a consultee within the same organization (Remley 1993). Because all parties involved are paid by the same employer, consideration does not exist within an in-house consultation situation. However, a contract *does* exist in the practical sense of the word—there is an offer and its acceptance—and fulfillment of the contract can have implications for an internal nurse consultant's performance evaluation and salary adjustments. Consequently, in internal nursing consultation situations, a written statement of understanding should be developed and signed by the parties involved.

Why Contract?

A formal contract represents agreement between the nurse consultant and consultee on key issues such as fees and their collection and goals for the nursing consultation relationship. As a result, a contract decreases the likelihood of future conflicts and legal problems arising from misperceptions and misunderstanding. A formal written contract also enhances a nurse consultant's image as a professional (Scott & Beare 1993).

Box 13-3. Checklist of Contract Components for Nurse Consultants

A complete formal contract for a nursing consultation project should address the following elements:

_____ General statement of project goals

_____ Avoidance of guaranteeing outcomes

_____ Work to be done by the nurse consultant—services to be provided, methods to be used

_____ Consultee responsibilities—tasks, supplies/resources to be provided

_____ Time line for consultation—number and length of sessions with consultee, desired date of final report

_____ Line of authority and to whom the nurse consultant is responsible; frequency of communication

_____ Procedures for auditing progress of work

_____ Criteria and methods of evaluation

_____ Confidentiality and its limits

_____ People and materials to which the nurse consultant has access

_____ Fees to be paid, reimbursement for expenses, terms of payment

_____ Process for modifying contract

_____ Process for terminating contract

_____ Signatures and date of acceptance

References: Dougherty, A. (1995). *Consultation: Practice and perspectives in school and community settings.* Pacific Grove, CA: Brooks-Cole; Remley, T. (1993). Consultation contracts. *Journal of Counseling and Development, 72,* 157-158; Scott, L., & Beare, P. (1993). Nurse consultants and professional liability, *Clinical Nurse Specialist, 7* (6), 331-334

Contract Components and Formats

Regardless of the format used for a nursing consultation contract, it should address the purpose of the consultation, methods for achieving this purpose, ground rules, expectations, resources needed to complete the consultation, and a time line (Kurpius, Fuqua, & Rozecki 1993). Box 13-3 provides a checklist of contract components for nursing consultation contracts.

Some consultants believe that written contracts are too "legalistic" and signify a distrust between the consultant and consultee that is antithetical to a productive consulting relationship (Schein 1987). However, contracts can vary in format from a relatively formal legal document with "legalese" (Figure 13-5) to a comparatively simple letter that is sent by one party (Figure 13-6) and signed and returned by the other (Figure 13-7). Most frequently, nurse consultants use a letter of agreement signed by both participants or a simple contract drafted by one party and signed by both (Remley 1993). Letters of understanding and memos (Figure 13-8) are also useful contract formats for internal consultation situations. When using a less formal format of contract, it is often easy to overlook the inclusion of essential contract components. The use of a checklist such as the one presented in Box 13-3 can help ensure that each contract has the components that are needed and appropriate for the specific consultation situation.

Perinatal Solutions, Inc.
Nursing Consultation Services

This is a contract between Mercy-West Home Health Care Agency, herein called the party of the first part, and Perinatal Solutions Inc., herein referred to as the party of the second part. This contract is entered into on the seventh day of September, 1999, as follows:

The party of the second part agrees to serve as a consultant between September 7 and October 19, 1997 by providing education and training concerning fetal assessment techniques for home health care nurses employed by the party of the first part. Specifically, the party of the second part agrees to serve as workshop facilitator and trainer for five days (each day from 9 AM to 4 PM): September 20, 25, 30, and October 5, 10 for a workshop to be entitled, "Teaching Home Care Nurses Fetal Assessment." The party of the second part further agrees to conduct evaluations of the workshop participants' learning relative to the goals of the workshop and, with the permission of the participants, to share those evaluations with the contact person designated by the party of the first part. The party of the second part agrees to uses Gladys Jackson, Director of Nurses at Mercy-West Home Health Care Agency, as the contact person for all matters pertaining to this consultation, including the possible use of additional consultants or the addition of other consultees as participants in the workshop.

The party of the first part agrees to pay the party of the second part a total of five thousand dollars ($5000) plus expenses for materials within 10 days of completion of the consultation services. The party of the second part also agrees to provide materials (including audiovisuals and handouts) as long as the request for such materials is made by September 15, 1999.

This contract is subject to renegotiation at any time and either party is free to terminate the agreement if either determines the consultation progress to be unsatisfactory. Fees (prorated) and expenses become immediately due and payable at such a time.

For Mercy-West Home Health Care Agency: For Perinatal Solutions, Inc.:

_____   _____

Title: _____   Title: _____

Date: _____   Date: _____

Perinatal Solutions, Inc.
Nursing Consultation Services

Partners for promoting healthy mothers, babies,
families, and communities

12703 125th Avenue, SE   Phone: (208) 546-9808
Bellevue, WA 98772   Fax: (208) 546-9888
                                email: peri.1342.aol.com

Figure 13-5. Sample Formal Contract
This contract is an example of a formal contract that has been generated by the nurse consultant.

Perinatal Solutions, Inc.
Nursing Consultation Services

12703 125th Avenue, SE
Bellevue, WA 98772

Margaret Planter, RN
Director of Community Health Services
MountainView Women's Clinic
North Avenue and C Street
Boise, Idaho 95443

July 12, 1999

Dear Ms. Planter,

I have had a chance to look over the packet of material that you sent and am eager to pursue a role working with your organization on the breast health awareness project. I think that breast health is an important and timely issue for women and your project looks like a good way to provide information as well as clarify some myths. I applaud your efforts in undertaking a project of this scope and think it is especially commendable that you have included evaluation plans in the project design.

The data analyses for this project would be pretty straightforward. I would look not only at test scores but at their relationship to demographic characteristics of the participants. The relationship between mammography utilization, breast self-exam, and these other characteristics could also be explored. This would give you information for further educational efforts.

I reviewed the questionnaires that you sent. You will note that I proposed some changes in wording and some additional items that I think would be worth reviewing. I would be happy to work with you to incorporate any of these items into the survey as well as to help you with format so that data can be entered directly from the survey into the computer.

If you do choose to involve me in this project, I would be willing to do all of the data processing and analyses as well as write a summary interpretive report. I would, of course, return all of the raw data and computer printouts to you either at the completion of the project or on an ongoing basis. I would like to discuss fee considerations and other contract details with you on the phone. I understand your financial constraints and am certain that I can work within your budget. I will want a portion of the total fee agreed upon at the time that I receive the first set of questionnaires for analyses. The remainder of my fee would be due at the time of submission of my final report. The time line you presented on the phone the other day would work out fine for me.

As you requested, I have enclosed a copy of my current curriculum vita. I look forward to hearing from you regarding this project. The best days to reach me in my office are Mondays and Tuesdays.

Sincerely,

Leslie Norton

Leslie Norton, RNC, MSN

Perinatal Solutions, Inc.
Nursing Consultation Services

Partners for promoting healthy mothers, babies,
families, and communities

12703 125th Avenue, SE
Bellevue, WA 98772

Phone: (208) 546-9808
Fax: (208) 546-9888
email: peri.1342.aol.com

Figure 13-6. Sample Offer of Nursing Consultation Services
This offer of services is less formal than a formal contract but, like a contract, establishes the parameters of a nursing consultation relationship. It requires acceptance and consideration before it is considered a contract.

MOUNTAINVIEW WOMEN'S CLINIC

North Avenue and C Street
Boise, Idaho 95443

Leslie Norton, RNC, MSN
c/o Perinatal Solutions, Inc.
12703 125th Avenue, SE
Bellevue, WA 98772

July 25, 1999

Dear Ms. Norton:

This correspondence serves as a letter of understanding regarding your offer to provide statistical analyses and final reporting of same in support of MountainView Women's Clinic's Breast Health Awareness project. As discussed, this project is being funded by a grant that was awarded to us by the State Health Division for purposes of planning, facilitating, and evaluating a project of health education to increase awareness and education among women about the personal and economic efficacy of early detection of breast cancer through better breast health practices.

As summarized in your letter, your services would include the following activities:
*   Formatting of the survey to facilitate data entry into your computer
*   Data processing and analyses
*   Provision of a written summary interpretive report

As we discussed, your fee for the above services is $2500, one-half to be paid at the time the first surveys are sent to you. The remainder of your fee will be paid to you at the time of our acceptance of your final written report. If these terms are acceptable, please sign below and return this letter to me. I will make certain that you receive a copy for your files.

Sincerely,

Margaret Planter

Margaret Planter, RN
Director of Community Health Services

I accept and agree to the conditions outlined in this Letter of Understanding.

Name: _____

Title: _____

Date: _____

Social Security #: _____

Figure 13-7. Sample Letter of Understanding
This letter is in response to an offer of services. Note that it delineates tasks and fees. The nurse consultant and consultee should both keep a copy of this document.

Jeanne Paulson, RNC, MSN
Pediatric Clinical Nurse Specialist
Mercy Medical Center

Corrine Raye, RN, CS
Director of Patient Care Services
Mercy Medical Center
1220 NW Mountain Blvd.
Bellevue, WA 98605

Dear Ms. Raye,

This memo serves as a letter of understanding about the nursing consultation services I will be providing for Mercy Medical Center.

The purpose of this consultation project is to work with employees of Mercy Medical Center to develop a plan for on-site child care services. As I understand the situation, I am to first conduct a needs assessment/interest survey and compile results. I also will conduct focus group interviews as a way of obtaining more in-depth responses from employees.

Once employees' interest in on-site child care is verified and I have obtained a sense of needs and preferences, I will visit other facilities that have on-site child care to observe how they operate. Finally, I will form a committee that represents a cross-section of interests in regard to this issue. I will work with this committee to develop a proposal to submit to Mercy Medical Center's administration and Board of Trustees.

My understanding is that 9 months have been allocated for this project and that I am to be released from my other responsibilities as Pediatric Clinical Nurse Specialist for up to 28 hours a week in order to provide this consultation. During these 9 months, I will continue to receive my regular salary (including any pay increases to which I am entitled during that period). Mercy Medical Center will make any needed travel arrangements and provide needed supplies and secretarial support services. Also, staff will be released from their regular duties with pay to participate in focus groups and committee meetings during their regular work hours. Staff who come in for a meeting during their off-shift hours will be compensated at their regular rate of pay.

As we agreed, I will report directly to you and we will have at least monthly progress meetings. Responses from employees will not be identified by name in any of my reports, nor will this information be made available without the participant's consent.

Would you please sign this letter and return it to me to indicate your acceptance of this project and its terms as outlined. Thank you for the opportunity to be involved in this project.

Sincerely,

Jeanne Paulson

Jeanne Paulson, RNC, MSN

Accepted:

Name: _____

Title: _____

Date: _____

Figure 13-8. Sample Memo of Understanding for an Internal Nursing Consultation Engagement
This memo identifies tasks, goals, and processes and requests acceptance of terms by the nurse-manager. The memo illustrates how contract components can be incorporated into an informal format of presentation.

Contracts with individual consultees are less likely to be written formally. The nurse consultant should keep in mind, however, that verbal contracts are often inadequate back-up for any misunderstandings that may develop in a nursing consultation relationship. Most consultants have learned from experience that a written agreement of some sort should be developed for every nursing consultation situation, even if it is just a brief memo (Kurpius et al. 1993; Metzger 1993). In all nursing consultation situations, it is essential that all signing parties (for example, the nurse consultant and consultee or representative of the client system) keep a copy of any signed contract and/or letter of acceptance.

Chapter Summary

As the services that nurse consultants can offer in today's health care environment gain recognition, more and more advanced practice nurses will opt to establish consultation practices. These nurse consultants will need to develop an additional knowledge base and take on a new set of skills—marketing, promotion, fees, and contracts—if they are to be successful. While nursing consultation has always been a part of advanced nursing practice, to a great extent, it remains an "emerging" role and profession. Nurses who wish to take advantage of the growing opportunities for nurse consultants need to develop "business savvy" and familiarity with business issues if they are to become recognized and valued as professional nurse consultants.

Applying Chapter Content

- Develop a consulting vita and capability statement that you could use for promoting nursing consultation services. Have a peer critique these for completeness and presentation.

- Critique the contracts that appear in Figures 13-5, 13-6, 13-7, and 13-8. What changes would you make in each of these contracts?

References

Barron, A. (1989). The CNS as consultant. In A. Hamric & J. Spross (Eds.), *The clinical nurse specialist in theory and practice* (2nd ed., pp. 125-146). Philadelphia: Saunders.

Cosier, R., & Dalton, D. (1993). Management consulting: Planning, entry, performance. *Journal of Counseling and Development, 72*, 191-197.

Dougherty, A. (1995). *Consultation: Practice and perspectives in school and community settings* (2nd ed.). Pacific Grove, CA: Brooks-Cole.

Finnigan, S. (1996). Getting started in business: From fantasy to reality. *Advanced Practice Nursing Quarterly, 2* (1), 1-8.

Franck, J. (1995, January). Know the who, what, and when of consulting clients. *Hospital Infection Control*, 10.

Frings, C. (1991, October). What it takes to be a successful consultant. *Medical Laboratory Observer*, 47-50.

Kurpius, D., Fuqua, D., & Rozecki, T. (1993). The consulting process: A multidimensional approach. *Journal of Counseling and Development, 71*, 601-606.

Lachmann, V. (1996). Positioning your business in the marketplace. *Advanced Practice Nursing Quarterly, 2* (1), 27-32.

Lanza, M. (1996). Money: Personal issues affect professional practice. *Clinical Nurse Specialist, 10* (6), 310-317.

Lewin, M. (1995). *The overnight consultant*. New York: John Wiley & Sons.

Lippitt, G., & Lippitt, R. (1986). *The consulting process in action* (2nd ed.). San Diego: University Associates.

Longworth, J., & DiNardo, E. (1995). Marketing your services. In M. Snyder & M. Mirr (eds.), *Advanced practice nursing: A guide to professional development* (pp. 241-251). New York: Springer Publishing.

Metzger, R. (1993). *Developing a consulting practice*. Newbury Park, CA: Sage.

Remley, T. (1993). Consultation contracts. *Journal of Counseling and Development*, 72, 157-158.

Schein, E. (1987). *Process consultation, volume II: Lessons for managers and consultants*. Reading, MA: Addison-Wesley.

Scott, L., & Beare, P. (1993). Nurse consultants and professional liability. *Clinical Nurse Specialist*, 7 (6), 331-334.

Tepper, R. (1985). *Become a top consultant: How the experts do it*. New York: John Wiley & Sons.

Additional Readings

Barron, A. (1989). The CNS as consultant. In A. Hamric & J. Spross (Eds.), *The clinical nurse specialist in theory and practice* (2nd ed., pp. 125-146). Philadelphia: Saunders.
This chapter includes useful strategies that can be used for promoting oneself as an internal nurse consultant.

Beare, P. (1988). The ABCs of external consultation. *Clinical Nurse Specialist*, 2 (1), 35-38.
This article provides a brief overview of how to establish oneself as a nurse consultant in private practice. Topics covered include finding consultation opportunities, contracting, and promotional services.

Cosier, R., & Dalton, D. (1993). Management consulting: Planning, entry, performance. *Journal of Counseling and Development*, 72, 191-197.
This article presents marketing and promotion strategies for prospective consultants. The emphasis is on management consultation using an expertise rather than a process approach. Particularly useful is the listing of associations and materials for prospective management consultants.

Cummins, R. (1994). Laying the foundation for a career in consulting. *Journal of AHIMA*, 65 (11), 38-43.
This article describes the author's development as a consultant from part-time ("moonlighting") to full-time in a business arrangement with a hospital to full-time as a member of a major consulting firm. The author also describes skills and attributes needed for successful consulting.

Finnigan, S. (1996). Getting started in business: From fantasy to reality. *Advanced Practice Nursing Quarterly*, 2 (1), 1-8.
This article provides excellent advice for potential entrepreneurs. Topics discussed include identifying clients, forming alliances, and setting and collecting fees.

Franck, J. (1995, January). Know the who, what, and when of consulting clients. *Hospital Infection Control*, 10.
This article presents a useful framework for defining a consultation market. Also useful is the discussion of providing free consultation services.

Frings, C. (1991, October). What it takes to be a successful consultant. *Medical Laboratory Observer*, 47-50.
Although this highly readable article is directed toward laboratory technicians who wish to become consultants, the advice given is also applicable to nurses. Particularly useful is the list of potential consultation opportunities which the article includes.

Kurpius, D., Fuqua, D., & Rozecki, T. (1993). The consulting process: A multidimensional approach. *Journal of Counseling and Development, 71,* 601-606.
  This article includes a brief discussion of fee setting and contracting in internal and external consultation situations.

Lachmann, V. (1996). Positioning your business in the marketplace. *Advanced Practice Nursing Quarterly, 2* (1), 27-32.
  This article presents an overview of basic marketing principles and the marketing process. It also presents numerous promotion ideas that could be used by nurse consultants. The author focuses particularly on marketing advanced practice nursing services in the managed care marketplace.

Lanza, M. (1996). Money: Personal issues affect professional practice. *Clinical Nurse Specialist, 10* (6), 310-317.
  This article explores conscious and unconscious issues surrounding money, case examples in nurse therapists' dilemmas in handling money issues, and implications for practice. Although directed toward nurses in direct patient care roles, the content in this article is also applicable to nurse consultants.

Lewin, M. (1995). *The overnight consultant.* New York: John Wiley & Sons.
  This book offers practical advice on developing a career as a consultant. Topics addressed include setting fees, organizing the business aspects of a consulting practice, marketing, and managing stress as a consultant. The book also includes examples of brochures, consulting agreements, and other types of correspondence.

Mackniesh, J. (1989). Issues and concerns of a health promotion consultant. *Occupational Therapy in Health Care, 5* (4), 101-113.
  This article describes the experiences of a health promotion consultant in private practice. It provides a realistic view of what is required to become self-supporting as a consultant in any discipline.

Metzger, R. (1993). *Developing a consulting practice.* Newbury Park, CA: Sage.
  This book is full of strategies for developing oneself as an independent consultant. In particular, it addresses how these issues can be handled by someone who does consulting on a part-time basis.

Remley, T. (1993). Consultation contracts. *Journal of Counseling and Development, 72,* 157-158.
  This is an excellent and thorough discussion of the dimensions of contracting. The author emphasizes that any written or verbal consultation agreement is a legal contract and suggests that taking the time to develop and agree to a written document can assist both parties in developing a clear understanding of the terms of the consultation relationship.

Rew, L. (1988). AFFIRM the role of clinical specialist in private practice. *Clinical Nurse Specialist, 2* (1), 39-43.
  The AFFIRM model is presented as a series of steps whereby a nurse can plan for a private nursing consultation practice.

Tepper, R. (1985). *Become a top consultant: How the experts do it.* New York: John Wiley & Sons.
  This book examines how ten of the most successful consultants from a variety of fields got into business and built their practices. It also describes the pitfalls they found and how they solved them.

~
14

Legal Aspects of Consulting

*The more one considers some of the legal ramifications
of the issues we've raised in this section, the clearer it
becomes that most matters are not neatly defined.*
(Corey, Corey, & Calanan 1984)

Key terms: liability, negligence, malpractice,
reasonable prudence, duty, tort

One of my first consulting experiences involved working with a physician to
develop data collection strategies and plan data analyses for a research project
about outcomes among women who had taken part in an inpatient substance abuse
treatment program while they were pregnant. I wrote a letter agreeing to this opportunity (initial contact had been made over the telephone) and outlining my fees and
reimbursement expectations for expenses. I then developed a series of data collection
instruments (the women were to be followed for 18 months) that the consultee
accepted. Following this, I traveled (a 400-mile round-trip by car) to meet with the
consultee and other involved individuals to finalize study protocols. When I returned
home, I submitted an itemized bill for my services and expenses to date. At the bot-
tom of this bill were the words "Net 15 days," the same terms that had been stated in
my original letter of understanding. Fifteen, thirty, sixty, and then ninety days passed
without receiving payment. Over the next 6 months, I shared my frustrations with
colleagues, made numerous telephone calls, and sent several registered letters to the
consultee. Finally, I was paid. I have not heard from the consultee since.

So, what did I learn from this experience? First, I learned that despite my initial
doubts, I *did* have a legal contract with the consultee. Second, I learned to *always* have
a mutually signed contract. Throughout this experience, however, I worried about liability issues related to confidentiality, breach of contract, abandonment, and fee collection. I also worried about the effect this incident would have on my reputation as a
beginning nurse consultant.

Professional liability is a fundamental issue all nurse consultants must consider in
order to be perceived as professionals as well as to protect professional and personal
interests. While nurses working as external consultants are most likely to have concerns about these issues, the same issues with just slight modification, also need attention by nurses who function as internal consultants.

This chapter introduces the legal issues with which nurse consultants are most
likely to contend. The chapter begins by reviewing basic legal concepts and terminology, and applying these concepts to the practice of nursing consultation. The next section discusses common causes of legal action against nurse consultants. Following
this, issues about which a nurse consultant might initiate legal action against a con-

sultee are considered. The final section explores self-protection strategies for nurse consultants. Think about the following questions as you read this chapter:

- How are the concepts of malpractice and confidentiality similar in clinical nursing practice and in nursing consultation? How are they different?

- In what ways are professional and legal standards of practice similar in clinical nursing practice and in nursing consultation? In what ways are they different?

- How are internal and external nursing consultation situations different in terms of risk of liability?

- How might self-protection strategies vary for internal and external nurse consultants?

Basic Legal Concepts and Terminology

Advanced roles in nursing practice, such as that of nurse consultant, promise increased autonomy for nurses. However, these roles also carry increased responsibility, accountability, and professional liability. As nurse consultants continue to gain recognition for their expertise and the positive contributions they make to health care delivery, they increasingly find themselves being held legally accountable for their specialized knowledge and problem-solving skills. The dilemma with this is that consultation in general, and nursing consultation in particular, is only an "emerging profession" (Dougherty 1995). Thus there are relatively few precedents to guide the courts when consultants encounter legal entanglements. Avoiding legal entanglements as a nurse consultant is facilitated by an awareness of the behaviors that can precipitate legal action. This requires an understanding of basic legal concepts and terminology.

Negligence and Malpractice

The terms "negligence" and "malpractice" are often used interchangeably. *Negligence* refers to the "omission to do something which a reasonable person guided by those ordinary considerations which ordinarily regulate human affairs, would do, or the doing of something a reasonable and prudent person would not do" (*Schneider v. Little Co., 1915*, cited in Gardner & Hagedorn 1997). Negligence, therefore, can take two forms: "crimes of omission" and "crimes of commission."

Malpractice refers to professional negligence or to misconduct by a professional (Gardner & Hagedorn 1996). In order for a charge of professional negligence or malpractice to be upheld, the plaintiff (for example, a consultee) must prove each of the following four elements:

1. Duty—the obligation toward another to comply with a particular standard of conduct. Duty can be demonstrated by a contract or implied by the nature of a relationship. In nursing consultation, the nurse consultant's duty may be toward the consultee, the client, a patient or patient group that is a stakeholder, the organizational contact person, the organization as a whole, and the nursing profession. Chapter 15 discusses ethical dilemmas related to the concept of duty.

2. Breach of duty—failure to uphold a contract. The contract can be actual or implied. When a breach of duty occurs, a promise has essentially been broken. Negligence is one form of breach of duty since the "promise" to act as a professional is not upheld when negligence occurs.

3. Harm or damages—suffering some sort of loss. Loss can be physical, emotional/psychological, or financial.

4. Causation—the existence of a causal link between the breach of duty and the damages suffered by the plaintiff (Dougherty 1995; Gardner & Hagedorn 1997; McCarthy & Sorenson 1993; Scott & Beare 1993.)

Embedded in the concepts of negligence and malpractice is the "reasonable person rule." That is, negligence represents departure of the defendant's behavior from that expected by a reasonably prudent person. In professional malpractice, the reasonably prudent person to whom a defendant is compared is another professional (in this case, a nurse consultant) who reflects the degree of knowledge and skill that is customary among other professionals practicing in the same area under the same or similar circumstances (Brent 1997; Corey et al. 1984; Dougherty 1995; Gardner & Hagedorn 1997). It is important to note that reasonable prudence is not a static concept but, rather, reflects the circumstances of the professional relationship as well as current research, technology, and social expectations.

To summarize, in nursing consultation, professional negligence (that is, malpractice) occurs when there is lack of "reasonable" or "ordinary" application of the nursing consultation process that results in injury to the consultee or client or another member of the client system. Professional negligence can arise from two types of situations:

- a failure to possess the requisite skill and knowledge to fulfill an accepted consultation contract or not knowing what to do when a reasonably prudent nurse consultant would, and

- a failure to use judgment in applying one's knowledge and exercising one's skills in the implementation of the nursing consultation process or knowing what to do but not doing it, or doing it carelessly (Brent 1997; Gardner & Hagedorn 1996).

Tort Law, Civil Law, and Criminal Law

A *tort* is a legal wrong, not involving a breach of contract, that causes injury to another and for which the person committing the wrong can be held liable for damages in a civil suit. Professional negligence is the legal wrong that most often results in damages (Brent 1997; Gardner & Hagedorn 1997).

Civil actions differ from criminal actions in terms of purpose, the courts of law in which they are tried, and the standard of proof that is required. The purpose of a civil action is to obtain monetary compensation for damages suffered. In contrast, the purpose of criminal action is to punish the wrongdoer and deter repeated offensive conduct. Civil damages are awarded on the basis of a preponderance of evidence or certainty (of guilt) as established by an expert witness who is "competent and qualified to render such an opinion" (Gardner & Hagedorn 1997). In nursing consultation, the expert witness would need to be another nurse consultant with similar expertise and credentials. By comparison, guilt in a criminal case requires proof beyond a reasonable doubt.

Professional negligence or malpractice reflects mistakes, inattention, and inexperience and is generally not considered a crime. In order to be considered a crime, malpractice needs to be accompanied by malice and/or wanton misconduct; that is, "an unconscious indifference to consequences" or "reckless disregard for the rights and safety of others" (Gardner & Hagedorn 1997).

Statutes of Limitations

A *statute of limitations* is "the time limit during which a person, having a cause of action for damages due to professional negligence, is required to file a lawsuit" (Gardner & Hagedorn 1997). After the statute of limitations has expired, a lawsuit may not be filed.

Time limits for statutes of limitations vary from state to state; most range from 1 to 6 years. The event to which the statute of limitations applies also varies by state. In some states, the statute of limitations is applied to the date of the activity that is alleged to have caused the injury. Other states apply the statute of limitations to the date of discovery of injury.

Usually, the *date of discovery* refers to the date that the plaintiff first knew or should have known of the injury. In some states, however, the date of discovery is applied to the date on which the plaintiff learned of the cause of the injury—for example, that it was linked to the nurse consultant's actions (Gardner & Hagedorn 1997). Because of variations in statutes of limitations as well as differences in terms of exactly to which event they apply, nurse consultants need to familiarize themselves with their state laws.

Causes of Legal Action against Nurse Consultants

Currently, there are no records (that is, case law and accompanying commentary) of legal action against nurse consultants. This could reflect several situations: (1) the actual lack of legal action against nurse consultants, (2) the possibility that nurse consultants identify themselves by other titles (for example, management consultant, educator-trainer, or clinical nurse specialist), or (3) out-of-court settlement of threatened legal actions against nurse consultants. Regardless, areas that are legally problematic for other advanced practice nurses and human resource consultants (that is, consultants who work with schools and social service agencies) are instructive and applicable to nurse consultants.

Among human service consultants, lack of skill is the most common cause of malpractice (Dougherty 1995). Other common causes of legal action against human service consultants are identified in Box 14-1. This list suggests that legal action can be brought against nurse consultants for behaviors related to implementation of the nursing consultation process as well as for behaviors related to the conduct of a nursing consultation (business) practice.

Box 14-1. Common Causes of Legal Action against Human Service Consultants

The following behaviors associated with legal problems for human service consultants can also create legal problems for nurse consultants:

- Use of improper assessment and diagnostic techniques
- Breach of contract
- Breach of confidentiality
- Misrepresentation of one's skills or credentials as a consultant
- Failure to consult with others about difficult cases
- Giving poor advice
- Failure to respect a consultee's integrity and privacy
- Inappropriate public statements
- Lack of informed consent
- Poor record keeping
- Use of inappropriate methods to collect fees

References: Corey, G., Corey, M., & Callanan, P. (1984). *Issues and ethics in the helping professions* (3rd ed.). Pacific Grove, CA: Brooks-Cole; and Dougherty, A. (1995). *Consultation: Practice and perspectives in school and community settings* (2nd ed.). Pacific Grove, CA: Brooks-Cole.

Behaviors Related to Implementation of the Nursing Consultation Process

The nursing consultation process is a systematic way of working with consultees to help them resolve problems related to the health status of clients and health care delivery. Conscientiously attending to the details of the nursing consultation process increases the likelihood of successful problem resolution and adherence to professional standards of practice. Behaviors related to implementation of the nursing consultation process that can prompt legal action against nurse consultants include malpractice, breach of contract, and breach of confidentiality.

Malpractice Charges of malpractice can be brought against a nurse consultant when ineffective or inappropriate implementation of the nursing consultation process has resulted in harm to the plaintiff. As mentioned earlier, the plaintiff in a malpractice suit against a nurse consultant could be the consultee, the client, the client system (a contracting organization, for example), or a stakeholder. Because one of the conditions necessary for a charge of malpractice to be valid is breach of contract, a malpractice suit is usually initiated by whomever signed the contract as the "consumer" of the nursing consultation services. Contracts, however, do not necessarily need to be written and can be implied by the nature of a professional relationship (for example, giving some sort of professional help). This opens up the possibility of malpractice charges by additional parties involved in the nursing consultation relationship.

Novice consultants are at particular risk for malpractice stemming from ineffective implementation of the nursing consultation process. This is because expertise in a clinical specialty area does not necessarily translate into expertise in the process or human process issues of nursing consultation (Alvarez 1993). Malpractice can result from actions or "mis-actions" during any phase of the nursing consultation process. Examples of actions in each phase of the nursing consultation process that could result in a charge of malpractice include the following:

- Gaining entry—contracting for consultation projects for which one is not qualified

- Problem identification—incomplete data collection, incomplete analysis, or inaccurate interpretation of assessment data

- Action planning—giving bad advice or proposing problem solutions that would cause harm to the client system if implemented (this often results from failure to assess or take into consideration the resources and culture of the client system)

- Evaluation—failure to monitor the consultation process (particularly for side effects) or to revise the nursing consultation process on the basis of evaluation feedback

- Disengagement—abandoning the consultee or client system without warning, failure to put continuity supports into place

Box 14-2 provides an example of ineffective implementation of the nursing consultation process.

Another potential source of malpractice action against nurse consultants is behaviors that reflect a possible confusion between ethical and legal duties. Activities that are legal or legally required may not seem ethical. Conversely, activities that seem ethical may not be legal. If a legal mandate applies to a problem or issue, however, it takes precedence over ethical or other concerns (McCarthy & Sorenson 1993). Ethical dilemmas in nursing consultation are discussed in Chapter 15.

Box 14-2. An Example of Ineffective Implementation of the Nursing Consultation Process

A nurse consultant accepts a contract from a home health care agency to develop a protocol for the assessment and management of clients on tocolytic therapy for preterm labor. At the time of the contract, the agency stated they were in the process of hiring staff with experience in obstetrical nursing. The nurse consultant developed a protocol based on the assumption that the nurses who would be caring for these patients would have obstetrical nursing backgrounds. Part of the protocol consisted of specifying situations in which a patient's physician should be notified immediately.

An agency nurse who did not have a background in obstetrics made a home visit to a woman on tocolytic therapy. She utilized the assessment protocol but made an inappropriate decision in terms of failing to notify a patient's physician. This resulted in an emergency situation for the patient.

The agency claimed that the nurse consultant had not specified that the protocol could only be effectively implemented by nurses with obstetrical experience. The agency also stated that at the time the protocol was written, most of their nurses providing care to perinatal patients did not have a clinical background in obstetrics. They also said they had wanted a protocol that could be used by any home health care nurse since they did not have specialty teams.

In this case, the base line knowledge and skills of agency staff who would be implementing the protocol were not adequately assessed. As a result, the nurse consultant did not have full information on which to develop the protocol. Furthermore, the nurse consultant had failed to communicate with the consultation contact person to verify what the agency really wanted. As a result, a patient was placed in danger, and the nurse consultant could be held legally responsible.

Breach of Contract Failure to adhere to the terms of the nursing consultation contract can also prompt legal action against a nurse consultant. Breach of contract may or may not constitute malpractice since negligence is only one form of breach of contract. Typical situations that result in claims of breach of contract (which would not be considered negligence or malpractice) include:

- Failure to adhere to the time line specified in the nursing consultation contract

- Cost overruns

- Failure to achieve promised results such as specified savings or increased productivity

- Failure to implement the nursing consultation process in the manner outlined in the contract; for example, not involving consultees when such involvement was specified in the contract

These situations point to the need for a contract to be written with some degree of flexibility rather than in absolute terms—for example, citing estimated or a range of costs and time needed. These situations also reinforce the need for including a revision clause in the contract and for regular progress reports to a designated person within the client system.

Breach of Confidentiality Breach of confidentiality as a cause of legal action against nurse consultants deserves special mention. Confidentiality is an ethical and professional as well as an actionable legal principle. In most states, breach of confidentiality is viewed as unprofessional conduct and can be grounds for revocation of certain types of professional licenses (McCarthy & Sorenson 1993). Nurse consultants need to be familiar with how the issue of confidentiality is addressed by both their state Nurse Practice Act and by any other licensing regulations under which they may be practicing (for example, dual licensure as a counselor, consultant, or social worker).

Nurses who are working as consultants also need to keep in mind and inform their consultees that confidentiality is not absolute. Disclosures may be both appropriate and required, as is the case with child abuse reporting requirements. In cases of known or suspected abuse, the nurse consultant's duty is to disclose information that was given in confidence; failure to disclose this information could precipitate legal action against the nurse consultant. Nurse consultants who work with parent or child consultee groups need to be particularly aware of this issue.

Nurse consultants who work with individual nurse or organizational consultees can also become privy to information (for example, ongoing fraud or plans for a strike) that, if not disclosed, could harm the client or other members of the client system. In this situation, however, confidentiality is an ethical rather than a legal obligation. That is, the nurse consultant is not duty bound to disclose this information. In situations such as this, which are probably more common in nursing consultation, the nurse consultant needs to weigh the risks and benefits of protecting and violating confidentiality. Chapter 15 discusses the ethical considerations related to confidentiality.

Behaviors Related to Conduct of a Nursing Consultation Practice

Legal action can also be brought against a nurse consultant because of consultee (or client or client system) dissatisfaction with the way in which a nurse consultant conducts the business aspect of nursing consultation. Misrepresentation and issues related to fees and their collection are particularly likely to create business-related legal entanglements for the nurse consultant.

Misrepresentation Misrepresentation is analogous to false advertising. Misrepresentation occurs when a nurse consultant gives inaccurate information about his/her credentials as a consultant, skills and abilities, and/or experience and "track record" as a consultant. Misrepresentation can create problems because it can lead a consultee to hire the wrong consultant for a project. For the nurse consultant, misrepresentation increases the likelihood of accepting a contract for which one is not qualified and setting in motion events that can ultimately lead to charges of professional negligence.

Another dimension of misrepresentation is inaccurately portraying how one conducts the nursing consultation process, including how charges are generated for services. For example, a nurse consultant could misrepresent a fee structure by quoting a "package price," but then billing extra for travel and other expenses.

Fees and Their Collection Misrepresentation is one way in which fees can create legal entanglements for nurse consultants. Fees can also prompt legal action when a nursing consultation relationship is terminated prematurely or when fee collection becomes problematic.

When a nursing consultation relationship is terminated prematurely, fees are generally prorated or otherwise based on work that has been completed to date. Difficulties with collection arise when there is disagreement or dissatisfaction about the calculation of "early termination fees," usually because there is disagreement about activities for which the nurse consultant should actually be reimbursed. Efforts can be made to prevent this situation by including a clearly written termination clause in the consultation contract, including specification of who will be responsible for prorating fees and determining what activities will be chargeable in an early termination situation. In a consultation relationship that will involve a longer period of time, the nurse consultant may want to bill the consultee on an ongoing basis rather than wait until the completion of the contract. This strategy helps a nurse consultant minimize losses should the consultation relationship end prematurely.

Fees can also create legal entanglements for nurse consultants when a consultee is dissatisfied with the collection methods being used (for example, a consultant expecting reimbursement within 15 days). This issue reinforces the need for the nursing consultation contract to clearly identify consultee responsibilities in regard to fees and for adherence to the terms of the contract. A consultee's dissatisfaction would be warranted if, for example, a contract merely stated that charges would be billed at the completion of the project without specifying a "due and payable" time frame, but the consultee received a statement that specified "net due in 15 days" and was expected and pressured (that is, charged interest or threatened with referral to a collection agency) to adhere to that time frame.

Nurse Consultants as Plaintiffs

Thus far, this chapter has focused on behaviors that can prompt legal action against nurse consultants. However, nurse consultants can also find themselves in situations in which they are considering initiating legal action against a consultee or client system. The situations in which nurse consultants are most likely to find themselves giving consideration to assuming the role of plaintiff involve issues related to consultee breach of contract, fees and their collection, and rights to materials generated in the course of the nursing consultation relationship.

Breach of Contract

A nursing consultation contract specifies behavioral expectations and responsibilities for all parties involved in the nursing consultation relationship. Thus consultees and other members of the client system as well as the nurse consultant have duties in regard to the nursing consultation relationship. Failure on the part of any party involved in the nursing consultation relationship to carry out agreed upon duties constitutes breach of contract.

Failure to make available previously agreed upon information is one situation that could prompt a charge of breach of contract against a consultee or client system. Withholding information can create problems for the nurse consultant because it means that problem identification and action planning is carried out without full knowledge of both the problem situation and the characteristics of the problem setting. This can cause a nurse consultant to formulate ineffective, and possibly harmful, problem solutions. Failure to provide promised resources (for example, personnel, meeting time, supplies) that are needed for completion of the nursing consultation contract also constitutes breach of contract.

While nurse consultants may not be able to prevent a consultee's breach of contract, they can avoid problems such as malpractice that can arise from the breach by terminating the nursing consultation relationship when a breach occurs, assuming the contract allows for this. Nurse consultants are probably most likely to initiate legal action for breach of contract only as a countersuit strategy against a consultee who has initiated malpractice charges. In other instances, breach of contract results only in termination of the nursing consultation relationship and legal action is avoided because of the possible negative effect it can have on the nurse consultant's reputation.

Fees and Their Collection

A consultee's failure to pay agreed upon fees or to adhere to an agreed upon payment schedule is another form of breach of contract. Problems with fee collection can be referred to a collection agency or pursued through small-claims court. Collection agencies are sometimes perceived by consultees as having more "clout" than the nurse consultant in terms of enforcing payment. Use of a collection agency also enables the consultant to avoid the time and hassle of repeated and often increasingly unpleasant follow-up telephone calls and letters. Collection agencies, however, charge for their services and generally keep 50% of whatever they collect for themselves.

After other collection strategies have been exhausted, nurse consultants can pursue collection of delinquent accounts through small-claims court. Because of attorney expenses and the time away from work that court action entails, most nurse consultants opt not to pursue fees in this manner. Taking a consultee to small-claims court is also associated with a certain amount of negative publicity that can adversely affect a nurse consultant's practice.

Most consultants accept that they will fail to collect on 10% of their accounts (Tepper 1985). Collection tends to be less of a problem in consulting than in other professions because failure to pay can have negative effects on both the reputation of the client system and the willingness of other consultants to work with them in the future. Strategies for avoiding collection problems were presented in Chapter 13. Billing consultees more frequently for smaller amounts is a particular strategy the nurse consultant can use for "testing" the client system. This practice also results in smaller losses for the nurse consultant if problems with fee collection do arise. The nurse consultant can also avoid escalating losses by stopping work on a project if an agreed upon payment plan is not adhered to. In general, despite the availability of legal recourse for collection problems, most consultants tend to take a loss as a bad debt and move on, wiser for the experience (Lewin 1995; Tepper 1985).

Rights to Materials

The third situation that may cause a nurse consultant to consider initiating legal action against a consultee or client system is disagreement about the ownership of materials (assessment tools and educational materials, for example) generated by the nurse consultant during the course of completing a consultation project. The typical point of disagreement is whether such material belongs to the nurse consultant as their creator or to the consultee or client system who paid the nurse consultant to solve a problem that necessitated the development of such materials. This dilemma arises when the consultation contract fails to identify to whom these materials belong after the consultation relationship is terminated. Nurse consultants who generate materials over which they want to maintain control in terms of access and use can consider copyrighting these materials (Lewin 1995).

The issue of rights to materials becomes more complicated when a subcontractor is involved in the nursing consultation relationship. Subcontractors are individuals hired by the nurse consultant to assist with a specific component of a consultation project. Subcontractors are generally used to "fill gaps" in the skills needed to complete the project. The issue of rights to materials arises when the subcontractor is hired to create materials for use in the project. The typical point of contention is whether these materials are the property of the subcontractor, the nurse consultant, or the client system. Nurse consultants should deal with this issue proactively by generating a contract or letter of agreement with the subcontractor that addresses this issue (Lewin 1995).

Self-Protection Strategies

Things can go awry during even the most carefully planned and implemented consultation relationship. Although consultation is a contracted and service-related relationship, it is also a human relationship. There will always be misunderstandings and disappointed consultees or client systems who blame the nurse consultant for an inevitable or unforeseen outcome, no matter how well a contract has been written. Depending on the consultee, these disappointments may result in litigation or in behavior that causes the nurse consultant to consider legal action against the consultee. In order to protect professional and personal interests in a litigious society, nurse consultants need to engage in self-protection strategies. Self-protection strategies for nurse consultants include preventive measures, legal counsel, and liability insurance.

Preventive Measures

A priori preventive strategies have been emphasized over after-the-fact legal action throughout this chapter. The recurring themes of strategies for avoiding legal entanglements are the following: establish and maintain open communication and a good working relationship with a consultee, know one's limits, have a written contract, and incorporate evaluation activities throughout the nursing consultation process (Alvarez 1993; Reinert & Buck 1989). Specific preventive measures related to these themes are presented in Box 14-3.

Open Communication   Maintaining open communication and a positive working relationship with a consultee and other members of a client system helps prevent legal problems that can arise as a result of simple misunderstandings. Consultation is more than applying expert knowledge; it is also the process of communicating that expert knowledge so that a consultee understands it, appreciates its importance, and feels empowered enough to use the information independently in the future (Alvarez 1993). Communication issues can create problems for a nursing consultation relationship when a consultee feels unheard and unserved. Open communication and a positive working relationship is facilitated by paying attention to the details of establishing psychological entry (see Chapter 8) during the gaining entry phase of the nursing consultation process. Open communication is further promoted by ongoing progress meetings with the consultee or organizational contact person.

Knowing One's Limits   Knowing and respecting one's limits as a nurse consultant can help the nurse consultant avoid becoming involved in problem situations that could ultimately result in charges of malpractice due to the nurse consultant's lack of knowledge or skill. Knowing and respecting one's limits also means subcontracting, consulting, and referring when a consultation situation progresses beyond the point of personal effectiveness. Finally, knowing and respecting personal limitations helps the nurse consultant avoid legal entanglements that can occur as a result of temptation to misrepresent one's knowledge and skills and accept inappropriate contracts.

Contracts   A contract provides legal protection by clearly delineating the expectations of both parties for the nursing consultation relationship. Thus a contract should clearly identify agreed upon outcomes as well as provide an opportunity to establish any limits of confidentiality, responsibilities of both the nurse consultant and consultee, and expectations related to fees and their payment. A written contract that is

Box 14-3. Avoiding Legal Entanglements as a Nurse Consultant

Experts agree that the following strategies are helpful for preventing legal action against consultants:

- Always act within your scope of competence; know your limits and seek consultation or make referrals appropriately
- Be sure that any promotional materials provide current and accurate information
- Be aware of local and state laws that limit your practice of consultation; be familiar with the policies of your employing agency and act within these sets of guidelines
- Engender positive feelings between yourself and your consultees; be open in your communication with consultees and take an active interest in their welfare; establish a personal consulting policy of personal and professional honesty and openness
- Establish realistic expectations
- Be aware of and communicate any limits of confidentiality
- Use a written and mutually signed contract to clarify your professional relationship with a consultee; present contract information in clear language
- Discuss fees and their payment at the outset of the nursing consultation relationship
- Systematically follow the nursing consultation process
- Provide high quality service and stand behind it; regularly seek and respond to feedback
- Keep adequate records; check how long they need to be retained
- Have access to an attorney for consultation in problematic matters

References: Corey, G., Corey, M., & Callanan, P. (1984). *Issues and ethics in the helping professions* (3rd ed.). Pacific Grove, CA: Brooks-Cole; Dougherty, A. (1995). *Consultation: Practice and perspectives in school and community settings* (2nd ed.). Pacific Grove, CA: Brooks-Cole. Reinert, B., & Buck, E. (1989). Issues in liability insurance and the nurse consultant. *Clinical Nurse Specialist,* 7 (6), 331-334.

signed by both the nurse consultant and the consultee provides evidence that these issues were discussed and agreed upon before the working part of the nursing consultation process got underway. Components and formats of contracts were discussed in Chapter 13.

Evaluation Evaluation acts as a device for both quality control and legal protection. An evaluation plan and evaluation data can be used in the event of legal action to demonstrate professionalism and fulfillment of contract obligations as well as document a nurse consultant's effectiveness during a project. Documentation of routine peer evaluation of one's consultation practices can also serve as evidence of a nurse consultant's concern for quality service and practicing within one's limits (Reinert & Buck 1989). Peer feedback in terms of the appropriateness of one's actions also helps establish adherence to professional, reasonable, and prudent standards of practice.

Legal Counsel

Nurse consultants should seek legal counsel whenever they are developing documents such as contracts for use in their consultation practice. Legal counsel should also be sought when a nurse consultant encounters difficulty implementing or enforcing consultee implementation of the conditions set forth in a contract, especially if such difficulties cannot be resolved by negotiation between the nurse consultant and consultee. Finally, nurse consultants should obtain legal advice when adverse outcomes are expected to occur or do occur as a result of premature and unilateral contract termination. In this case, legal counsel should be sought *before* any legal action against a consultee is initiated.

Liability Insurance

Although professional liability insurance cannot prevent charges of malpractice from arising, when legal action does occur, liability insurance can help the nurse consultant prevent devastating financial loss. Insurance carriers view nurses who are practicing in advanced practice roles (such as that of consultant) as independent practitioners and raise premiums accordingly (Scott & Beare 1993). The specific type and amount of insurance a nurse consultant will need depends on the structure of the nursing consultation practice.

Nurses who negotiate a contract for their consultation services and are paid directly are considered self-employed and generally need more extensive and expensive coverage. Nurse consultants who have independent consultation practices may also need business or premise liability insurance (for example, to protect against a lawsuit that could result from injuries a consultee sustains in a fall on the nurse consultant's business premises) in addition to malpractice insurance (Reinert & Buck 1989).

Nurses who are practicing as internal consultants may be covered by standard personal professional liability policies. Traditionally, standard professional policies have covered nurses for any duties that are assigned to them by their employer as long as they are functioning within the scope of their state Nurse Practice Act, professional scope of practice, and institutional policies and procedures (Scott & Beare 1989).

The laws relating to nursing practice and the availability of malpractice insurance and what it covers are changing rapidly as the health care environment is undergoing reforms. Nurses who are practicing in extended or advanced practice roles need to check the parameters of their coverage with their carrier. Box 14-4 presents common terms that are used in malpractice insurance contracts. Liability insurance designed specifically for consultants in other disciplines does exist. This insurance is usually available through professional organizations such as the American Psychological Association and the American Management Association. Some nurse consultants hold membership in these or other professional organizations that specifically include consultants so that they can take advantage of the group's malpractice insurance.

Chapter Summary

In today's litigious society, nurse consultants are naive if they believe that they don't need to worry about legal entanglements. Protecting oneself from legal action directly and effectively involves taking preventive measures. Another dimension of professional and personal self-protection is knowledge of legal terms and appreciation of the types of situations most likely to prompt legal action. Because the health care and legal environments are constantly and rapidly changing, staying informed and adapting one's practice of nursing consultation are important means of maintaining professional standards of practice and avoiding legal entanglements.

Box 14-4. Terms Used in Malpractice Insurance Contracts

Claims-made insurance—this type of insurance policy offers protection against claims that are filed only while the policy is in effect; that is, only while the professional is practicing her/his profession. A "tail" must be purchased to provide coverage against claims based on incidents that occurred during the policy period but filed when the policy is no longer in effect (for example, after the policyholder has retired). Claims-made insurance is generally less expensive to purchase than is occurrence coverage since the insurance company is assuming risk only for the duration of the policy.

Occurrence coverage—this type of insurance policy covers claims if the policy was in effect at the time of the incident. The claim itself can be filed after the policy is no longer in effect (for example, the policyholder has retired from practice or changes insurance carrier) and the policyholder will still be covered. Occurrence coverage is more expensive to purchase than is claims-made coverage since the coverage is for a longer period of time. However, because of inflation, original coverage limits may be inadequate to cover a claim requesting damages in current amounts.

Declarations—the section of an insurance policy that states the limits of liability and the amount of coverage per claim.

Insuring agreements—identification of what specifically is covered by the policy.

Conditions—events that must be satisfied before the insurer is obligated to pay for any losses.

Provisions for cancellation—specification of how the insurance contract can be cancelled by either the insured or the carrier.

Reference: Reinert, B., & Buck, E. (1989). Issues in liability insurance and the nurse consultant. *Clinical Nurse Specialist, 3* (1), 42-45; Scott, L., & Beare, P. (1993). Nurse consultants and professional liability. *Clinical Nurse Specialist, 7* (6), 331-334.

Applying Chapter Content

- Analyze the scenario presented in Box 14-2. Critique the nurse consultant's actions and liability issues. Rewrite the scenario to adhere to suggestions for legally protective behavior.

- Investigate the statute of limitations for professional negligence in your state. What is the time frame for the statue of limitations? To what event is it applied?

- Look at your own professional liability insurance policy. Would it cover you (a) as an internal nurse consultant and (b) as an external nurse consultant?

References

Alvarez, C. (1993). Potential liability in good consultative practice. *Clinical Nurse Specialist, 7* (6), 330.

Brent, N. (1997) *Nurses and the law: A guide to principles and applications.* Philadelphia: Saunders.

Corey, G., Corey, M., & Callanan, P. (1984). *Issues and ethics in the helping professions* (3rd ed.). Pacific Grove, CA: Brooks-Cole.

Dougherty, A. (1995). *Consultation: Practice and perspectives in school and community settings* (2nd ed.). Pacific Grove, CA: Brooks-Cole.

Gardner, S., & Hagedorn, M. (1997). *Legal aspects of maternal-child nursing practice.* Menlo Park, CA: Addison-Wesley.

Lewin, M. (1995). *The overnight consultant.* New York: John Wiley & Sons.

McCarthy, M., & Sorenson, G. (1993). School counselors and consultants: Legal duties and liabilities. *Journal of Counseling and Development, 72,* 159-167.

Reinert, B., & Buck, E. (1989). Issues in liability insurance and the nurse consultant. *Clinical Nurse Specialist, 3* (1), 42-45.

Scott, L., & Beare, P. (1993). Nurse consultants and professional liability. *Clinical Nurse Specialist, 7* (6), 331-334.

Tepper, R. (1985). *Become a top consultant.* New York: John Wiley & Sons.

Additional Readings

Alvarez, C. (1993). Potential liability in good consultative practice. *Clinical Nurse Specialist, 7* (6), 330.

This commentary identifies problems that may arise during nursing consultation and precipitate legal action against a nurse consultant. These problems are linked to different phases in the nursing consultation process and to human process issues that can arise during a nursing consultation relationship.

Corey, G., Corey, M., & Callanan, P. (1984). *Issues and ethics in the helping professions* (3rd ed.). Pacific Grove, CA: Brooks-Cole.

Although this text is written primarily for counselors, much of the discussion is applicable to consultants. Chapter 6 describes legal issues related to confidentiality. Chapter 7 includes a discussion of malpractice issues in the helping professions.

Dougherty, A. (1995). *Consultation: Practice and perspectives in school and community settings* (2nd ed.). Pacific Grove, CA: Brooks-Cole.

Chapter 7 has a brief but useful section on the consultant and the law. Although the discussion is directed toward school-based consultants and "human service" professionals, the points are transferable to nursing consultation.

Finnigan, S. (1996). Getting started in business: From fantasy to reality. *Advanced Practice Nursing Quarterly, 2* (1), 1-8.

This article provides excellent advice for potential entrepreneurs. Topics discussed include setting and collecting fees.

Lewin, M. (1995). *The overnight consultant.* New York: John Wiley & Sons.

This book includes a useful discussion on how to protect materials that one develops as a consultant.

McCarthy, M., & Sorenson, G. (1993). School counselors and consultants: Legal duties and liabilities. *Journal of Counseling and Development, 72,* 159-167.

Legal issues discussed in this article include privacy, privilege, and confidentiality. Among the legal liabilities discussed are those arising from contract, tort, and criminal law. Although directed at counselors and consultants who work in educational systems, much of the content in this article can be applied to health care settings.

Metzger, R. (1993). *Developing a consulting practice.* Newbury Park, CA: Sage.

This book is full of strategies for developing oneself as an independent consultant. In particular, it addresses how these issues can be handled by someone who does consulting on a part-time basis.

Reinert, B., & Buck, E. (1989). Issues in liability insurance and the nurse consultant. *Clinical Nurse Specialist, 3* (1), 42-45.

   This article provides an excellent discussion of professional liability as it relates to nursing consultation. The article also gives general guidelines for purchasing liability insurance.

Scott, L., & Beare, P. (1993). Nurse consultants and professional liability. *Clinical Nurse Specialist, 7* (6), 331-334.

   This article presents issues to consider when choosing insurance to protect against professional liability issues that can arise in consultative practice.

Ethical Issues in
Nursing Consultation

The complex nature of consultation requires a
significant extension of even the most basic ethical
principles. (Newman 1993)

Key terms: professional ethics, moral philosophy, values,
dual relationship, confidentiality, anonymity

Nurses are well accustomed to dealing with ethical dilemmas in clinical practice: being caught between the wishes of a patient or the patient's family and those of the attending physician, being asked by a parent to divulge information given in confidence by an adolescent, and using "floats" as a response to inadequate staffing. Nurse consultants deal with parallel dilemmas: being caught between the needs of a consultee and those of the client system as a whole, being asked by an organizational contact person to divulge information given in confidence by a consultee, and being expected to solve a problem with inadequate resources. The common element in all of these situations is the sense of unease and uncertainty about the rightness of one's decision. This sense of unease reflects that the decision means choosing between competing values. When a problematic situation has these characteristics, it is considered an ethical dilemma.

Members of the helping professions such as nurses and consultants are particularly likely to face ethical dilemmas because they work with individuals who are in somewhat vulnerable or needy positions. Ethical dilemmas also arise for both nurses and consultants because they work in situations involving more than one individual, each of whom has different needs and trusts that these needs will be met. Ethical dilemmas can be particularly burdensome for nurse consultants because of the potentially large number of people (a patient group, entire organization, or community, for instance) who can be directly and indirectly affected by the nurse consultant's values, interpretation of ethical principles, and decisions.

This chapter does not seek to provide answers to ethical dilemmas. Rather, it focuses on the ethical issues and dilemmas that nurse consultants are most likely to confront in practice and offers suggestions for dealing with these dilemmas. The chapter begins with a brief overview of basic ethical concepts. Next, the ethics of consultation, specifically ethical guidelines for consultants, are considered. The third section of the chapter explores the ethically problematic situations that are most likely to arise in a nursing consultation relationship. The chapter ends by offering strategies nurse consultants can use to deal with ethical dilemmas. The following are questions to think about as you read this chapter:

- What ethical obligations do nurse consultants have beyond those to their consultees?

- What examples can you think of in which legal and ethical obligations in nursing consultation might conflict with one another?

- In what ways are nurse consultants most likely to violate the rights of consultees? Why do you think this might occur?

- To what extent is the American Nurses Association *Code for Nurses* useful as a guide to ethical behavior in nursing consultation? What are its limitations?

- What system of beliefs do you use to guide decisions when faced with an ethical dilemma? What implications might this have for your practice of nursing consultation?

Basic Ethical Concepts

Ethics is the study and definition of values concerning how one ought to live (Kimbrough 1985). Because ethics focuses on "oughts," it encompasses norms and beliefs about right and wrong as well as good and bad behavior. The ethics of any group has its roots in the group's value system. Ethics defines for members of a group the everyday judgments they are expected to make in terms of behavior, apart from the provisions of the law and written policy (Kimbrough 1985).

Professional ethics is the system of moral principles or standards that govern professional conduct (Dougherty 1995). Professional ethics, therefore, define professionally acceptable behavior. A professional is considered "ethical" when his/her behavior conforms to the standards of conduct of the particular professional group.

The ethics of any group is characterized by recurring themes of expectations, or *obligations of form*. (Kimbrough 1985). Obligations of form can be worded as "thou shalt" statements or ethical propositions—specific statements about duties, obligations, and responsibilities toward others. Obligations of form for consultants in general and for nurse consultants in particular, are discussed in a later section of this chapter.

Ethical Dilemmas

An ethical dilemma is said to exist when a decision necessitates choosing between competing needs and values. For example, the ethical dilemma in the clinical nursing situation of being asked by a patient not to reveal a diagnosis to her/his family reflects the tension between supporting values concerning autonomy, privacy, and others' rights to know. Nurse consultants can experience this same type of tension, and thus experience an ethical dilemma, when a consultee shares information in confidence (as an extreme example, knowledge of embezzlement) that has implications for the entire client system.

Ethical dilemmas are often manifested as a sense of unease or uncertainty about the decision one needs to make. This reflects that ethical dilemmas frequently represent a "gray zone" in which there is no absolutely right or wrong solution. This sense of unease also reflects that responses to ethical dilemmas threaten compliance with a group's obligations of form. Thus ethical dilemmas present a "tug of war" between competing perspectives of what constitutes right and wrong behavior and a good or bad outcome.

Ethical Decision Making

Most, if not all, decisions in nursing consultation have an ethical component. That is, decisions made in nursing consultation, like those in clinical nursing, involve applying one's values and making value judgments about what constitutes "best" behavior and outcomes. The process of ethical decision making entails applying one's personal values, those core beliefs that "one holds most dear" and uses to guide behavior, as well as the values reflected in the ethics of one's profession, to the decision at hand. Most of us can readily articulate at least some of our personal values—honesty, fairness, and service to others, for example. However, even these values can have different interpretations and applications; what is "fair" in one situation may not seem fair in another or may not be perceived as fair by everyone in the same situation. How one applies one's values reflects a more fundamental and overarching belief system that is influenced by family and friends, life experiences, reading, and contemplation. This overarching belief system constitutes one's moral philosophy—the most fundamental beliefs about how one ought to live, what counts as good reasons for acting one way or another, and what constitutes a good life for human beings (Norman 1983). Understanding one's own moral philosophy as well as that which shapes the ethics of one's profession provides one with decision criteria for responding to ethical dilemmas and making routine decisions. Understanding one's moral philosophy is important because it reveals the biases one brings to problem situations. Traditionally, six major schools of moral philosophy have been recognized; these are summarized briefly in Box 15-1. The relationship between moral philosophy, values, ethics, and ethical decision making is illustrated in Figure 15-1.

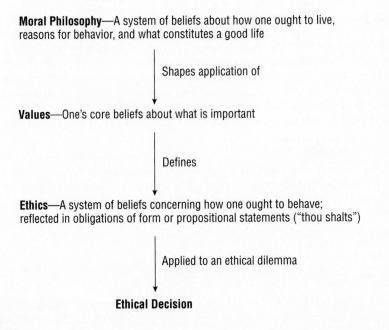

Moral Philosophy—A system of beliefs about how one ought to live, reasons for behavior, and what constitutes a good life

Shapes application of

Values—One's core beliefs about what is important

Defines

Ethics—A system of beliefs concerning how one ought to behave; reflected in obligations of form or propositional statements ("thou shalts")

Applied to an ethical dilemma

Ethical Decision

Figure 15-1.
Relationship between Moral Philosophy, Values, Ethics, and Ethical Decision Making
One's moral philosophy is the foundation of ethical decision making because it shapes the application of one's values and defines how these values will be packaged into a system of beliefs about obligations and how one ought to live.

Box 15-1. Major Schools of Moral Philosophy

Idealism—"Right" behavior is behavior that "naturally" brings happiness; according to idealists, ends justify means

Kantian ethics—Behavior should be guided by categorical imperatives or independent moral obligations that are derived from pure reason and reflect duty and conscience; behavior is judged right or wrong independent of its consequences

Utilitarianism—Proper decisions, actions, or behaviors are those that bring the greatest good to the greatest number; moral values are those that maximize pleasure and minimize pain

Situation ethics—Ethical decisions reflect the spirit of the loving and caring thing to do

Ethical relativism—There is no one set of ethics that is correct for all societies; what is good or right is determined by the cultural context in which a decision is being made

Ethical egoism—Good acts are those that promote a person's self interest.

References: Kimbrough, R. (1985). *Ethics: A course of study for educational leaders*. Arlington, VA: American Association of Counseling and Development; Norman, R. (1983). *The moral philosophers: An introduction to ethics*. Oxford: Clarendon Press.

Ethics and Consultation

Human service professionals such as nurses and consultants are expected by society to interact with their consumers (patients and consultees) according to certain standards of behavior. These standards of conduct are made explicit in each state's Nurse Practice Act and in the standards of practice and codes of ethics developed by different professional organizations. Codes of ethics make explicit the values, assumptions, and expectations a profession has about the form the behavior of its members should take.

Obligations of Form

Obligations of form were defined earlier in this chapter as the recurring themes in a group's ethics. Obligations of form reflect general rules of behavior that are stated more specifically in a profession's code of ethics. The following obligations of form can be identified in codes of ethics (and state Nurse Practice Acts) for nurses and consultants:

- The duty to uphold human rights
- The duty to fulfill commitments
- The duty to practice one's profession competently

Upholding Human Rights   The profession of nursing recognizes the basic human rights of self-determination, freedom from harm, privacy, and fair treatment (American Nurses' Association [ANA] 1985).

Self-Determination   Self-determination is the right of an individual to have a say in his/her own future (ANA 1985). Self-determination encompasses the concepts of willing participation and informed consent. In nursing consultation, the right to self-determination translates into freedom to choose to be a part of the consultation relationship and understanding what involvement in the relationship will entail. In nursing consultation, the consultation contract is the primary vehicle for informed consent.

Freedom from Harm Freedom from harm is the right of a consultee to expect that things will not get worse as a result of participation in the nursing consultation relationship. Nurse consultants need to consider possible physical, emotional, and financial harm to consultees. Consideration needs to be given to harm or side effects that are more likely to be immediate as well as to those that might be delayed. This obligation of form ("do no harm") intertwines with that of self-determination in that part of informed consent involves making consultees aware of possible adverse side effects of the nursing consultation relationship.

In nursing consultation, consideration of a risk/benefit ratio often replaces the absolute obligation to do no harm. For example, a hospital may choose to incur a short-term financial loss while planning and implementing a new program in the hopes of gaining a more competitive market position in the long run.

Privacy The right to privacy addresses expectations about sharing information. Confidentiality is an explicit promise to reveal nothing about an individual except under conditions the individual has agreed to (Corey, Corey, & Callanan 1984; Dougherty 1995). The intent of the right to privacy and confidentiality is to protect individuals from harm.

Fair Treatment Fair treatment refers to providing services that protect human dignity. In nursing consultation, fair treatment encompasses fostering consultee self-sufficiency rather than dependency and acting in the consultee's best interest rather than promoting one's own interests.

Fulfilling Commitments The second obligation of form for nurse consultants is the responsibility to fulfill commitments. In other words, nurse consultants are ethically bound to fulfill the terms set forth in the consultation contract. From an ethical perspective, fulfilling a contract overlaps with a consultee's right to fair treatment. As discussed in Chapter 14, this obligation of form also has a legal component.

Competence Nurses and consultants are expected to practice their profession competently. This obligation of form encompasses the expectation that nurse consultants participate in continuing education as well as in ongoing evaluation of their practice (ANA 1985). A second dimension of the expectation of competence is knowing one's limitations and restricting consultation activities to those compatible with one's skills and expertise.

Ethical Guidelines for Consultants

A profession embodies its obligations of form in its code of ethics and standards of practice. A code of ethics provides general guidelines for acting as a professional and fulfilling the responsibilities associated with being a professional. Ethical codes provide a professional with minimal appropriate behavioral standards for their conduct and relationships with others in carrying out their professional role. By adhering to one's professional code of ethics, one should be safe from both legal action and professional censure (Corey et al. 1984). A code of ethics signifies the maturity of a profession and its attempts to engage in self-regulation. A code of ethics prevents a professional from bending behavior with the exigencies of volatile economics, difficult consultees, and "crass opportunism" (Lewin 1995).

Like other professions, consultation has an ethic, or sense of right and wrong, of its own. However, consultation lacks a codified body of knowledge or a quality control

---

Box 15-2. Ethical Standards for Nurse Consultants: Guidelines from Non-Nursing Helping Professions

Statements from the codes of ethics of non-nursing professional organizations offer the following guidelines for implementing the consultant role:

1. Consultants put the welfare and needs of their consultees and clients ahead of their own.
2. Consultants inform consultees about the nature of the consultation process, including its risks and benefits.
3. Consultants do not accept contracts for activities for which they lack skill or training.
4. Consultants avoid dual relationships that create conflicts of interest and interfere with their effectiveness.
5. Consultants avoid manipulating consultees and creating dependency. Instead, they assist a consultee to develop autonomy in problem solving.
6. Consultants establish contracts with well defined limits and adhere to their contracts.
7. Consultants clarify the nature and purposes of data gathering activities at the outset of the consultation relationship.
8. Consultants choose assessment strategies that are consistent with the needs and purposes of the consultee.
9. Consultants only propose actions for consideration. These actions should fit the needs, values, and resources of the client system.
10. Consultants evaluate the outcomes of their services. They ask for feedback from consultees and peers on a regular basis.
11. Consultants respect the privacy of consultees. This entails informing them of confidentiality and its limits. This also means that participation in consultation activities is voluntary. Consultants respect a consultee's freedom to decline involvement in activities that require disclosure of feelings, values, and personal issues.
12. Consultants are continually involved in professional and personal development activities for the purpose of increasing their knowledge and skills.

Reference: Corey, G., Corey, M., & Callanan, P. (1984). *Issues and ethics in the helping professions* (3rd ed.). Pacific Grove, CA: Brooks-Cole.

---

body (Metzger 1993). This situation stems, in part, from the fact that consultation is generally regarded as an "emerging" profession. It also reflects that consultants come from many disciplines and that consultation encompasses a variety of services provided to individuals and groups with diverse problems across a range of settings. Consequently, many consultants argue that no single code of ethics will ever work for all consultants. Nurse consultants are left then, with applying and adapting the code of ethics of the nursing profession (including the standards of practice established by its specialty organizations) and ethical codes from other helping professions to situations and types of relationships that differ from those for which the codes were intended (Dougherty 1995).

Some professional organizations such as the American Psychological Association, the American Society for Training and Development, the Institute of Management

---

Box 15-3. Ethical Standards for Nurse Consultants: Guidelines from the American Nurses' Association Code for Nurses

The following statements from the American Nurses' Association *Code for Nurses* (1985) seem particularly applicable as guidelines for implementing the role of nurse consultant:

The nurse provides services with respect for human dignity and the uniqueness of the client...
Application to nursing consultation:
• Involve consultees in the nursing consultation process
• Provide informed consent about what the consultation relationship will involve
• Individualize consultation activities
• Foster consultee self-reliance

The nurse safeguards the client's right to privacy by judiciously protecting information of a confidential nature.
Application to nursing consultation:
• Be clear about limits of confidentiality
• Use professional judgment and discretion
• Provide anonymity when information must be shared

The nurse assumes responsibility and accountability for individual nursing judgments and actions.
Application to nursing consultation:
• Areas of responsibility for a nurse consultant are problem identification, action planning, evaluation, and disengagement
• Be aware of the limits of one's competence
• Evaluate the effectiveness of one's performance as a nurse consultant as well as the effectiveness of specific interactions and interventions

The nurse maintains competence in nursing.
Application to nursing consultation:
• Engage in personal and professional development activities
• Seek feedback from peers about one's skills

The nurse exercises informed judgment and uses individual competence as qualifications and criteria in seeking consultation and accepting responsibilities.
Application to nursing consultation:
• Know and respect personal limits in knowledge and skills
• Seek consultation and refer when appropriate
• Avoid misrepresentation of abilities and qualifications

Reference: American Nurses Association. (1985). *Code for nurses with interpretive statements.* Kansas City, MO: Author

---

Consultants, and the American Association of Counseling and Development do provide specific guidelines for consultation activities that organizational members might undertake. Selected statements from the ethical codes of these non-nursing helping organizations are shown in Box 15-2.

The American Nurses Association *Code for Nurses* (1985) offers guidelines primarily for direct care nursing activities. As discussed in Chapter 1, however, nursing consultation is an indirect care activity and only selected statements from the ANA *Code* seem particularly applicable to nursing consultation activities. These statements and their application to nursing consultation are highlighted in Box 15-3 on the previous page.

To summarize, formal guidelines for the ethical practice of consultation, specifically nursing consultation, are not currently available. At the same time, existing codes of ethics provide only limited guidance for the practice of nursing consultation. As a result, nurse consultants bear heavy personal responsibility for the consequences of their decisions and actions as professional nurse consultants (Newman 1993).

Ethically Problematic Situations for Nurse Consultants

The consultation relationship has been defined as a tripartite, voluntary, peer relationship that focuses on work-related rather than personal problems of consultees. These characteristics of the nursing consultation relationship give rise to ethical dilemmas about responsibility, power, and dual relationships.

Responsibility Dilemmas

The tripartite nature of the consultation relationship can create problems in terms of determining to whom the nurse consultant's responsibility extends. Responsibility dilemmas reflect tension in terms of fulfilling obligations of form related to protecting human rights, freedom from harm and fair treatment.

Usually, a nurse consultant's primary responsibility is considered to be to the consultee with whom the consultant is directly working in the consultation relationship. It is often difficult to conceptualize responsibility to the client since clients do not usually take an active part in the consultation process and do not have an opportunity to voice and advance their goals and priorities. In cases where the client is an individual patient or type of patient (a group defined by a particular illness, for example), it is unlikely that the client is even aware that consultation on his/her behalf is taking place. Clients are affected by consultation then, but without the benefit of participating in the consultation process (this creates an additional dilemma around the right to self-determination).

One response or view to responsibility dilemmas is that a consultant's responsibility extends to clients as well as to others who may be victims or beneficiaries of the nursing consultation relationship. This view of responsibility is consistent with that proposed in Chapter 1 of this text. That is, nurse consultants need to consider the risks and benefits of any nursing consultation action on actual and potential patients, because patients—who can be either clients or stakeholders—are always the ultimate beneficiaries of a nursing consultation relationship. The ethical dilemma associated with this view of responsibility is determining how much responsibility is then owed to consultees. Also, if patients are only stakeholders, how much responsibility is owed to them as compared to the client (who might be an organization)?

Another view of responsibility in nursing consultation is that a consultant's primary responsibility is to the client and that responsibility to the consultee and stakeholders (including patients) is only a secondary obligation. The situation becomes even more confusing when the consultation has been arranged by a contact person such as an administrator in the client organization. In these situations, is the nurse consultant responsible to the contact person, the organization, the client, or the consultee?

In summary, the implications and difficulty of the tripartite nature of nursing consultation relationships is that nurse consultants are responsible for the impact of their

---

Box 15-4. A Potential Misuse of Expert Power: The "Halo Effect"

A family nurse practitioner (FNP) is asked to provide consultation to a school district about a comprehensive health education curriculum. The curriculum is to include topics such as AIDS, eating disorders, violence, substance abuse, depression, and suicide. The school district also wants the FNP to identify and develop teachers for this curriculum. The FNP was offered this opportunity because of a reputation of being a skilled and empathetic clinician who is "good with teens." The FNP accepts the consultation opportunity because of a desire to help.

- Was there a misuse of expert power in this situation?

---

services on individuals with whom they may have little contact (Herlihy & Corey 1992). The nature of the nursing consultation relationship can create ethical dilemmas in terms of target of responsibility. These dilemmas occur because of tension upholding the human rights of fair treatment and freedom from harm.

Misuse of Power

The power relationship between a nurse consultant and consultee is complex. The consultation relationship is intended to be one of peers; the nurse consultant shares expertise and knowledge and works with a consultee to resolve a problem. At the same time, the nurse consultant-consultee relationship is inherently one of unequal power. The fact that the consultee is seeking help implies that the consultee is lacking and in need of something (knowledge or skills) that the nurse consultant has (Herlihy & Corey 1995; Sneed 1991). Nurse consultants need to be aware of the potential for misusing their power and the possibility of manipulating and inappropriately influencing a needy consultee's attitudes and behavior. Misuse of power can create dependency and conflicts of interest and create tension in terms of satisfying obligations of form related to providing fair treatment, freedom from harm, and fulfilling commitments.

Recall from Chapter 5 that nurse consultants are most likely to have expert power (related to specialized and needed knowledge and skills) and personal power (related to the ability to develop followers through personal characteristics such as charisma and friendship tactics). These forms of power can be blatantly as well as more subtly misused.

Misuse of Expert Power Perceived expertise is usually the reason for asking a specific nurse to provide consultation. The appropriate and ethical use of expertise is to help consultees increase their own problem-solving abilities. Expertise is misused when knowledge of problem-solving skills is withheld to keep a consultee in a dependent position. Nurse consultants may also foster consultee dependency and prolong a consultation relationship in order to meet financial needs or to gain personal gratification through a sense of significance (Corey et al. 1984; Newman 1993). These actions violate obligations of form related to self-determination, fair treatment, freedom from harm, and fulfilling contracts. Professional codes of ethics (for example, those of the American Association of Counseling and Development) speak specifically against creating dependency.

Expert power can create further ethical dilemmas due to its "halo effect." That is, consultees (and nurse consultants themselves) may generalize a consultant's expertise in one area to other areas. This violates obligations of form related to competence.

Box 15-5. Potential Misuse of Personal Power: Promoting Self-Interests

A nurse consultant is working with the nurse-managers in a large health maintenance organization (HMO) to help them develop a telephone triage system. Over the course of several weeks, the nurse consultant develops rapport and a friendly, trusting relationship with several of the nurse-managers. While the nurse consultant and the nurse-managers are having coffee after one of the work sessions, one of the nurse-managers reveals rumors about the impending resignation of two top administrators at the same time that an opening is planned for a major satellite clinic in the HMO system. Based on this information, the nurse consultant schedules an appointment with the chief administrative officer of the HMO to discuss interest in pursuing administrative level full-time employment in the system.

• Was there a misuse of personal power in this situation?

Expert power is also misused when nurse consultants allow their qualifications to be misrepresented or attempt to intervene in areas outside their scope of competence. In addition to being unethical, attempting to exercise expert power in areas outside of one's actual range of expertise can "backfire" and decrease a nurse consultant's perceived power if consultation efforts are unsuccessful (Sneed 1991). Furthermore, as mentioned in Chapter 14, practicing nursing consultation in areas outside of one's expertise can result in legal action against the nurse consultant for malpractice or breach of contract. Box 15-4 on the previous page presents a scenario illustrating the problem of the "halo effect."

Misuse of Personal Power   A second source of power for nurse consultants is personal power. Personal power is useful in nursing consultation because it facilitates the establishment of trust and rapport between a nurse consultant and consultee. Personal power is misused, however, when a nurse consultant uses charisma and friendship tactics to enter into or use a consultation relationship for reasons of self-interest. These actions create a conflict of interest and may cause the nurse consultant to lose objectivity about the consultation situation. Misusing one's personal power to advance self-interests in a nursing consultation relationship violates obligations of form regarding self-determination, protection from harm, fair treatment, and fulfilling commitments. Box 15-5 presents a situation that involves a potential misuse of personal power.

Dual Relationships

A dual relationship occurs when "a professional assumes two roles simultaneously or sequentially with a person seeking help" (Herlihy & Corey 1992). Assuming a dual role reflects trying to accommodate a professional role plus a personal, social, or financial relationship, or to fill two conflicting professional roles. It is easy for nurse consultants to end up in dual relationships because consultation interventions can be difficult to define and often encompass a variety of intertwined needs and issues. Dual relationships tend to create conflicts of interest and, therefore, violate obligations of form related to protection from harm, fair treatment, and fulfilling commitments.

Dual relationships also cause incompatible behavioral expectations for both the consultee and nurse consultant. Combining a social or financial relationship with a professional relationship such as that of nurse consultant, for example, can result in decisions and actions that promote the consultant's self-interest but collide with what

---

Box 15-6. "Blurred Boundaries" in Nursing Consultation

An independent nurse consultant with a background in management and psychiatric nursing (including experience with group therapy) is hired to facilitate a team-building retreat with the nursing staff of two recently merged air ambulance services. As the retreat gets underway and the nurse consultant is assessing the needs of the group, it becomes apparent that many of the nurses have unresolved feelings about the merger and how it has affected them on a personal level. For some workers, feelings of grief over loss of former coworkers has triggered unfinished business in regard to grieving other losses. For other nurses, the key issues have to do with loss of trust, betrayal, financial impact of decreased work hours, and job insecurity. The nurse consultant decides it is more important to focus on these individual needs rather than on team building. During the remainder of the retreat, the nurse consultant meets with staff individually and in small groups to deal with these issues.

- Did this nurse consultant take on a dual role? If so, was it justified?

---

would be in the best interest of a consultee or client. Dual relationships can cause low morale within a consultee group if one group member is singled out for special treatment by the nurse consultant. Dual relationships can also undermine the credibility of the nurse consultant (and the entire profession) if they are perceived as "cheating" the client system of full attention and loyalty (Herlihy & Corey 1992). The dual relationships that are particularly likely to be problematic for nurse consultants are those of consultant/supervisor, consultant/counselor, and consultant/clinician (caregiver).

Nurse Consultant/Supervisor The potential for a nurse consultant to take on a second role as supervisor exists because it is often hard to determine when the feedback given to consultees as a part of the nursing consultation process becomes supervisory evaluation (Herlihy & Corey 1992). This can be especially problematic in internal consultation situations because internal nurse consultants often hold administrative or managerial roles within the client system.

Assuming a supervisory role while providing nursing consultation services violates the peer nature of the consultation relationship as supervision involves making judgments about and having control over a supervisee (Dougherty 1995). By the same token, the consultation relationship is built on values of consultee growth and formative evaluation and feedback.

The dual role of nurse consultant/supervisor creates further dilemmas because a supervisor is expected to serve not only the supervisee's interests (such as fair performance evaluation and facilitation or protection of continued employment) but the interests of the employing agency and the public (such as safe practice and cost-containment). Finally, the dual role of nurse consultant/supervisor creates an ethical dilemma related to expectations to share information with parties at interest and yet maintain the confidentiality of the consultation relationship (Herlihy & Corey 1992).

Nurse Consultant/Counselor Because nurses have a personal helping orientation, it can be difficult for them to draw the line between consulting and counseling when they are acting as nurse consultants. Indeed, there is often a fine line between consultation interventions and counseling. When, for example, does acknowledging a consultee's negative emotions become counseling about these emotions? Also, in many nursing consultation situations, the boundaries between personal and work-related

---

Box 15-7. An Ethically Mandated Dual Relationship

A clinical nurse specialist (CNS) is asked by nursing staff to help them develop interventions for dealing with a post-myocardial infarction patient's delirium and disorientation. The staff insists these conditions are just normal psychological reactions to adjusting to the seriousness of the medical condition. The staff further insists that the patient is medically stable and just needs some cognitive interventions such as "those that are used in nursing homes." The CNS, however, recognizes that these reactions of the patient may signal a change in medical condition or an adverse reaction to a medication the patient is taking. Accordingly, the CNS immediately orders some laboratory studies, conducts a neurological screening assessment, and contacts the patient's physician rather than proceed to work with staff to develop cognitive interventions.

• Was assuming a dual role justified in this situation?

---

issues are blurred. The problem of blurred boundaries and a potential dual relationship is illustrated in the scenario presented in Box 15-6 on the previous page.

Assuming a dual role as nurse consultant and counselor can be problematic for several reasons. First, focusing on a consultee's emotional needs and issues tends to disrupt the peer relationship on which effective consultation practice is built and emphasize instead, the neediness and vulnerability of the consultee; this creates a hierarchical or uneven relationship. Secondly, adding the role of counselor to that of nurse consultant contaminates, de-emphasizes, and possibly dislocates, the work-related focus of the consultation relationship. In some cases, this change in emphasis from work-related to personal problems can be interpreted as a breach of contract and as cheating a client system of the work-related problem-solving services for which it contracted. This type of dual relationship, therefore, violates obligations of form related to fulfilling commitments.

Nurse Consultant/Clinician Nurse consultants who are providing consultation about patient care issues may face the dilemma of needing to determine when it is appropriate and inappropriate to assume the simultaneous role of clinician and direct caregiver. While the nurse consultant usually needs to step back and help nursing staff learn to problem solve a patient care problem on its own, there are times when patient safety issues warrant stepping in and taking on this dual role. In consulting situations where patient care is seriously compromised and the nurse consultee is not able to make the decisions or provide the care needed, the nurse consultant is legally and ethically bound to step in and assume clinical responsibility for the patient (Barron 1989). Box 15-7 illustrates an extreme situation in which a nurse consultant needs to assume a dual role on a temporary basis.

Confidentiality

While confidentiality is a professional expectation and obligation of form for consultants, how it is enacted is increasingly being determined by the law. Child abuse reporting laws and the duty to warn and protect potential victims are just two of the legal limits that have been set in regard to confidentiality. In nursing consultation situations, any limits to confidentiality should be explicitly identified in the nursing consultation contract. The contract should identify what information can be shared and how it is to be shared (for example, only verbally), as well as with whom it can be

---

Box 15-8. An Ethical Dilemma Associated with Confidentiality

A nurse consultant is asked to work with the nurse-managers in a large medical center to help them implement a plan for restructuring the organization. Specific interventions include working with the nurse-managers to develop communication, decision-making, and delegation skills. At the outset of the consultation, it was agreed that the nurse consultant would not be asked to give opinions about the performance of any of the consultees. It was also agreed that all aspects of the consultation would remain confidential.

A couple months into the consultation relationship, the chief administrator (who was the initial contact for the consultation and who signed the contract) asks the nurse consultant about the performance of one particular nurse-manager to whom they are considering offering a promotion. The administrator assures the nurse consultant that this information will go no further. When the nurse consultant reminds the administrator that sharing this type of information is strictly precluded by the consultation contract, the administrator becomes angry, demands that the information be shared, and threatens to terminate the consultation relationship if it is not.

---

shared and under what circumstances (for example, only "in emergency" or at the completion of the consultation engagement).

Confidentiality can present the nurse consultant with the ethical dilemma of having important information but not being able to use it. It is not uncommon that during the course of a nursing consultation relationship, a consultee will develop enough trust and rapport with a nurse consultant that information is shared with the nurse consultant on a private basis. Accepting information under these conditions may place the nurse consultant in the uncomfortable position of having information that is important to the consultation process or the well-being of the client system but not being able to use it. Accepting this information also supports a system's norm of secrecy and is antithetical to the desired openness of the nursing consultation relationship. On the other hand, if the information is rejected, the nurse consultant may miss valuable information and compromise the trust relationship that has been established with the consultee.

To deal with this type of dilemma, consultants frequently substitute a promise of anonymity for one of confidentiality. Anonymity allows information to be used as long as its source is protected (Dougherty 1995). Anonymity, therefore, has the advantage of facilitating the flow of information critical to successful consultation. A typical dilemma presented by obligations of form related to confidentiality forms the basis for the scenario presented in Box 15-8.

Informed Consent and Voluntary Participation

Informed consent means that participation in a nursing consultation relationship is voluntary and based on full awareness of the purpose, nature, risks, benefits, and potential outcomes of the relationship (Newman 1993). Informed consent implies the freedom to choose from among alternatives, including nonparticipation. As mentioned earlier, the nursing consultation contract is the primary vehicle for informed consent in a nursing consultation relationship. Two types of liability can arise from failure to obtain informed consent: negligence/malpractice and breach of contract (Corey et al. 1984).

Trying to uphold obligations of form related to informed consent and self-determination can create ethical dilemmas for a nurse consultant. For example, in organizational consulting situations (where the organization is the client and initial contact has been made by someone in the administrative hierarchy of the organization), administration may require workers (consultees) to participate in the nursing consultation process. Workers (for example, nursing staff) fear negative consequences if they refuse, so they participate when they would rather not. Nurse consultants who decline a consultation opportunity in this type of situation forego the opportunity to become involved in helping (and learning from helping) the consultees and client system. On the other hand, proceeding with a nursing consultation engagement in a situation where the consultees are not truly voluntary participants undermines the obligation of form related to self-determination. It also creates the challenge of needing to overcome consultee resistance in order to develop an effective problem-solving relationship. In situations where there is less than voluntary participation in the nursing consultation process, the nurse consultant should, at the very least, openly acknowledge the dilemma and discuss the accompanying issues with the consultees.

In nursing consultation, informed consent and self-determination also means that consultees have the freedom to do whatever they wish with a nurse consultant's opinions and recommendations. The positive aspect of self-determination and informed consent is that it relieves the nurse consultant of any responsibility for the consultee's behavior. This relief may be more perceived than real, however. For example, what (and to whom) is a nurse consultant's responsibility when a consultee's refusal to participate could bring harm to the client or client system?

Dealing with Ethical Dilemmas

Thus far, the discussion in this chapter has focused on "consciousness-raising" or increasing awareness about the types of situations that can create ethical dilemmas for nurse consultants. Unfortunately, there is no way of avoiding these situations and dilemmas and there are no absolute strategies for resolving them. Nurse consultants can, however, rely on some general guidelines—in addition to state Nurse Practice Acts, standards of practice, and existing professional codes of ethics—when formulating a response to an ethical dilemma.

Earlier in this chapter, an ethical dilemma was defined as occurring when the need to make a decision about an appropriate course of action arouses feelings of unease or uncertainty because the decision entails choosing between competing values. The following steps can be used to facilitate decision making in these situations:

1. Identify the problem or dilemma.

2. Identify the ethical issues involved. Specifically, what obligations of form are being threatened?

3. Review relevant professional guidelines (for example, state Nurse Practice Acts and organizational policies).

4. Identify possible courses of action and the most likely consequences of each.

5. Obtain consultation from a colleague.

6. Determine the best course of action for the circumstances (Corey et al. 1984; Dougherty 1995).

From a legal perspective, the fifth step in this process ("consult with a colleague") is particularly important. If a colleague agrees with the course of action that has been taken, there is an increased likelihood of being able to demonstrate that a decision was both made in good faith and was reasonably prudent.

Lewin (1995) offers additional "tests" that can be applied when one has doubts about actions in regard to an ethical dilemma. First, validate actions for consistency with one's professional codes. If uncertainty about one's actions remains, apply the *"New York Times* rule": Don't do anything you wouldn't want to read about in the banner headlines of the *New York Times*. If, after this test, "right" or "best" actions are still ambiguous, err on the side of omission rather than commission. That is, don't do something that might be interpreted as ethically ambiguous. As a final guideline for dealing with ethical dilemmas, the following is worth keeping in mind:

> The ethical basis of consulting boils down to the eternal Golden Rule: Do unto others as you would have them to unto you. That means show your clients [consultees] respect, discretion, honesty, and appropriateness as we would have them do unto us. (Lewin 1995).

A nurse consultant can minimize the likelihood of making an inappropriate or unethical decision by objectively confronting each consultation task and situation. Incorporating values of consultee self-determination, growth, and learning into one's practice of nursing consultation can help to prevent the misuse of power, creation of dependency, and manipulation of the consultee and consultation relationship for personal gain. Making use of all available resources, including assessment data and consultation with colleagues, to help determine an appropriate course of action can help the nurse consultant identify the issues and consequences associated with different behaviors and interventions. Finally, engaging in reflection of one's own moral philosophy, self-evaluation, and professional growth activities sensitizes a nurse consultant to personal values and biases that can precipitate an ethical dilemma (Lippitt & Lippitt 1986).

Chapter Summary

In nursing consultation, ethical dilemmas arise because consultation is a tripartite helping relationship that entails competing needs of consultees, clients, stakeholders, and the nurse consultant. Ethically problematic situations rarely occur in isolation and instead, tend to arise from and present as a set of intertwined issues and dilemmas. Likewise, ethical obligations can intertwine or conflict with other professional and legal obligations. Nurse consultants are faced with dealing with ethical dilemmas by translating and applying ethical standards from related helping professions and the direct care-oriented *Code for Nurses*, seeking consultation from peers, and assuming personal values of self-evaluation and professional growth.

Applying Chapter Content

- Analyze the scenarios presented in Boxes 15-4, 15-5, 15-6, 15-7, and 15-8 and answer the following questions:

  What are the specific ethical issues, potential violations of obligations of form, and other potential problems in the scenario?

  Critique the nurse consultant's response to the situation. Identify the moral philosophy that is reflected in the response.

  What possible harm could result from the nurse consultant's response?

  Develop an ethically acceptable alternative course of action. Identify the moral philosophy that underpins this course of action.

- What potential ethical issues and dilemmas are you most likely to face in your own practice of nursing consultation? What kind of harm might arise from these issues? How would you respond to these dilemmas?

References

American Nurses Association. (1985). *Code for nurses with interpretive statements.* Kansas City, MO: Author.

Barron, A. (1989). The CNS as consultant. In A. Hamric & J. Spross (Eds.), *The clinical nurse specialist in theory and practice* (2nd ed., pp. 125-146). Philadelphia: Saunders.

Corey, G., Corey, M., & Callanan, P. (1984). *Issues and ethics in the helping professions* (3rd ed.). Pacific Grove, CA: Brooks-Cole.

Dougherty, A. (1995). *Consultation: Practice and perspectives in school and community settings* (2nd ed.). Pacific Grove, CA: Brooks-Cole.

Herlihy, B., & Corey, G. (1992). *Dual relationships in counseling.* Alexandria, VA: American Association of Counseling and Development.

Kimbrough, R. (1985). *Ethics: A course of study for educational leaders.* Arlington, VA: American Association for School Administrators.

Lewin, M. (1995). *The overnight consultant.* New York: John Wiley & Sons.

Lippitt, G., & Lippitt, R. (1986). *The consulting process in action* (2nd ed.). San Diego: University Associates.

Metzger, R. (1993). *Developing a consulting practice.* Newbury Park, CA: Sage.

Newman, J. (1993). Ethical issues in consultation. *Journal of Counseling and Development, 72,* 148-156.

Norman, R. (1983). *The moral philosophers: An introduction to ethics.* Oxford: Clarendon Press.

Sneed, N. (1991). Power: Its use and potential for misuse by nurse consultants. *Clinical Nurse Specialist, 5* (1), 58-62.

Additional Readings

Corey, G., Corey, M., & Callanan, P. (1984). *Issues and ethics in the helping professions* (3rd ed.). Pacific Grove, CA: Brooks-Cole.
While this text primarily addresses ethical issues that are likely to be encountered by counselors, much of the discussion is applicable to consultants. The discussions of confidentiality (Chapter 6), dual relationships (Chapter 7), and working with groups (Chapter 11) are especially pertinent to consultation.

Dougherty, A. (1995). *Consultation: Practice and perspectives in school and community settings* (2nd ed.). Pacific Grove, CA: Brooks-Cole.
Chapter 7 provides an in-depth discussion of ethical dilemmas faced by human service consultants. Case studies and examples of these different dilemmas are included.

Herlihy, B., & Corey, G. (1992). *Dual relationships in counseling.* Alexandria, VA: American Association of Counseling and Development.
Chapter 1 of this book gives an overview of different types of dual relationships and the potential problems they can create. Chapter 11 specifically addresses dual relationships that can confound the consultation process.

Lewin, M. (1995). *The overnight consultant.* New York: John Wiley & Sons.
Chapter 9 of this book offers guidelines for dealing with ethical dilemmas.

Lippitt, G., & Lippitt, R. (1986). *The consulting process in action* (2nd ed.). San Diego: University Associates.

Chapter 5 presents an excellent discussion of common ethical dilemmas in consulting. The authors also propose a code of ethics for consultants and share decision-making processes that underlie resolving a specific ethical dilemma.

Newman, J. (1993). Ethical issues in consultation. *Journal of Counseling and Development, 72,* 148-156.

This article emphasizes the complex nature of consulting relationships and addresses ethical issues as they relate to four aspects of consultation: relationship issues, the role of values, consultant competence, and consultation interventions.

Norman, R. (1983). *The moral philosophers: An introduction to ethics.* Oxford: Clarendon Press.

This text offers a comprehensive overview of different schools of ethical thought.

Schein, E. (1987). *Process consultation, volume II: Lessons for managers and consultants.* Reading, MA: Addison-Wesley.

Chapter 11 discusses the ethical dilemma of balancing the competing interests of different members of a client system. The chapter includes a case study of this type of dilemma occurring in an organizational consultation situation.

Sneed, N. (1991). Power: Its use and potential for misuse by nurse consultants. *Clinical Nurse Specialist, 5* (1), 58-62.

This article provides an excellent review of the types of power a nurse consultant has as well as examples of how these different types of power can be misused in a consultative relationship.

Ulschak, F., & SnowAntle, S. (1990). *Consultation skills for health care professionals.* San Francisco: Jossey-Bass.

Chapter 10 discusses ethical issues and common pitfalls that are encountered in internal consulting situations.

16

Nurses as Legal Consultants

*The use of nurses as legal consultants represents
an untapped resource for the attorney trying a case
involving an injured party.* (Faherty 1991b)

Key terms: defendant, plaintiff, expert witness, malpractice,
negligence, tort, standard of care

A nurse practitioner receives a call from an attorney who is defending another nurse practitioner against charges of malpractice. At issue is whether the nurse practitioner failed to diagnose and properly treat a patient with bacterial meningitis. As a result of the disease, the 12-year-old patient lost both legs. The attorney wants the plaintiff's medical records reviewed in order to determine whether the care given by the nurse practitioner (defendant) was consistent with current standards of practice. In this same case, the plaintiff's attorney is seeking consultation from a nurse with rehabilitation expertise for help in determining the amount of financial compensation that should be sought for the plaintiff's loss. In both of these scenarios, nurses are being asked to serve as expert witnesses and nurse legal consultants.

At the beginning of this text, nursing consultation was defined as "working with individuals and groups to help them resolve actual or potential problems related to the health status of clients or health care delivery." Nurse legal consultants (NLCs) are registered nurses who use their clinical knowledge and expertise to assist attorneys in the evaluation of cases where health care delivery and legal issues overlap, so that the trier of fact (a judge or jury) will be convinced of the validity of the client's position ("Scope and Standards" 1995; Wetther 1993). More specifically, NLCs work with attorneys to help them resolve cases that involve charges of loss (change in health status) that have been suffered as a result of the delivery of allegedly inappropriate or substandard nursing care, injury, or exposure to hazardous products or environmental conditions.

Legal consulting by nurses is presented in this chapter as an example of nurses working as entrepreneurs with professionals in other disciplines to uphold standards of nursing care and protect the public's health. Thus the practice of legal consulting is an example of interdisciplinary external nursing consultation. The interactions and activities of NLCs highlight the unique and varied expertise of nurses and illustrate how nurses can contribute their expertise in consulting relationships with professionals from other disciplines to help resolve health-related issues.

This chapter begins with a description of how NLCs approach consulting relationships and define their goals and objectives. It also explores interventions that are typical of NLCs and the types of practice patterns in which NLCs tend to be engaged. The next section focuses on how NLCs implement the consultation process. The final portion of the chapter identifies opportunities and challenges for NLCs. As you read this chapter, think about the following questions:

- How could your own expertise be used in medical/nursing-legal cases?

- What are your feelings about working for attorneys of plaintiffs versus attorneys of defendants in medical-legal cases? How might this affect your ability to be an effective nurse legal consultant?

- For what types of issues or cases might the services of a nurse legal consultant be useful in your own practice situation?

Approach to Consultation

Nurse legal consulting is defined by a characteristic consultation relationship and a distinct set of goals and objectives. In addition to giving advice, NLCs perform a variety of activities or interventions. Nurse legal consultants implement the consultation process through a variety of practice patterns. The manner in which NLCs approach the consultation relationship and the consultation process is shaped by the unique characteristics of the problems with which they tend to become involved. Box 16-1 provides an overview of nurse legal consulting and highlights characteristics of this specialized area of consultation practice.

The Nursing Consultation Relationship

The consultation triad in the nurse legal consulting relationship most frequently consists of the NLC, the attorney (who is the consultee), and the attorney's client. Less frequently, a nurse consultant may be appointed to serve as an expert witness by the court. In this situation, the court becomes the consultee. In nurse legal consulting, the client system is redefined and excludes the consultee. The client system in the nurse legal consulting relationship is comprised of the client and other individuals such as family members or coworkers who are also affected by the problem situation.

Nurse legal consultants are external consultants. That is, they are not members of the client system. In nurse legal consulting, internal consultation would create a conflict of interest and dual relationship and could appear to compromise objectivity. While it is tempting to think of NLCs who work in-house as members of an attorney's staff as internal consultants, because they are not members of the *client* system they are still functioning as external consultants.

Goals and Objectives

The ultimate goal of nurse legal consultation is to help the employing attorney's client obtain justice. For a defendant, justice means being found not guilty on charges of malpractice, negligence, or having otherwise inflicted harm. Justice for a plaintiff is a remedy or compensation commensurate with losses that have been incurred. An intermediate goal or immediate objective of a NLC is to provide an attorney with an objective analysis of the nursing care issues in a case so that they can achieve justice for their client. Figure 16-1 illustrates the nurse legal consulting relationship and its goals and objectives.

Interventions

In many nursing consultation relationships, the nurse consultant is an option-giver who develops an action plan for implementation by the consultee. While NLCs may

---

Box 16-1. Overview of Nurse Legal Consulting

The specialty role of nurse legal consultant has only been recognized since the 1980s. It was in 1990 that the American Association of Legal Nurse Consultants was established (Wetther 1993). There is increasing recognition among the legal community, however, of the comprehensive nature of NLCs' contributions to legal actions that involve nursing and health care delivery issues.

Nurse legal consultants are involved primarily in civil rather than criminal cases. They essentially serve as expert witnesses and are employed by either a plaintiff's or defendant's attorney to assist in legal actions where explanations or interpretations of medical evidence or nursing practice is necessary (Perry 1992). As an expert witness, a NLC may provide in-court testimony as well as out-of-court consultation. Providing testimony may be the most visible part of the NLC role. However, most work of NLCs is actually done "behind-the-scenes." Less than 1% of all medical-legal cases actually go to trial, and educating attorneys is considered a major role for NLCs (Faherty 1991b).

The information developed by a NLC may help an attorney decide whether to pursue a case or not. It may also enable a case to be settled without having to go to trial. In malpractice cases, a nurse expert witness can protect a nurse defendant from unjust accusations or can help a plaintiff obtain justice (frequently in the form of financial compensation for harm attributable to allegedly substandard or inappropriate nursing care). In either situation, the NLC is ultimately protecting standards of practice and serving as an advocate for the nursing profession and patients (the public). In other cases such as product liability and toxic tort litigation, the NLC protects society by helping to call attention to specific health risks.

Currently, there are no established programs for specifically preparing nurses to function as legal consultants. Most NLCs "fall into" the role and gain needed knowledge and skills through on-the-job training, self-study, and continuing education programs.

General agreement exists that current clinical experience and expertise is the most important credential for a NLC (Faherty 1991b, 1995; Perry 1992; Wetther 1993). The best NLC for any case is one whose current clinical experience involves assessing, planning, and implementing care for patients similar to the plaintiff. Generally, a minimum of five years of clinical experience in more than one clinical setting is considered necessary for establishing expert credentials (Perry 1992). In addition to current clinical experience, recommended evidence for qualification as an expert includes educational preparation, professional association memberships, evidence of continuing education, and specialty

---

limit their activities to giving advice and making recommendations (a solution-prescription or doctor-patient interaction pattern), in many cases they are also actively involved in implementing the agreed upon interventions. This is consistent with the solution-provision or purchase of expertise interaction pattern that was described in Chapter 3.

The interventions in which NLCs are involved are primarily educational, investigational, interpretive, and organizational in nature. Key activities of NLCs are

Box 16-1. *(continued)*

certification (Faherty 1995). NLCs also need to be familiar with health care regulations and statutes that govern the specific segment of the health care industry (for example, long-term care, acute care settings, health maintenance organizations) about which they are providing consultation (Schabes 1992). Being a member of a nursing faculty, especially if one's responsibilities include the clinical supervision of students, is considered a particularly strong credential since it implies clinical competence as well as familiarity with current standards of nursing practice and health care delivery (Faherty 1991b).

A general understanding and working knowledge of the legal system is considered a helpful but not crucial credential for a NLC (Davis 1991; Faherty 1991b, 1995; Perry 1992). The employing attorney should be willing to provide the necessary legal and procedural guidance. More important than legal experience are personal traits such as analytic and organizational skills, self-direction, creativity, objectivity, communication and interpersonal skills, and the ability to work with people under difficult and trying circumstances (Wetther 1993).

Finally, to be effective, NLCs must have a clear sense of ethical standards of behavior, be clear regarding the limits of their expertise, and avoid offering opinions about issues that fall outside of their area of expertise or scope of knowledge ("Scope and Standards" 1995). For example, it would be inappropriate for a nurse with trauma expertise to help determine a client's long-term needs for health care services, rehabilitation, and medical equipment. Likewise, it is not appropriate for a nurse to estimate life expectancy; this should be done instead by an actuary or medical consultant. Nurse legal consultants should also avoid involvement in cases involving institutions with whom they have a current or previous employment or consulting relationship, as this could raise questions about a conflict of interest ("Scope and Standards" 1995). Finally, NLCs need to recognize that they can offer expert opinion on nursing care—but not the physician-delivered medical care—of a given case.

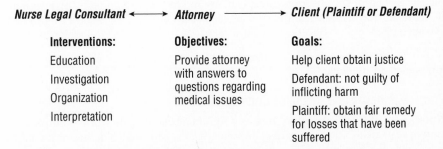

Figure 16-1. The Nurse Legal Consulting Relationship and its Goals and Objectives

The NLC's educational, investigational, organizational, and interpretive interventions help provide an attorney with answers to questions regarding the medical issues in a case. This, in turn, helps the attorney achieve a favorable outcome for the client. For both a plaintiff and a defendant, a favorable outcome is intended to represent the ultimate goal of justice.

screening cases, interpreting caregiving activities, and organizing and reviewing records.

Screening Cases Nurse legal consultants can screen a case to help an attorney decide whether to pursue the case as well as whether to try to reach an out-of-court resolution or take a case to trial. Nurse legal consultants can help a defendant's attorney identify a potentially problematic case. Likewise, NLCs can help a plaintiff's attorney understand weaknesses in their case or strengths of the defense's case. Screening cases also involves recommending potential (additional) defendants. For a defendant, this means identifying another party who shares liability and can decrease the defendant's share of blame. Screening cases involves reviewing a complete set of medical records and usually takes 1–6 hours of time (Milazzo 1993).

Interpreting Caregiving Activities In malpractice cases, a major contribution of NLCs is defining deviations from and adherence to acceptable standards of nursing care. Educating an attorney about actions that represent adherence to standards of care or acceptable variations in operating style enables the attorney to determine the merits of a negligence or malpractice case and to avoid arguing about actions that can be easily defended. Interpreting standards of care can involve reviewing the client's medical record, conducting interviews with coworkers and experts, as well as reviewing nurse practice acts, specialty organization standards of practice, agency policies and procedures, and nursing textbooks (Perry 1992). Additional dimensions of interpreting the adherence of care to acceptable standards are discussed later in this chapter.

Organizing and Reviewing Records In addition to a patient's medical record, records of interest in medical-legal cases can include deposition transcripts and institutional policies and procedures. A purpose of reviewing medical records is to educate attorneys about the meaning and significance of entries and alert them to areas that need additional investigation. Organizing records involves translating them so that they are meaningful and compiling them so that the information they contain is easily retrievable. Strategies a NLC can use to organize records include creating a chronology of events, cross-referencing entries so that later findings can be linked to initial events, and creating a daily record of all activities carried out by a given provider.

Nurse legal consultants review records not only for their content, but for quality of entries: legibility (which could cause an entry to be misunderstood), erasures, omissions, insertions, and adherence to standards regarding timeliness and completeness of entries. Transcripts of depositions and testimony should be reviewed for inaccuracies, inconsistencies, and statements that strengthen or weaken a client's case (Milazzo 1993).

Box 16-2 provides additional examples of the wide variety of activities in which NLCs may be involved.

Practice Patterns and Business Considerations

Nurses who practice legal consulting on a full-time basis usually work in-house as an employee of an attorney or group of attorneys (Davis 1991). Much of the work they do is like that of a paralegal. Nurse legal consultants also work for hospitals and insurance companies as well as in private practice. Most nurses who work strictly as an expert witness do so on a part-time or "moonlighting" basis and continue to be actively involved in clinical practice.

In 1993, typical fees for NLCs ranged from $60-100 per hour (Perry & Vogel 1993). Actual fees vary according to community standards as well as a NLC's background, experience, expertise, education, communication skills, and nature of the case. Fees

Box 16-2. Activities and Interventions of Nurse Legal Consultants

A nurse legal consultant's interventions are primarily educational, investigational, interpretive, and organizational in nature. These interventions will vary according to the nature of a particular case. In addition, different activities tend to predominate during different phases of the litigation process.

Prelitigation Phase

This phase of the litigation process precedes the filing of a lawsuit. During this phase, activities focus on ensuring that the case has merit and is worth pursuing. Typical activities include:

- interviewing the plaintiff or defendent
- researching standards of care
- screening medical records to determine adherence to standards of care, who is negligent, and proximate cause
- identifying the primary medical issues in the case
- consulting with appropriate medical personnel
- assisting in the preparation of a complaint or response

Discovery Phase

During this pretrial phase, attorneys who represent the involved parties can examine relevant materials and interrogate parties who can provide information about the case. This is typically the most active phase of the litigation process for nurse legal consultants. Activities might include:

- reviewing a complaint and providing an opinion regarding its strengths and weaknesses from a medical perspective
- analyzing records
- summarizing and interpreting records; preparing chronologies of events
- library research
- attending depositions and reviewing the transcripts that are generated
- locating, retaining, and conferring with experts
- educating the employing attorney about the medical issues involved in a case
- observing independent medical examinations
- assisting with the identification and preparation of witnesses
- assisting the attorney to prepare medically accurate reports or correspondence
- assisting with the development of case strategies

Trial Phase

Less than 1% of all medical issue cases go to trial. The nurse who is working as a behind-the-scenes consultant rather than as a testifying expert consultant might be involved in the following activities:

- providing input into jury selection
- coordinating the schedule of testifying witnesses
- listening to testimony in order to detect inconsistencies
- reviewing the primary issues of the case with expert witnesses

References: Perry, S. (1992). The clinical nurse specialist as expert witness. *Clinical Nurse Specialist, 6* (2), 121-127; Perry, S., & Vogel, J. (1993). The business of being an expert witness and legal consultant. *Clinical Nurse Specialist, 7* (3), 154-161; Wetther, K. (1993). Forensic responsibilities of the legal nurse consultant. *Journal of Psychosocial Nursing, 31* (11), 21-25.

also tend to differ for behind-the-scenes and trial work. Fees are generally higher for giving a deposition and making court appearances since these activities are more stressful and must be carried out during regular work hours rather than at the NLC's convenience. If asked what charges would be for a specific service or activity, a NLC should avoid quoting a firm total price and instead quote an hourly rate plus a range of time typically needed for the activity. This protects the NLC from not being reimbursed for extra time that was needed for a case due to unforeseen variables.

Nurse legal consultants sometimes work on a retainer basis. NLCs who work under a retainer are paid to be available to provide consultation to an attorney as needed. However, they receive additional reimbursement for their actual consultation services. Placing a NLC on retainer assures an attorney of the NLC's availability for appropriate cases. It also precludes the NLC from involvement in cases brought against clients represented by the retaining attorney. For example, if a NLC worked under retainer for Attorney X, the NLC could not become involved with another attorney in a case against Hospital A which is represented by Attorney X.

Nurse legal consultants are generally advised to avoid contingency fees (reimbursement that is based on the outcome of a case). Contingency fees tend to erode a NLC's credibility because they create the appearance of having a financial interest in the outcome of a case. In addition, nurses who practice nurse legal consulting on a moonlighting basis but derive a significant proportion of their total income from work as a NLC may be viewed as biased. When questioned, all NLCs need to clarify that they are being reimbursed for the *time* spent testifying or providing expert consultation and are not "being paid to testify" since the latter implies being bought and told what to say (Perry 1992).

In addition to charging for consulting activities and court appearances, NLCs also charge for time spent traveling, making telephone calls, doing library research, and writing requested reports. As discussed in Chapter 13, when submitting a bill, consultation-related activities should be itemized and other reimbursable expenses (copying, postage, mileage, parking, and so forth) should be detailed separately (Perry & Vogel 1993).

Utilization of Nurse Legal Consultants

Before proceeding with a discussion of how NLCs implement each phase of the nursing consultation process, it is helpful to have an idea of some of the types of cases in which NLCs are involved. As mentioned earlier, nurse legal consultants work for attorneys of both plaintiffs and defendants. When working for a plaintiff's attorney, a NLC assists the attorney in substantiating a client's claim of harm and damages due for losses attributable to incurring the harm. When working for a defendant's attorney, a NLC assists the attorney in establishing that the client's actions are not the proximate cause of the plaintiff's losses. Some NLCs limit their practice to work on behalf of either plaintiffs or defendants. Additional career alternatives for NLCs are identified in Box 16-3.

Working on Behalf of Plaintiffs

One example of the type of work a NLC may perform on behalf of a plaintiff is development of a life care plan. A life care plan is a proposal for present and future health care rehabilitation, home modification, and equipment and community support service needs of an injured client (Wetther 1993). A life care plan provides the basis for some of the compensation an attorney seeks on behalf of a client. In these cases, a NLC's activities may include client, home, and community assessment; development

---

Box 16-3. Career Alternatives for Nurse Legal Consultants

Nurse legal consultants use their clinical expertise to assist attorneys with cases that involve health care delivery issues. Roles and career alternatives for nurse legal consultants include:

- Expert witness
- Court-appointed expert
- Court-appointed patient advocate
- Independent medical examiner
- Outcome analyst for clinical specialty area or specific procedures
- Claims adjuster
- Utilization manager
- Risk manager

---

and "costing out" of the proposed care plan; and serving as an interim case manager (Faherty 1991a, 1991b).

When a NLC is providing consultation in a life care plan case, the purpose of assessment activities is to document losses and gather information about services and resources that can return a client to as normal a life as possible, given their current deficits. The NLC's ability to conduct a holistic assessment that is based on a nursing framework (such as Orem's framework of self-care deficits or Gordon's functional health patterns framework) increases the reliability and validity of subsequent recommendations for care. An assessment based on a nursing framework also gives the trier of fact increased insight into the philosophy behind the life care plan and prevents the plan from appearing arbitrary and biased (Faherty 1991b).

Developing the actual life care plan involves detailing and explaining each recommendation as well as identifying a schedule for recommended services. Appropriate care providers and needed equipment need to be identified. Recommendations should take into consideration family caregiver burden and caregiving abilities as well as community limitations to providing services. Costing out services is based on the ability to develop a likely trajectory of a client's condition and adjusting the schedule of services as the client's condition changes.

Nurse legal consultants sometimes serve as a case manager for a life care plan client pending the outcome of litigation. In carrying out case management activities, the NLC facilitates the provision of needed services in order to prevent further deterioration of the client's condition. This demonstrates the attorney's interest in not only the financial aspects of the case, but in the client's well-being as well. Also, case management allows the true nature of a client's condition and potential to manifest and provides support for recommendations for future care. Box 16-4 provides additional examples of the types of cases in which a NLC might provide expertise on behalf of a plaintiff.

Working on Behalf of Defendants

Much of the work NLCs do for attorneys of defendants is in regard to nursing negligence and malpractice cases (malpractice and negligence are differentiated in Chapter 14). A central activity of NLCs in these types of cases is assisting the attorney to demonstrate that the defendant's actions were consistent with standards of nursing care in operation at the time of the incident and/or did not cause the plaintiff's loss. "Standard of care" (see Chapter 14) refers to the expected actions of a reasonably

Box 16-4. Areas of Practice for Nurse Legal Consultants

Nurse legal consultants may be involved in cases where a plaintiff believes loss has been suffered and is seeking to obtain a "remedy." The desired remedy is usually financial recovery that will purchase needed care and equipment; compensate for loss of past, present, and future income; and/or compensate for physical as well as emotional pain and suffering that has been incurred. These cases may involve any the following health care issues:

- Personal injury: cases that arise from incidents such as motor vehicle accidents, falls, swimming pool accidents, and so forth
- Malpractice: cases that arise from claims of harm due to a breach of professional nursing duty
- Negligence: cases that arise from charges of substandard nursing care
- Product liability: cases that arise from claims of harm due to nonmedical and medical products (including medications)
- Toxic tort litigation: cases that arise from claims of harm attributed to exposure to toxic substances such as asbestos, smoke from commercial grass burning, and so forth
- Worker's compensation: cases that involve claims of work-related injuries

prudent nurse in the same or similar circumstances (Kjervik 1990; Perry 1992). Standards of care are established by means of expert opinion. A NLC working on a malpractice case, therefore, often functions as an expert witness who offers an opinion about the consistency of a defendant's actions with accepted standards of care.

Some of the investigative activities a NLC may need to carry out during a negligence or malpractice case were described earlier in this chapter. Once the needed information about standards of care has been identified and accessed, an NLC's interpretive work begins. For example, a NLC needs to determine whether published standards represent minimum expectations for care or ideal behavior. In addition, a NLC must determine what part of care or what specific activities are essential if care is to be classified as meeting the standard of safe practice. Finally, NLCs working on negligence or malpractice cases can contribute their opinion about the relationship between a defendant's actions and the plaintiff's loss. In some cases, substandard care may have been given, but was not the cause of a plaintiff's loss. For instance, a patient's anaphylactic reaction to a medication can be attributed to receiving the offending drug, but is not necessarily attributable to a nurse's administration of the drug (Perry 1992). The plaintiff may have failed to report a drug allergy or may have experienced anaphylaxis after being given the drug for the first time.

Implementation of the Nursing Consultation Process

The preceding illustrations of the types of cases in which NLCs are involved are useful for depicting the range of activities that NLCs undertake as they implement each phase of the nursing consultation process.

Gaining Entry

Nurses are usually contacted about providing consultation in medical-legal cases by word of mouth referrals. For example, a hospital administrator or dean of a school of nursing may be asked to provide names of nurses with certain types of expertise. Sometimes, an attorney's client may suggest a nurse to serve as an expert witness. In other cases, an attorney may contact a nurse who is a personal acquaintance. Because initial contact tends to take place in this manner, it is important that environmental scanning verifies that there is no conflict of interest for the NLC (or even the appearance of one) and that there is a fit between the NLC's expertise and experience and that required by the case. It should go without saying that a NLC would avoid providing an opinion in a case in which the attorney's client is an acquaintance. Another key issue to address during environmental scanning is time expectations related to the case: can the required work be done during the NLC's "off-hours" from a "regular" job, how much time will be involved, and what is the urgency of the case.

Nurse legal consultants should work under formal contract with their employing attorney. In addition to the usual contract components (these are outlined in Chapter 13), the NLC will want to make sure that the contract clearly identifies the nature of the activities in which the NLC is to be involved. For example, is the NLC being asked to work only behind-the-scenes, or is courtroom testimony also an expectation? Because NLCs often vary their fees for different consultation activities, reimbursement expectations need to be clearly detailed at the outset of the consultation relationship.

Physical entry should consist of the employing attorney introducing the NLC to staff in his/her office with whom the NLC may need to interact. Physical entry should also include orientation to physical facilities, support services, and resources such as paralegals and legal references. If the NLC will be interacting with the client, the employing attorney should facilitate this introduction, too.

A nursing consultation relationship is most likely to be productive when there is trust and rapport among all the parties involved. The NLC needs to establish trust and rapport with the attorney and, in many cases, with the client. Establishing psychological entry with clients in a legal consulting case can be challenging; plaintiffs (patients) may be concerned that a NLC is naturally biased in favor of a nurse defendant, and nurse defendants may expect a NLC to discard objectivity in their favor. These dilemmas can be handled by emphasizing to clients that the ultimate goal of the case is justice and protection of professional standards of nursing practice.

Problem Identification

The goal of the problem identification phase of the nursing consultation process is to determine the cause of the problem that prompted the request for nursing consultation. In nurse legal consulting, the tasks of the problem identification phase remain the same. However, the goal of these tasks is to determine the relationship between a defendant's activities (for example, nursing care or product performance) and a plaintiff's injuries.

Assessment activities in legal consulting consist primarily of document review. Depending on the nature of the case, witnesses, the client, and other members of the client system may be interviewed. For example, in a case involving charges of negligence against a nurse, other nurses working on the same unit as the defendant might be interviewed. Because plaintiffs and defendants are often called to testify in negligence and malpractice cases, it is important that the NLC interview the hiring attorney's client for their version and interpretation of the events in question. In toxic tort litigation or product liability cases, the NLC may be asked to conduct research of the offending product or agent. In a case involving personal injury or worker's compensation, the NLC might interview the plaintiff's family or coworkers in an effort to determine the actual extent and impact of the injury. In any case, the challenge for the NLC is to remain impartial and objective. This can be particularly difficult when the

NLC identifies with a nurse defendant and the circumstances surrounding the problem situation.

The problem diagnosis in legal consulting is a conclusion about the standard of care practiced and the link between the defendant's actions (or product) and the plaintiff's injuries. This conclusion is usually communicated to the consultee (attorney) in a written report. The conclusion may also be communicated to the court through testimony.

Action Planning

In legal consulting, action planning often occurs at two points in time. First, an action planning phase may occur prior to problem identification activities. More specifically, NLCs often find it helpful to meet with the consultee and, possibly the client, to establish specific goals and strategies for the problem identification phase of the consultation process. As an example, a NLC working with the defense attorney in a malpractice case may need to meet with both the attorney and defendant to plan who it would be appropriate to interview and what to ask them, what policies and standards would be important to review, and so forth.

Action planning also takes place in a legal consulting relationship after the assessment and diagnostic activities of the problem identification phase have been completed. During this second action planning phase, the NLC may work with the attorney and client to determine what to do with the information and conclusions generated through the problem identification process. In some cases, the action plan may be to drop the case. In other cases, a plan might be made to attempt to settle out of court or to proceed to trial.

If a NLC is working on behalf of a plaintiff in a case where financial compensation is being sought, it is likely that the amount of compensation will be determined during the action planning phase. Nurse legal consultants with the appropriate expertise can provide valuable information about long-term care needs and a plaintiff's potential for rehabilitation—data that are considered when financial compensation is requested. Action planning for requesting financial compensation for a life care plan will necessitate recycling to the problem identification phase and gathering additional information about caregiver abilities, availability of community services, and the anticipated trajectory of a client's condition and rehabilitation. As mentioned earlier in this chapter, an action plan might also be developed for the NLC to serve as case manager for a plaintiff, pending the outcome of litigation.

Evaluation

Evaluation is as important in legal consulting as it is in other nursing consultation relationships. However, because the goal of legal consulting is not a change in behavior but rather justice, a legal consulting relationship is often evaluated only in terms of the outcome of the legal proceedings. That is, there is a tendency to judge legal consulting effective only if the consultee (attorney) wins the related case. Summative evaluation of legal consulting relationships can, however, provide a broader perspective. For example, it might make sense to judge a legal consulting relationship "effective" if it prevented a consultee from taking a weak case to trial. As in other consulting relationships, summative evaluation of the services provided by a NLC should also address adherence to the terms of the consultation contract (especially time line and budget) and satisfaction with the interpersonal interactions which occurred during the consultation process.

Nurse legal consultants should also make an effort to gather formative evaluation information so that interaction patterns and consultation activities can be revised if they are not facilitating accomplishment of necessary tasks. Formative evaluation could reveal, for example, problems with secretarial or paralegal support that are hindering the NLC's review of records and other necessary documents.

Disengagement

In most legal consulting relationships, the disengagement phase will be very brief. There is usually no need to develop a system of continuity supports and decreased contact with the consultee tends to occur naturally once the NLC offers an opinion about the case.

In most legal consulting relationships, disengagement will center around termination activities. At the very least, the NLC should try to arrange a conference with the consultee to bring closure to the consultation relationship and, if appropriate, to express interest in providing consultation in the future. When it is not possible to arrange a closing conference, the NLC can terminate the consultation relationship by letter. Often, NLCs will also request a summary letter from the consultee verifying the nature of the NLC's contribution to the case.

Challenges and Opportunities

Reforms in both health care and the legal system present new opportunities and challenges for NLCs. For example, as tort reform progresses, NLCs may find themselves contributing their expertise to medical-legal cases that are focused on arbitration rather than costly litigation.

Changing patterns of health care delivery will also create new medical-legal issues in which NLCs can become involved. As increasing numbers of nurses take on advanced practice roles as primary care providers, NLCs will find themselves involved in more cases related to practicing outside one's scope of practice (for example, "practicing medicine without a license"). As unlicensed assistive personnel assume more and more tasks that have traditionally been performed by nurses, NLCs are likely to find opportunities for involvement in cases that deal with delegation and supervision issues. The challenge for NLCs will be to keep current on changing professional practice acts, related statutes and regulations, and standards of care.

New medical technologies will challenge NLCs to be able to interpret reasonable patient expectations for outcomes. Technology and improved care that increases the survival rate for victims of serious accidents will provide growing opportunities for NLCs to be involved in developing life care plans. To date, NLCs have tended to provide legal consultation services on a reactive basis. As nursing care delivery becomes more complex, entrepreneurial opportunities may arise for NLCs to develop practices around proactive advice or anticipatory guidance.

Other changes in society will also provide opportunities for NLCs. Increased consumerism will most likely create expanded opportunities for NLCs to be involved in product liability cases. Current concerns about environmental issues may correspond to an increase in toxic tort litigation.

As the types of issues in which NLCs are involved become more diverse and complex, consideration will need to be given to role preparation and documentation of role qualifications. The nursing profession as a whole and nurse legal consultants in particular will need to decide whether there is a need for standardized educational preparation as well as what content it should include and what form it should take. Nurse legal consultants will also need to tackle the issue of credentialing as a means of quality control and regulating the profession.

Chapter Summary

Nurse legal consultants exemplify interdisciplinary external nursing consultation that addresses problems in client health status and health care delivery. As the health care delivery and legal systems continue to undergo reform, nurse legal consultants will be presented with new challenges and opportunities. In today's litigious society, individuals are inclined to seek compensation whenever adverse outcomes occur, whether due to malpractice, product liability, or environmental circumstances. This mindset shows no signs of changing soon. As expert witnesses, nurse legal consultants can help place medical events and outcomes in their proper perspective. In doing so, they function as patient advocates, uphold standards of nursing practice, and protect society from actual and potential threats to health.

Applying Chapter Content

- Review the scenario from the opening of this chapter. Identify issues that a nurse legal consultant would need to attend to during each phase of the nursing consultation process.

- Identify medical-legal issues in your own practice situation as a clinician, educator, or manager for which you might need the services of a nurse legal consultant. Analyze the availability of these services in your community.

- Critique your own ability to provide nursing legal consultation services.

References

Davis, S. (1991). The functions of a nurse legal consultant. *Rehabilitation Nursing, 16* (4), 234.

Faherty, B. (1991a). Preparing case reports as a nurse legal consultant. *Rehabilitation Nursing, 16* (2), 77-81, 84.

Faherty, B. (1991b). The nurse legal consultant and disabling injuries. *Rehabilitation Nursing, 16* (1), 30-33.

Faherty, B. (1995). Legal nurse consultants: Who are they? *Journal of Nursing Law, 2* (1), 37-49.

Kjervik, D. (1990). Law and ethics consultation. *Journal of Professional Nursing, 6* (4), 193, 246.

Milazzo, V. (1993). Why would an attorney hire a nurse? *American Journal of Nursing, 93* (2), 22-23, 25-26.

Perry, S. (1992). The clinical nurse specialist as expert witness. *Clinical Nurse Specialist, 6* (2), 121-127.

Perry, S., & Vogel, J. (1993). The business of being an expert witness and legal consultant. *Clinical Nurse Specialist, 7* (3), 154-161.

Schabes, A. (1992, November/December). Selecting a legal consultant in today's troubled waters. *Nursing Homes,* 10-11.

Wetther, K. (1993). Forensic responsibilities of the legal nurse consultant. *Journal of Psychosocial Nursing, 31* (11), 21-25.

Additional Readings—Professional and Practice Issues

Ehrlich, C. (1995). Certification developments. *Journal of Legal Nurse Consultants,*
   6 (1), 6-9.
   The author reviews the status of current efforts to develop certification processes for nurse
   legal consultants.
Faherty, B. (1991a). Preparing case reports as a nurse legal consultant. *Rehabilitation*
   Nursing, 16 (2), 77-81, 84.
   This article details the composition of a report about a client's health care needs. Such a
   report may be used in personal injury, worker's compensation, or malpractice litigation
   to help establish the financial settlement that is requested on behalf of a client.
Faherty, B. (1991b). The nurse legal consultant and disabling injuries. *Rehabilitation*
   Nursing, 16 (1), 30-33.
   This article discusses six different ways in which a nurse legal consultant can provide
   assistance to an attorney. Recommended qualifications for a nurse legal consultant are
   also identified.
Heydlauff, A. (1995a). Applying the standards of practice. *Journal of Legal Nurse*
   Consultants, 6 (4), 72.
   Standards of practice for nurse legal consultants are identified in this article.
Lobb, M., Riley, G., & Clemens, A. (1994). The legal nurse consultant's role on the
   defense team in a medical malpractice lawsuit. *Network: News for the Legal Nurse*
   Consultant, 5 (4), 3-7.
   The authors outline activities that nurse legal consultants undertake when working on
   behalf of defendants.
Magnusson, J. (1995). Standards of practice for the legal nurse consultant. *Journal*
   of Legal Nurse Consultants, 6 (3), 19.
   This article reviews standards of practice for nurse legal consultants.
Mason, M. (1994, Spring/Summer). Nurse on the case: Legal nurse consultants
   provide attorneys with the inside view in medical litigation. *Advanced Practice*
   Nurse, 35-37.
   The author discusses some of the services that nurse legal consultants can provide to
   attorneys.
Perry, S. (1992). The clinical nurse specialist as expert witness. *Clinical Nurse Special-*
   ist, 6 (2), 121-127.
   The author describes the variety of roles that may be assumed by a nurse legal consultant.
   Specific guidelines for reviewing records, giving a deposition, and providing testimony
   are shared.
Perry, S., & Vogel, J. (1993). The business of being an expert witness and legal con-
   sultant. *Clinical Nurse Specialist, 7* (3), 154-161.
   This article describes the roles nurse consultants may play in legal actions. Establishing
   fees for legal consultation, marketing oneself as a legal consultant, and business consider-
   ations related to an entrepreneurial role as a nurse legal consultant are also discussed.
Quigley, F. (1991). Responsibilities of the consultant and expert witness. *Focus on*
   Critical Care, 18 (3), 238-239.
   The author differentiates the roles of expert witness and consultant.
Scope and standards for the legal nurse consulting practice. (1995). *Journal of Legal*
   Nurse Consultants, 6 (4), 24-27.
   This article discusses the scope of practice for nurse legal consultants.

Wetther, K. (1993). Forensic responsibilities of the legal nurse consultant. *Journal of Psychosocial Nursing, 31* (11), 21-25.
Roles of the nurse legal consultant during the prelitigation, discovery, and trial phases of legal action are identified. Characteristics of successful nurse legal consultants are described.

Additional Readings—Career Alternatives

Bogart, J., & Beerman, J. (1995). Expert fact witness: A testifying role for the legal nurse consultant. *Journal of Legal Nurse Consultants, 6* (4), 2-8.

Clemens, A., & Woo, P. (1992). The role of the legal nurse consultant in toxic tort litigation. *National Medical Legal Journal, 3* (2), 1, 6-7.

Davis, S. (1992). The nurse consultant's role in products liability litigation. *National Medical Legal Journal, 3* (1), 1, 6-7.

Heydlauff, A. (1995b). The independent medical examination and the legal nurse consultant. *Journal of Legal Nurse Consultants, 6* (3), 2-4, 15.

Ismark, D. (1994). Career alternatives for the legal nurse consultant: Claims adjuster. *Network: News for the Legal Nurse Consultant, 5* (3), 16-17.

Lauer, M., & Levin, N. (1994). Career alternatives for the legal nurse consultant: Utilization management consultants. *Network: News for the Legal Nurse Consultant, 5* (2), 15-16.

Orr, M. (1994). The role of the legal nurse consultant in assisting with a toxic tort case. *Network: News for the Legal Nurse Consultant, 5* (2), 9-10.

Sarff, L. (1994). Career alternatives for the legal nurse consultant: Perinatal outcome analyst. *Network: News for the Legal Nurse Consultant, 5* (3), 16, 29.

Sloan, M. (1991). The legal nurse consultant's role in product liability cases. *National Medical Legal Journal, 2* (4), 3.

Turner, N. (1995). The legal nurse consultant as a court-appointed expert. *Journal of Legal Nurse Consultants, 6* (1), 12-14.

Woo, P., & Clemens, A. (1991). Trial support: The legal nurse consultant's role. *Network: News for the Legal Nurse Consultant, 2* (4), 5.

Nurses as Ethics Consultants

*The philosophical role of an ethics consultant is to provide
health care providers with a full understanding of the conceptual, epistemological, and metaphysical issues, sometimes
supplying answers and at other times clarifying why an
unequivocal answer is not possible.* (Kjervik 1993)

Key terms: ethics, morals, norms, values,
humanism, surrogate decision maker

An 89-year-old man suffers a cardiac arrest during cardiac catheterization. He has
an emergency quadruple bypass operation that is followed by a stormy postop-
erative course. Should his spouse be allowed to have his life-sustaining treatment
discontinued? Should an HIV+ woman be denied infertility services? Should a
woman who is having preterm labor at 30 weeks gestation be allowed to refuse
tocolytic therapy?

Nurse ethics consultants (sometimes referred to as nurse ethicists) are nurses with
specialized training and expertise that equips them to identify, analyze, and help
resolve problems that arise in the care of individual patients, such as those problems
illustrated in the previous paragraph (LaPuma & Scheidermayer 1991). Nurse ethics
consultants (NECs) work with health care providers and/or family caregivers to help
them make difficult choices in situations where valid differences in value systems are
obstacles to decision making (Spike & Greenlaw 1994). At the heart of the situations in
which NECs are asked to intervene is the challenge of protecting a patient's or surrogate decision maker's autonomy while balancing the needs and interests of other
involved parties such as nurses, physicians, family members, payers, and the institution. Ethics consultation has been recognized as "an expedient way to open discussion
and promote patient-centered decisions" (Bosek 1993).

Nurse ethics consultants exemplify the consultant role of option-giver. That is,
rather than present a consultee with a single problem solution (which is unrealistic
since a problem often reflects issues on which society has not reached consensus), a
NEC presents all legally and morally permissible options for consideration (Fry-Revere
1994). The role of a NEC also serves as an example of patient-centered interdisciplinary
internal nursing consultation. As such, implementation of the consultation process by
NECs illustrates nurses working within an institutional setting with all members of a
health care team to protect and promote a patient's interests. Nurse ethics consultants
serve as role models for other nurses implementing the nursing consultation process in
similarly complex situations.

This chapter begins by describing the nursing consultation relationship, goals and
objectives, interventions, and practice patterns that characterize nurse ethics consultants. Next, how NECs implement each phase of the nursing consultation process is

illustrated. The final section of this chapter considers challenges and opportunities for NECs. As you read this chapter, think about the following questions:

- What types of ethical dilemmas do you encounter most frequently in your own practice setting? How do you usually respond to these dilemmas?

- What resources are available in your work setting for help with ethical dilemmas? How satisfactory are these resources? What do you think contributes to their effectiveness or ineffectiveness?

- What opportunities do you see for implementing nurse ethics consulting as an external consultation service?

Approach to Consultation

Nurse ethics consultants, like other specialty consultants (such as psychiatric consultation-liaison nurses and nurse legal consultants), implement the consultation process in their own unique way. They are guided by a specific set of goals and objectives, use a common approach or interaction pattern, and rely on a characteristic set of interventions for resolving problems. The consultation process itself is implemented through a variety of practice patterns. An overview of nurse ethics consultation is presented in Box 17-1.

The Nursing Consultation Relationship

The consultation triad in a nurse ethics consultation relationship includes the NEC, the caregiver(s), and the patient or surrogate decision maker. Caregivers, who typically are the consultee in this relationship, may be physicians, nursing staff, or family members. Common stakeholders in a nurse ethics consultation relationship include family members, the institution, the patient's payer system, and other patients with similar problems. Less frequently, a nurse ethics consultation relationship is dyadic and the patient is both consultee and client.

Goals and Objectives

The ultimate goals of a NEC are to provide a clearer understanding of the patient's or surrogate decision maker's perspective of an ethically problematic situation and to help disagreeing parties come to a morally permissible problem solution (Bosek 1993; Edinger 1992; LaPuma & Scheidermayer 1991). Nurse ethics consultants, therefore, function as patient advocates. The more immediate objectives or intermediate goals of a NEC are to assist caregivers (physicians and nursing staff) to recognize actual or potential ethical issues in a situation and to develop structured, coherent, and humane strategies for analyzing and resolving ethical dilemmas (LaPuma & Scheidermayer 1991). Thus another major role of a NEC is that of educator. The basic ethical concepts and principles with which NECs need to be familiar are reviewed in Chapter 15. Figure 17-1 illustrates the consultation relationship in nurse ethics consultation and its goals and objectives.

Interventions

A nurse ethics consultant's interactions with a caregiver are primarily educational and supportive in nature. A specific intervention that is commonly used by nurse ethics consultants is the "opinion paper" (Bosek 1993; Spike & Greenlaw 1995). An opinion paper summarizes a case's ethical issues and identifies possible problem solutions. An opinion paper also details the current normative perspective (for example, legal

> ## Box 17-1. Overview of Nursing Ethics Consultation Services
>
> Ethics consultation is a relatively recent professional service. However, because of the increasingly complex issues that are confronted in the delivery of health care and because of social and regulatory pressures, ethics committees and ethics consultants have now become the norm for hospitals. They are also becoming more common in other health care settings. The increased demand for ethics consultation services provides unique opportunities for nurses who wish to develop an advanced practice role as a nurse consultant.
>
> Hospital-based ethics consultation was first implemented at several large university affiliated medical centers and the National Institutes of Health in the 1960s and 1970s (LaPuma & Scheidermayer 1991). During the late 1970s, a series of papers outlining a role for clinical ethics as a special field of expertise in medicine were published. In 1982, the first handbook on clinical ethics was published and, in 1990, the first issue of a journal devoted to clinical medical ethics (*The Journal of Clinical Ethics*) made its appearance.
>
> Since 1986, there has been increased pressure from both the government and private regulatory bodies for health care institutions to form institutional ethics consultation services. In 1991, the Joint Commission on Accreditation of Healthcare Organizations asserted that hospitals need to have a mechanism in place for assisting patients and staff in dealing with ethical issues. This same mandate was extended to home health care agencies in 1992. Other pressures that have encouraged the development of ethics consultation services include providers' concerns about liability and payers' concerns about the cost of care (LaPuma & Scheidermayer 1991). In addition, there is growing recognition by the health care community that nurses who continue to experience ethical burdens without having the opportunity to also experience resolution are at increased risk for burnout (Bosek 1993).
>
> More than 90% of all hospitals were found to have some sort of formal ethics consultation service in place just two years after JCAHO made its recommendations (Fry-Revere 1994). Ethics consultation services have been identified by nursing staff as "very" or "somewhat" important in identifying ethical issues in 94% of referred cases. Ethics consultation has been credited with effecting a "considerable change" in management in 40-50% of cases (LaPuma & Scheidermayer 1991).
>
> Nurses' clinical expertise, familiarity with the dynamics of health care delivery, and skills in interpersonal processes provide them with much of the foundation that is needed for providing effective consultation about ethical issues. Nurse ethics consultants also need expertise in moral reasoning, a working knowledge of medical law and relevant legal precedents, and an awareness of current opinions on ethical issues (Edinger 1992).

statutes and formal position statements) about the ethical issue. Dissenting opinions regarding each problem solution, recommendations regarding the moral permissibility of each option, and potential issues to address later are also identified. Copies of the opinion paper are provided to the patient or surrogate decision maker and the patient's primary physician. A copy is also placed in the patient's chart. The advantage of an opinion paper as an educational intervention is that it avoids the appear-

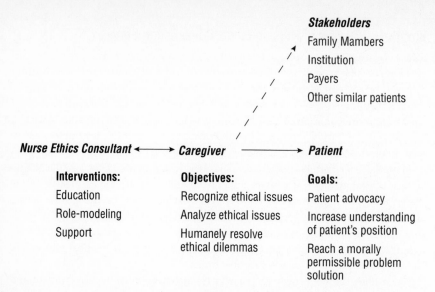

Figure 17-1. The Nurse Ethics Consultation Relationship and its Goals and Objectives
The nurse ethics consultant uses educational and supportive interventions to help a caregiver (physician, nursing staff, or family member) learn to recognize, systematically analyze, and humanely resolve ethical dilemmas. This facilitates achieving the ultimate consultation goal of patient advocacy.

ance of any infringement by the NEC in the decision-making process (Spike & Greenlaw, 1995). References that can be consulted for developing ethics opinion papers are identified in Box 17-2.

In addition to providing consultation on individual cases, NECs engage in other activities that address ethical issues related to patient care. For example, NECs often serve as members of a hospital's ethics committee. In this position, NECs can share their expertise, work with members of other disciplines to reflect on trends in ethical issues, and help in the development of institutional policies. Membership on an institution's ethics committee also provides NECs with the opportunity to receive multi-disciplinary critiques of their work. Nurse ethics consultants also frequently serve as members of institutional review boards for research projects.

A major activity of most NECs is staff education. Educational interventions take place not only through role-modeling and case specific consultation; NECs are frequently expected to provide formal in-service education programs and conduct ethics "grand rounds." A proactive educational and support intervention that is used by some NECs is ethics discussion groups. These ongoing groups provide a forum in which caregivers can discuss their feelings and beliefs about ethical issues and develop decision-making skills.

In some institutions, the role of NEC is paired with that of bereavement counselor (Murphy 1993). In this role, the NEC is available to provide follow-up support, brief counseling, and referral services to family members and staff after a patient's death.

Practice Patterns

Most nurse ethics consultants practice as internal consultants within hospitals, home health care agencies, or long-term care facilities. Reporting relationships and the spe-

---

Box 17-2. Resources for Developing Ethics Opinion Papers

The following resources can provide references for current perspectives on medical ethical issues. Note that professional codes of ethics only provide general guidelines for daily professional conduct; they are not intended to provide the means for resolving all ethical questions.

- Reports from national commissions such as the President's Commission for the Study of Ethical Problems in Medicine
- Publications from institutions that have been established for the study of ethical problems; the Hastings Center and the Kennedy Institute of Ethics are two examples
- Professional codes of ethics: the American Nurses Association *Code for Nurses*, the American Medical Association's *Principles of Medical Ethics*, and *The Patient's Bill of Rights* developed by the American Hospital Association

Reference: Edinger, W. (1992). Which opinion should a clinical ethicist give? Personal viewpoint or professional consensus? *Theoretical Medicine, 13*, 23-29.

---

cific lines of authority under which a NEC operates will differ according to institutional structure and mission. Nurse ethics consultants may have a reporting relationship to a facility's medical staff, nursing services department, chief executive officer, or board of trustees. Regardless of to whom they are officially accountable, NECs recognize that their ultimate accountability is to patients and patients' caregivers.

For a NEC, there are distinct advantages to being a member of an institution's nursing services department. Nurse ethics consultants who are aligned with nursing services are more accessible to staff nurses because they are readily identified as nurses (this presumes common background and experiences) and because their services come out of the same budget (so nursing services won't be charged for consultation provided by another department). Also, in most institutions nursing services is one of the larger bureaucracies. This means that nurse ethics consultants who work under nursing services have the ability to access the "engines of institutional influence" for the purpose of promoting their role and services (Murphy 1993).

Implementation of the Nursing Consultation Process

Nurse ethics consultants work with caregivers to address ethical dilemmas that arise in the course of making decisions about and providing patient care. The knowledge and skills used by NECs as they implement the nursing consultation process are described in Box 17-3.

Gaining Entry

The request for an ethics consultation is usually initiated by a staff nurse or physician. The request reflects a personal patient-centered ethical dilemma or difficulty working with a patient or family confronting an ethical decision. Depending on the practice pattern in place at an institution, the request for consultation services may be made formally or informally. Common reasons for seeking consultation from a NEC are identified in Box 17-4.

During the environmental scanning activities that take place during the gaining entry phase, the NEC obtains answers to the following questions:

Box 17-3. Knowledge and Skills for Nurse Ethics Consultants

Nurse ethics consultants (NECs) are asked to provide opinions about ethically responsible behavior, to intervene in problems that have developed because of a lack of open communication between a health care provider and patient, and to resolve conflicts in complex, emotionally charged situations. The roles a NEC assumes include professional colleague, negotiator, patient advocate, and educator.

The knowledge needed for effective implementation of the NEC role include:
- Moral reasoning processes
- Frameworks for ethical decision making
- Medical humanism and humanistic behavior (integrity, compassion, caring, respect)
- Clinical psychology and strategies for evaluating decision-making abilities
- Sociology of health care delivery, relationships among health care providers
- Health care law; case and statutory law related to issues such as life-sustaining treatment, advanced directives, and surrogate decision making
- Ethical standards of professional practice and ethically responsible behavior
- Adult education theory

Some of the skills needed for effective implementation of the NEC role include:
- Ability to identify and analyze ethical problems
- Ability to use reasonable clinical judgment
- Communication skills
- Negotiation and mediation skills
- Teaching skills
- Conflict resolution skills
- Ability to recognize and consider the interests of varied stakeholders
- Ability to provide support to persons under stress

- What ethical issues does this problem situation represent? In one study (La Puma et al. 1988), ethics consultants were found to identify an average of 3.0 ethical issues in each referred case.

- Are there other confounding issues in this situation?

- What actions have already been undertaken in an effort to resolve this problem?

- What type of help (information, education, or support) is wanted?

- What other types of help (for example, help with communication processes) are needed?

- What is the urgency of the situation?

- Can I be objective in this case? (Bosek 1993)

Because NECs are internal nurse consultants, they usually don't have the luxury of turning down a case on the basis of "poor fit." However, a NEC should determine possible problems related to dual relationships or overidentification with a problem situation, as well as need for additional expertise and resources.

Box 17-4. Reasons for Seeking Ethics Consultation

Ethics consultation is sought when a patient's family or nursing staff is uncertain about how to proceed in a situation that involves questions about morals, values, and doing the right thing. Situations that tend to prompt a request for ethics consultation include:

- Disagreement about whether actions are ethically justifiable (for example, discontinuing life-sustaining treatment or using life support on terminally ill patients)
- Valid differences in value systems are creating obstacles to either decision making or providing optimum patient care
- A designated decision maker feels a need for support
- A family and patient need help discussing end of life decisions
- A care provider (physician or nurse) needs help discussing ethical issues with a patient or family
- A caregiver (physician) needs reassurance that allowing a patient to die does not constitute abandonment
- Issues related to needing to provide care to offensive or noncompliant patients, patients who wish to reject nursing care measures, and patients who represent a risk to the caregiver's health

---

Consider the following scenario: A 17-year-old with cystic fibrosis is admitted in respiratory failure and refuses to be intubated. The patient's family, however, refuses to sign a DNR (Do Not Resuscitate) order and, by state law, the patient is too young to sign such an order. The physician both feels the patient is mentally competent and wants to respect the patient's wishes. The staff nurses are not sure what to do, so they request an ethics consultation.

During environmental scanning, the NEC determines the following:

- The ethical issues represented by the case are self-determination and nonmaleficence (do no harm).

- Confounding issues are parental rights and the patient's legal status as a minor.

- The action undertaken thus far to resolve this problem has been a frank discussion between the physician, the patient, and the patient's parents. The physician has discussed the probable trajectory of the patient's condition with and without intubation. Another physician was also present for this discussion.

- The type of help wanted by the physician and nurses is reassurance about the legal safety and moral acceptability of acting in accordance with the patient's wishes.

- The NEC identifies that other types of help that might be needed in this case are help with parent-child communication and grieving.

- The urgency of the situation is high; the patient's oxygen saturation levels are hovering around 90%.

Gaining entry also includes establishing physical entry and initiating psychological entry. Because NECs are usually internal consultants, physical entry into the problem setting has most likely been established. Psychological entry involves establishing rapport, trust, and credibility. Nurse ethics consultants can facilitate the development of psychological entry by listening objectively and expressing empathy for the difficulty of the situation. It is particularly important that the NEC clarify issues surrounding confidentiality with any staff who are involved in the problem situation. Nursing staff involved with the patient who has cystic fibrosis, for example, might fear reprisal or ostracism for their actions and opinions, especially if their opinions are not consistent with those of the majority or could be viewed as legally questionable.

Problem Identification

During the problem identification phase of an ethics consultation, the NEC gathers additional information about (1) the patient's medical problem, (2) relevant social history, (3) the values, beliefs, and assumptions of those involved in the situation, and (4) the variables that triggered the present consultation request. In the example scenario, the NEC might want to gather information about the patient's prior hospitalizations, experiences with intubation and resuscitation, and other medical problems. Relevant social history would include asking about other family members with cystic fibrosis and other experiences with loss and grief. It would also be important to clarify points of consistency and inconsistency in relation to beliefs about the purpose of life, quality of life, and self-determination held by the patient, the patient's parents, and the involved caregivers. This information can help determine potential barriers to problem solving, as well as illuminate factors that might facilitate decision making. Variables that might have triggered the consultation request might be the patient's rapidly deteriorating condition and caregiver confusion about legally required and morally permissible actions.

Assessment activities may or may not include a bedside assessment of the patient. While a bedside assessment is sometimes considered intrusive, among the advantages of performing a bedside assessment are that it . . .

- enables a NEC to see the patient holistically—as a person with beliefs, fears, and hopes as well as medical problems,

- allows observation of the relationship among the patient, family, and caregivers,

- facilitates determination of a patient's understanding of the situation and decision-making capacity, and

- protects against abstraction, moral posturing, and paternalism (LaPuma & Scheidermayer 1990).

Action Planning

In a nurse ethics consultation relationship, action planning involves describing all possible options for responding to the problem and the likely outcome of each response. The ethical principles, legal statutes, and current perspectives that support or negate each option should be detailed and referenced. The ultimate goal of the action planning phase is to identify who should make the decision about a problem's solution. In the example scenario, possible responses to the situation include full resuscitation efforts when needed, no intervention, or partial intervention (for example, oxygen by nasal cannula, suctioning, hydration, and other comfort measures). Potential decision makers in this scenario include the patient, the patient's parents, or the court. Because of the legal issues that complicate this case (the patient's status as a minor), it is likely that regardless of the problem solution or who is accepted as decision-maker, legal consultation—most likely from the hospital's attorney—would also be obtained.

Evaluation

Because ethics consultation frequently occurs under conditions of urgency as in the example scenario, it can be difficult to engage in any kind of formative evaluation. The NEC should, however, monitor the consultation relationship to make sure that all parties are being heard, adequate information is being gathered, and all possible action options are being considered. In short, the NEC needs to monitor for the development of "groupthink" (the phenomenon of groupthink is described in Chapter 6).

Summative evaluation can take place either in debriefing sessions or by anonymous survey once the problem situation is resolved. Among the questions a NEC might use as a framework for a summative evaluation of the consultation relationship are:

- Did the consultees have opportunities to express their concerns?

- Did the consultees feel that they were objectively listened to?

- Did the consultees feel that they were kept informed of how the problem-solving process was progressing?

- Was there opportunity to discuss the advantages, disadvantages, and implications of the different possible problem solutions?

- Did the consultees understand the reason for the recommended course of action?

Disengagement

Because NECs are members of the problem setting in which the consultation relationship occurs, they often find it difficult to accomplish disengagement. Frequently, a NEC will find that there are emotional issues—anger and grief, in particular—that linger after a particularly difficult problem situation. In these situations, the NEC may schedule educational and debriefing sessions as one strategy for decreasing involvement with the client system. In other situations, the NEC might determine that it is appropriate to enlist the help of a psychiatric consultation-liaison nurse to work with staff to resolve their feeling and provide support.

Challenges and Opportunities

A potentially problematic issue for NECs is that of dual loyalties. While NECs recognize that their client is the patient, they often find themselves involved in cases where the patient's interests are threatened by the wishes of family, the wishes or policies of the institution, and financial constraints. Nurse ethics consultants may find themselves in the uncomfortable position of pursuing legal appeals as well as confronting the family, medical and nursing staff, hospital administration, and insurance companies in order to fulfill their role as patient advocate.

Related to the issue of dual loyalties is the pressure a NEC may feel to assume other roles in a case. Nurse ethics consultants may find themselves being asked to be the case conscience, the case legal counselor, the case quality reviewer, the case psychoanalyst, or the case clergy. Clearly, NECs need to adhere to ethical standards of practice and avoid practicing outside their scope of expertise. As consultants, NECs must also recognize that the consultation relationship will be undermined if a dual role is assumed.

Issues that threaten role viability for NECs include their unknown risk for legal liability and their lack of income generation for an institution. While health care facilities are mandated to provide access to some sort of resource for ethics consultation, in the present environment of cost-consciousness and downsizing, it seems possible that

NECs could be asked to assume additional income-generating roles and provide ethics consultation as just one part of their role. The trend of cost-containment, therefore, challenges NECs to document outcomes and cost-effectiveness and to become active in efforts directed toward obtaining third-party reimbursement for their services.

An additional challenge for NECs is keeping current with ethical issues, opinions, and related legal statutes. As technology raises more ethical issues and health care reform attempts to set limits on who can receive what kinds of interventions, NECs are faced with the need to read widely and follow trends and issues.

A final challenge for NECs is that of preventing their own burnout. As the need for ethics consultations increases, cases become more complex, and conflict among stakeholders more pronounced, the risk is very real for NECs to succumb to the stresses of their role and become apathetic, judgmental, and ineffective. Institutions must provide supportive resources for NECs and NECs must provide this support to one another.

While to date, NECs have worked almost exclusively as internal consultants, opportunities also exist for NECs as external consultants. Nurse ethics consultants can, for example, make their services available on a contractual basis to facilities that are too small to have a NEC on staff full time. Nurse ethics consultants can also provide consultation to larger institutions that are interested in developing an ethics consultation service. Schools of nursing that are interested in adding health care ethics to their curriculum or in developing a special program of study for role preparation in ethics consultation could also benefit from the expertise of a NEC.

Chapter Summary

Nurse ethics consultants are a valuable resource for patients and caregivers who face illness-related ethical dilemmas. As health care technology and health care reform continue to evolve, so too will the role of the NEC. Nurse ethics consultants are an example of how nurses can use expertise they develop in other disciplines to address and resolve problems that arise during the course of health care delivery. NECs can serve as role models to other nurses who wish to incorporate expertise from areas other than nursing into their contributions to patient well-being.

Applying Chapter Content

- Read the following case studies:

  Spike, J., & Greenlaw, J. (1994). Case study: Ethics consultation. *Journal of Law, Medicine, & Ethics, 22* (4), 347-350.
  This case study focuses on a request for infertility services by a woman who is HIV+.
  Spike, J., & Greenlaw, J. (1995). Ethics consultation: Refusal of beneficial treatment by a surrogate decision-maker. *Journal of Law, Medicine, & Ethics, 23* (2), 202-204.

- Critique the ethics consultation that was provided in each of these cases. Specifically consider the following issues:
  1. Identify how each phase in the consultation process was implemented.
  2. What ethical issues were represented in each case?
  3. How do you think each of these cases might have been approached differently by a *nurse* ethics consultant?
  4. How would you have handled this case?

- Review the scenarios that were used in the chapter opening. As a nurse ethics consultant, how would you implement the nursing consultation process in each of these scenarios?

- Conduct an assessment of resources that are available for ethics consultation in your community. What gaps in services (and service accessibility) can you identify? What limitations do you see in these services?

References

Bosek, M. (1993). What to expect from an ethics consultation. *MEDSURG Nursing, 2* (5), 408-409.

Edinger, W. (1992). Which opinion should a clinical ethicist give: Personal viewpoint or professional consensus? *Theoretical Medicine, 13,* 23-29.

Fry-Revere, S. (1994). Ethics consultation: An update on accountability. *Pediatric Nursing, 20* (1), 95-98.

Kjervik, D. (1990). Law and ethics consultation. *Journal of Professional Nursing, 6* (4), 193, 246.

LaPuma, J., & Scheidermayer, D. (1990). Must the ethics consultant see the patient? *Journal of Clinical Ethics, 1,* 56-59.

LaPuma, J., & Scheidermayer, D. (1991). Ethics consultation: Skills, roles, and training. *Annals of Internal Medicine, 114* (2), 155-160.

LaPuma, J., Stocking, C., Silverstein, M., DiMartini, A., & Siegler, M. (1988). An ethics consultation service in a teaching hospital: Utilization and evaluation. *JAMA, 260* (6), 808-811.

Murphy, P. (1993). A nurse-ethicist model of ethics consultation. *Trends in Health Care, Law, & Ethics, 8* (4), 23-24.

Nursing Ethics Committee. (1989). The ethics survey: An important step in promoting nursing ethics. *Journal of the New York State Nurses Association, 20* (4), 4-8.

Spike, J., & Greenlaw, J. (1994). Case study: Ethics consultation. *Journal of Law, Medicine, & Ethics, 22* (4), 347-350.

Spike, J., & Greenlaw, J. (1995). Ethics consultation: Refusal of beneficial treatment by a surrogate decision-maker. *Journal of Law, Medicine, & Ethics, 23* (2), 202-204.

Additional Readings

Bernal, E. (1995, January/February). Ethics consultation is not therapy. *Neonatal Intensive Care,* 26-27.
This article differentiates the roles of ethics consultant and family therapist. An ethics consultant's loyalty is to the standards of bioethics whereas the family therapist's primary loyalty is to the family.

Fowler, M. (1990). Reflections on ethics consultation in critical care settings. *Critical Care Nursing Clinics of North America, 2* (3), 431-435.
The author describes issues that are settled, unsettled, and unsettling in ethics consultation.

Ingersoll, G., & Jones, L. (1992). The art of the consultation note. *Clinical Nurse Specialist, 6* (4), 218-220.
The guidelines provided for documenting consultation activities in this article can be applied to documenting ethics consultation. An outline for the format of a consultation note is provided.

Nebraska Nurses' Association. (1995). Focus on ethics: Care for the dying patient— ethical guidelines. *Nebraska Nurse, 28* (2), 34.
This position paper presents guidelines to support nurses in their role as advocates for dying patients and their families. Included in these guidelines are roles for a nurse ethics consultant.

Rubin, S., & Zoloth-Dorfman, L. (1995, March/April). First person plural: Community and method in ethics consultation. *Neonatal Intensive Care, 29-34.*

The authors differentiate psychotherapy and ethics consultation and describe the danger of trying to approach ethical dilemmas from a psychotherapeutic model of intervention.

Watne, K., & Donner, T. (1995). Distinguishing between life-saving and life-sustaining treatments: When the physician and spouse disagree. *Dimensions of Critical Care Nursing, 14* (6), 42-47.

This article discusses roles for an ethics consultation service or nurse ethicist in regard to situations where a patient's physician and surrogate decision-maker disagree.

The Future and
Nursing Consultation

*Consultation is not a profession itself, but a way of
practicing one.* (Frings 1991)

Key terms: entrepreneur, intrapreneur, trend,
inductive reasoning, deductive reasoning

Nursing consultation is a way of practicing the profession of nursing: working
with individuals and groups to help them solve actual or potential problems
related to the health status of clients or health care delivery. Advanced practice
nurses' knowledge and competence as clinicians, managers, educators, and
researchers provide them with both the content expertise and essential skills needed
for success as nurse consultants (Hazelton, Boyum, & Frost 1993). Skill as a clinician
facilitates an advanced practice nurse's ability to assess and identify nursing consultation problems. Management skills help a nurse manage time and resources during
the nursing consultation process. Education skills are used when a nurse consultant
interacts with consultees to help them learn problem-solving skills. Research skills
facilitate an advanced practice nurse's ability to interpret assessment data and evaluate the nursing consultation process. Advanced practice nurses, thus, have the foundation needed to serve as consultants to anyone who seeks assistance with a problem
or concern that is within the scope of their expertise.

So far, this text has presented a description of the nursing consultation process
(Chapters 1-4 and 8-12) and a discussion of the contextual basis (Chapters 5-7) and
professional issues (Chapters 13-15) associated with nursing consultation. Examples
of different ways in which nurses implement the nursing consultation process (Chapters 16 and 17) have also been presented. In this final chapter, the focus is on envisioning how nursing consultation can become a part of one's personal practice of
advanced practice nursing. In a sense, the content in this chapter is a way of wrap-
ping up, tying together, and moving into the future everything that has come before.

This chapter begins with an overview of strategies that can be used for envisioning
opportunities in nursing consultation. Next, these strategies are applied to intrapreneurial and entrepreneurial practice patterns of nursing consultation. The final section
of this chapter considers what is needed to turn a vision of consultation practice into
a reality. As you read this chapter, think about the following questions:

- How are the trends identified in this chapter currently reflected in health care?

- What other trends can you identify? What are the implications of these trends for
  health care?

- What opportunities do these trends suggest for nursing consultation? What
  opportunities do they present for you personally as a nurse consultant?

The Art of Futurethink for Nurse Consultants

You have to remember to stop and think. And think ahead.
Or else you lose track of the future. (Popcorn 1992)

"Futurethink" is the art of envisioning realistic opportunities. Futurethink means systematically identifying trends and speculating about alternate possible futures so that one's product or service will meet the likely needs and desires of its intended consumers. Services—such as nursing consultation—that are developed on the basis of futurethink have a greater chance of viability and longevity than do those based on hunches or meeting one's own personal needs.

Identifying Trends

Trends are pervasive ways of thinking and patterns of behavior that have a common underlying theme or meaning. Trends last an average of 10 years or more and appeal to the mainstream rather than just specific groups, although trends may be stronger in some groups than in others (Popcorn 1992). When considered together, trends provide a clear profile of the marketplace: what's starting to happen now and what will be happening in the immediate as well as more distant future (Popcorn & Marigold 1996). Trends serve as predictors of what will be sought, what types of problems will need to be solved, and what types of problem solutions will be most desired. Trends also indicate where present need gaps are. In a very real sense, the ability to recognize trends is the ability to recognize the future (James 1996).

Identifying trends means finding new patterns in everyday occurrences. It also means scanning the present culture for signs of the future. Cultural indicators of emerging trends can be found in children's literature, science fiction, television sitcoms, news magazines, symbols (clothes, jewelry, hair styles), new stores, and language (James 1996). Often, "people messing with the rules" (Barker 1992) can be an initial and early indicator of an evolving trend.

Identifying trends then, involves applying inductive reasoning to specific observations to reach general conclusions about the observation's economic, social, political, and consumer significance (James 1996). For nurse consultants, relevant trends are identified from observations of health care delivery practices as well as more general social and political patterns of behaving and thinking.

Becoming familiar with the thinking of current futurists is another way to get ideas about general trends as well as those that can be applied to health care and nursing consultation. It is important, however, to become familiar with the trends identified by a variety of futurists because every futurist tends to view the world differently and come to different conclusions about the future. Naisbitt and Aburdane (1990), for example, take a macro-environmental approach and focus on global trends. The "mega-trends" they have identified are presented in Box 18-1. In contrast, Popcorn (1992) and Popcorn and Marigold (1996) focus on social trends that are reflected in everyday behavior. The social trends that they identify are highlighted in Box 18-2. As a third perspective on trends, Schwartz (1996) identifies "driving forces" (see Box 18-3) that can be used to speculate about needed goods, services, and modes of service delivery. Celente (1997) identifies two trends that have particular significance for health care providers: "Survival Strategies"—an emphasis on staying healthy and living longer, and "New Millennium Medicine"—recognition of the mind-body connection, acceptance of alternative treatment modalities, and an emphasis on nutrition, vitamins, and "clean food."

Box 18-1. Global Trends in the 1990s

Naisbitt and Aburdane (1990) identify the following global trends. As you scan this list, ask yourself about (1) the implications of the trend for health care and (2) opportunities this trend could create for nurse consultants.

- A booming global economy—an increasing amount of disposable income
- A renaissance in the arts—a growing appreciation for the importance of the cultural side of life
- Emergence of free market socialism—the opening of new consumer markets in formerly socially and politically restrictive environments
- Global lifestyles and cultural nationalism—cultural blending and homogenization rather than isolated diversity
- Privatization of the welfare state—changes in funding sources for social welfare programs
- Rise of the Pacific Rim—growing importance of Asian markets as both consumers and producers
- The decade of women in leadership—increasing opportunities in the upper echelons of management for women
- The age of biology—increasing use of and advances in biotechnology
- Religious revival—increasing emphasis on the spiritual dimension of life
- Triumph of the individual—greater emphasis on and respect for individual rights

Reference: Naisbitt, J., & Aburdane, J. (1990). *Megatrends 2000: Ten new directions for the 1990s.* New York: Avon Books.

Other strategies that can be used for gathering information about emerging trends include talking with "key players," reading widely both within one's discipline and in the popular literature, and travel (Popcorn & Marigold 1996). Identifying trends and their implications also requires a certain type of mindset. Hamel and Prahalad (1994) describe this mindset as having the following characteristics:

- curiosity
- willingness to challenge assumptions
- humility and willingness to engage in speculation
- a valuing of eclecticism
- a belief in the need to be "customer-led"
- contrariness
- empathy

The implications of any identified trend for health care in general, and particularly for nursing consultation opportunities, can be speculated on by using deductive reasoning skills. That is, questions can be asked about how a specific trend is reflected in present patterns of health care delivery and how a trend might drive health care delivery to change. A nurse consultant can use these observations and predictions about emerging patterns of changes in health care delivery to identify the types of problems

---

Box 18-2. Social Trends for the 1990s and Beyond

Popcorn and Marigold (1996) identify the following 16 social trends. As you look at this list, consider how these trends might be reflected in health care needs and health delivery issues. How are these trends reflected in the current health care system? What do these trends suggest in terms of health care delivery "wants" and potential problems? What ideas do these trends present for nursing consultation opportunities? What types of nursing consultation interventions do these trends suggest will be most successful?

- 99 Lives—the pressure to assume multiple roles
- Anchoring—reaching back to what was comfortable in the past
- Being alive—increasing awareness of the concept of wellness
- Cashing out—questioning personal satisfaction and goals and opting for simpler living
- Clanning—the inclination to "hang out" with groups of like kinds that can provide security and validation of one's own belief system
- Cocooning—strategies to protect oneself from the harsh realities of the outside world
- Down-aging—a nostalgia for childhood that is reflected in a lightness in adult lives
- Ego-nomics—looking for ways to make a personal statement
- Fantasy adventure—seeking excitement in risk-free adventures as a break from modern tension
- Femalethink—an increasing emphasis on caring, sharing, and familial values
- Icon toppling—active rejection of the monuments of government and business and the pillars of society
- Mancipation—a new way of thinking for men that embraces the feeling of being an individual
- Pleasure revenge—cutting loose and seeking "forbidden" pleasures
- Small indulgences—rewarding oneself with small luxuries
- SOS (Save Our Society)—a rediscovery of a social consciousness, including environmentalism
- Vigilante consumer—an increased emphasis on consumerism: value, quality, safety

Reference: Popcorn, F., & Marigold, L. (1996). *Clicking: 16 trends to fit your life, your work, and your business.* New York: HarperCollins.

---

and issues that might arise as a result of these changes. Trends can also give direction about how to package possible problem solutions. These possible problems and solutions can then be used to shape nursing consultation services. Serious futurists systematically keep a journal of their observations and thoughts about the implications of what they are observing.

Building Scenarios

Scenarios are myths about the future or stories about how the world might turn out (Schwartz 1996). Scenarios can be thought of as alternate packages or combinations of trends. Scenarios help one recognize to what one will need to adapt. By so doing, sce-

Box 18-3. Driving Forces for the Next Two Decades

"Driving forces" refer to the evolving realities of the business world. Driving forces occur in both the micro- and macro-environment. Schwartz (1996) identifies the following as the driving forces of the next two decades. Which of these forces could keep the health care system going on as it is and which could influence it to change? What are the implications for these forces for nursing consultation services?

- Shuffling political alignments
- The technology explosion
- Global pragmatism ("whatever works") as a new political ideology
- Demographics—an increasing number of elders and teens; the number and proportion of teens will increase markedly in Asia, Africa, and South America
- Increasingly cautious energy consumption because of efficiency and perceived risk to the environment
- Public concern about the environment
- A global information economy—the possession of information will become the new measure of wealth

Reference: Schwartz, P. (1996). *The art of the long view: Planning for the future in an uncertain world*. New York: Currency-Doubleday.

narios can function as tools for "taking the long view in a period of uncertainty" (Schwartz 1996). For nurse consultants, scenarios, like trends, can be used to identify what health care delivery might look like, what types of problems will most likely need solving, and, consequently, what types of nursing consultation services will be needed. Scenarios can help nurse consultants strategically position themselves and their services for the future.

Scenario-building is most productive when a diverse group of people become involved in the envisioning process. Nurse consultants, for example, might want to consider the opinions of nurses, physicians, hospital administrators, patients, educators, legislators, and insurance executives in the development of scenarios. The first step in building a scenario is identifying forces in both the near and more remote environments that would support or hinder the success of a proposed service. These forces are then ranked in terms of their importance and their degree of certainty or uncertainty. The two or three most important driving forces are then put together in various combinations or themes to form a scenario. Themes around which scenarios tend to be built include:

- Winners and losers—a scenario of increasingly scarce resources and increasingly aggressive competition

- Evolution—a scenario of slow change that allows plenty of time for adaptation

- Revolution—a scenario of sudden and dramatic change

- Challenge and response—a scenario of serial unpredictable events, each calling for a different response

- Infinite possibilities—an optimistic scenario of increased resources

- The "lone ranger"—a scenario of the individual (or "little guy") versus the system (Schwartz 1996)

Nursing Consultation, Intrapreneurship, and Entrepreneurship

[Insight is] the ability to look at the same landscape as someone else and see something original. (Popcorn & Marigold 1996)

Intra- and Entrepreneurial Practice Patterns

Both intrapreneurship and entrepreneurship imply that a nurse consultant is a risk taker who is offering an innovative service and responding to a current or anticipated future need gap in some sort of unique way. An intrapreneur is an "intracorporate entrepreneur" (Brandiet 1995). That is, a nurse consultant who is an intrapreneur is employed by an organization such as a hospital and offers consultation services to both internal and external client systems. Intrapreneurs have the freedom and flexibility to autonomously innovate while being able to take advantage of their employing organization's financial and resource supports and assuming little, if any, personal financial risk. In contrast, nurse consultants who are entrepreneurs are self-employed and assume full responsibility, accountability, and financial risk for the services they offer. An advantage, however, of being an entrepreneur is the opportunity to earn financial rewards that are commensurate with one's efforts and performance.

Nurse consultants who assume intra- and entrepreneurial practice patterns accelerate the evolution of the nursing profession by expanding its scope, territory, and visibility (Hazelton et al. 1993). Nurse consultants in entrepreneurial roles such as that of nurse legal consultant (discussed in Chapter 16) are often more visible than are nurse intrapreneurs. Intrapreneurial consultation practice, however, can be equally impressive. Malone's (1989) description of how clinical nurse specialists at one hospital established a consulting service is one example of an intrapreneurial practice pattern for nursing consultation. As consultants, the clinical nurse specialists secured internal and external consulting contracts with the hospital's nursing services department, private industries, community agencies, physicians, and a school of nursing. In just three years, the consulting income generated by the clinical nurse specialists reached $450,000.00. The ability of the clinical nurse specialists to become revenue generators saved their role by offsetting the cost of their salaries to nursing services and the hospital's overall budget.

Applying Trends

Trends can be used to identify and develop potential intra- and entrepreneurial nursing consultation (and other career) opportunities. For example, trends can be used to identify which services are likely to have the most profitable future. These trends can then be used to shape a consultation career. Trends can also be used to identify what visions and fantasies for an entrepreneurial nursing consultation practice are worth incubating as a "spare-time" business until the practice is strong enough to provide full-time income. Trends can be used to provide direction for how to reshape services already being offered so that they continue to be viable and profitable. Finally, nurse consultants can use trends to shape the problem solutions and advice they offer to consultees.

The exercise of "Clickscreen" or "trend discontinuity analysis" (Popcorn & Marigold 1996) is a methodology that can be used for measuring a proposed nursing consultation service against trends. The purpose of this analysis is to determine a proposed service's fit with trends and maximize its likelihood of success. Trend discontinuity analysis essentially serves as a screening device for "go" versus "no go" decisions and should be carried out before going on to the logistics of establishing a service.

One method for carrying out a trend discontinuity analysis is to list identified trends down the left-hand side of a page and then set up columns labeled "Yes," "No," "Maybe," and "Possible change." A proposed nursing consultation service or intervention is then evaluated against each trend. A service's likelihood of success is increased when it is driven by at least one trend and supported by at least three or four others (Popcorn & Marigold 1996). If the proposed service or intervention is a poor fit with trends, consideration can be given as to how trend-supporting elements can be added (the process of "trend-bending"). In a similar way, existing nursing consultation services can be measured against trends and reshaped ("twisting the familiar") to make them more trend-consistent and increase their longevity and success. Box 18-4 illustrates how trend discontinuity analysis (based on the trends identified in Box 18-2) could be used to help a nurse design a consultation practice.

Strategic Planning with Scenarios

Scenarios can also be used for strategically planning nursing consultation services. A proposed service or intervention is tested against a scenario to identify its strengths and vulnerabilities. Of additional interest is how many different scenarios a proposed service fits. Driving forces, inevitabilities, and uncertainties in each scenario are then identified and used to shape a proposed service so that it will be responsive to the widest possible variety of future situations. The process of using scenarios to plan a consulting service is illustrated in Box 18-5.

Making It Work

Trend-worthiness and scenario viability are only two of the factors needed for a nursing consultation service to be successful. Careful planning, adequate support, and the right mindset are other factors that will influence the success of a nursing consultation venture.

For planning purposes, the AFFIRM model (Rew 1988) provides the following checklist of factors to consider when developing a consultation service:

- Availability—Are the proposed services already available? If yes, how will these additional services be unique? If no, are the proposed services needed? Are the resources needed to offer the proposed service available? Institutional resources needed in order for an intrapreneurial consultation venture to be successful include strong administrative support for autonomous nursing practice and for generating new sources of revenue (Brandiet 1995).

- Formulation—Exactly what will the proposed service look like? What will it cost? To whom will it be offered and under what circumstances? Where will it be offered?

- Factual Information—What information and skills are needed to develop and maintain the consultation service?

- Referrals—From whom will the consultation service receive referrals? To whom, in turn, will it refer? Realizing the limitations of one's services and forming strategic alliances and complementary collaborative relationships with others is key to a successful consultation practice.

- Monitoring—How will the success of the consultation service as a whole be determined?

Other issues such as setting fees and marketing that are part of planning either an intra- or entrepreneurial nursing consultation practice were discussed in Chapter 13.

Box 18-4. Trend Discontinuity Analysis: Developing a Consultation Practice

Proposed Service: A nursing consultation service that specializes in research development, research facilitation, data analysis and interpretation, and packaging research findings for publication and presentation. The target market is health care providers.

Trend	Yes	No	Maybe
99 Lives	X		

Comments: This service could help busy health care providers respond to pressures to discover and disseminate new knowledge.

Anchoring		X	
Being Alive	X		

Comments: This service offers health care providers opportunities to increase understanding and teach others about wellness and health promotion.

Cashing Out			X

Comments: Health care providers can simplify their lives by turning research responsibilities over to someone else.

Clanning			X

Comments: Research may offer health care providers an opportunity to network with others who have similar interests

Cocooning		X	
Down-Aging		X	
Ego-nomics	X		

Comments: Interpreting and presenting research findings is one way of making a personal statement. There is a certain amount of prestige associated with doing research.

Fantasy Adventure			X

Comments: The adventure of learning new skills and making discoveries?

Femalethink			X

Comments: Could doing research be one way to promote this agenda?

Icon-Toppling	X		

Comments: The opportunity to discover new knowledge that can "knock-down" old ways of practicing medicine.

Mancipation			X

Comments: As is the case with Femalethink, research could offer opportunities to promote this agenda.

Pleasure Revenge		X	
Small Indulgences			X

Comments: Doing "something different" (for example, research) and having help with it might be perceived as a luxury

Save Our Society	X		

Comments: Research is a social and professional responsibility.

Vigilante Consumer	X		

Comments: Research is a strategy for informing consumers about safety, values, and quality of health care.

Box 18-4. *(continued)*

Conclusion: This proposed consultation service stands a good chance of success since it is driven by six trends and supported by six others. "Trend-bending" can be used to strengthen the service even more by developing promotion strategies that emphasize consistency of the service with trends that received only a "maybe" rating.

Box 18-5. Using Scenarios to Plan a Nursing Consultation Service

Proposed service:
Consultation services that specialize in working with health care providers and health care delivery systems to resolve issues such as poor morale, staff burnout, and communication problems. The service will be based on a philosophy that emphasizes a process consultation interaction pattern.

Relevant environmental forces:
- Local emphasis on cost-containment and "belt-tightening"
- Needs for these services are currently met by out-of-town consultants
- A local hospital and home health care agency are talking about merging their administrative services and nursing staff
- The local nursing programs have experienced decreasing enrollments the past couple of years; this means that there is almost no back-up pool of new potential workers

Scenario #1—Winners and losers
As competition becomes fiercer among local health care providers, morale problems and burnout are likely to increase. Since there is only a minimal pool of back-up workers, this scenario would support the consultation service.

Scenario #2—Evolution
With a slow, steady change in health care delivery practices, health care workers would have time to adjust to changes on their own. This scenario might not support the proposed consultation service.

Scenario #3—Revolution
In a scenario of sudden and dramatic upheaval, there is likely to be morale and communication problems. However, there might not be enough time to resolve these problems with a process consultation interaction pattern. The proposed service might not be realistic for this scenario.

Scenario #4—Infinite Possibilities
In a scenario of increasing resources, there would be little or no need for the proposed services.

Conclusion:
1. The environment needs to be monitored for indicators of each impending scenario.
2. The nurse consultant needs to consider redesigning the proposed services so that they would be responsive to more possible scenarios.

Nurses who want to establish intrapreneurial nursing consultation services also need to plan how their time will be divided between revenue-generating and non-revenue-generating activities so that nonbillable institutional needs such as providing consultation to nursing staff don't go unmet. As an example of addressing this issue, Malone (1989) describes an arrangement where clinical nurse specialists' time was allocated to nonbillable clinical services (50%), building and developing the structure and processes of hospital-based nursing consultation services (20%), external consultation and revenue-generating activities (20%), and professional development (10%).

Just as identifying trends and their implications takes a certain mindset, so too, does taking advantage of opportunities the future holds for nursing consultation. Nurses planning careers as nurse consultants need characteristics such as flexibility, ingenuity, fast footwork, and the ability to balance multiple agendas (James 1996). They also need a strong sense of self-worth and a belief that their services are needed and valuable—and they must be able to communicate this sense of worth to others (Brandiet 1995).

Closing Thoughts (Summary)

Hard work, long hours, and perseverance are necessary prerequisites in this undertaking and will help prepare the determined professional to assume the challenge of success, achievement, and life balance. (Mackniesh 1989)

Incorporating the consultation process into one's practice of nursing provides additional opportunities for responding to both current health care needs and emerging health care delivery issues. Futurethink—consideration of the implications of health care reform, global ("mega") trends, social trends, possible futures, and driving forces—can be used to identify opportunities for nursing consultation services and shape them to be successful. Careful planning, creativity, and motivation that is based on both a desire for challenge and a desire to fill a void will help to further ensure the success of one's practice of nursing consultation.

Applying Chapter Content

Consider the following scenarios:

- **Scenario #1:** You are a nurse-manager who has been asked to work with two home health care agencies that are considering a merger. Use trend discontinuity analysis to speculate on the likely success of this merger. Based on this analysis, what advice would you share with these agencies about this proposed merger? Based on a consideration of trends, how would you suggest that they carry out this merger? What specific interventions and strategies would you propose to enhance the success of the merger?

- **Scenario #2:** You are consulting with a group of nurse practitioners who want to establish an independent nurse practitioner clinic. Besides considering the usual economic factors, you do a trend discontinuity analysis to predict the likely success of this clinic. What do you think your findings would show? How could you apply "trend-bending" to this situation? Are there any specific or additional services you would suggest that the nurse practitioners offer?

- **Scenario #3:** You are a nurse practitioner who is consulting with a family about how to support lifestyle changes needed by the father (age 48) who has just suffered a stroke. How could you used trend discontinuity analysis in this situation? How could "trend-bending" and "twisting the familiar" be used?

- **Scenario #4:** You are a nurse-educator who is providing consultation to a school of nursing that wants to revise their baccalaureate curriculum and develop a master's program. Based on a consideration of possible scenarios and emerging social trends as well as trends in health care, what types of curriculum revisions do you suggest they consider? What types of graduate programs do you recommend that they offer?

References

Barker, J. (1992). *Paradigms: The business of discovering the future.* New York: Harper-Business.

Brandiet, L. (1995). Entrepreneurial and intrapreneurial initiatives. In M. Snyder & M. Mirr (Eds.), *Advanced practice nursing: A guide to professional development* (pp. 271-285). New York: Springer Publishing.

Celente, G. (1997). *Trends 2000.* New York: Warner Books.

Frings, C. (1991, October). What it takes to be a successful consultant. *Medical Laboratory Observer,* 47-50.

Hamel, G., & Prahalad, C. (1994). *Competing for the future.* Boston: Harvard Business School Press.

Hazelton, J., Boyum, C., & Frost, M. (1993). Clinical nurse specialist subroles: Foundations for entrepreneurship. *Clinical Nurse Specialist, 7* (1), 40-45.

James, J. (1996). *Thinking in the future tense: Leadership skills for a new age.* New York: Simon & Schuster.

Mackniesh, J. (1989). Issues and concerns of a health promotion consultant. *Occupational Therapy in Health Care, 5* (4), 101-113.

Malone, B. (1989). The CNS in a consultation department. In A. Hamric & J. Spross (Eds.), *The clinical nurse specialist in theory and practice* (2nd ed., pp. 397-413). Philadelphia: Saunders.

Naisbitt, J., & Aburdane, J. (1990). *Megatrends 2000: Ten new directions for the 1990s.* New York: Avon Books.

Popcorn, F. (1992). *The Popcorn report.* New York: HarperBusiness.

Popcorn, F., & Marigold, L. (1996). *Clicking: 16 trends to fit your life, your work, and your business.* New York: HarperCollins

Rew, L. (1988). AFFIRM the role of clinical nurse specialist in private practice. *Clinical Nurse Specialist, 2* (1), 39-43.

Schwartz, P. (1996). *The art of the long view: Planning for the future in an uncertain world.* New York: Currency-Doubleday

Additional Readings

Beare, P. (1988). The ABCs of external consultation. *Clinical Nurse Specialist, 2* (1), 35-38. *The author discusses how clinical nurse specialists can develop a new role as community-based (external) consultants.*

Cerne, F. (1993, September 5). A call for consultants. *Hospitals & Health Networks,* 32-35. *Consulting opportunities related to health care reform are described. Nurse consultants are qualified to respond to many of these opportunities.*

Cummins, R. (1994). Laying the foundation for a career in consulting. *Journal of AHIMA, 65* (11), 38-40.

Consulting opportunities related to health information management are discussed. While directed toward health information specialists, many of these opportunities could also be taken advantage of by nurse consultants.

Finnigan, S. (1996). Getting started in business: From fantasy to reality. *Advanced Practice Nursing Quarterly, 2* (1), 1-8.

This article discusses the practical business realities that influence a venture's success or failure. Specific topics addressed include examining motives, applying commonsense approaches, demonstrating value, and achieving and sustaining profitability.

Hesslebein, F., Goldsmith, M., & Beckhard, R. (Eds.). (1997). *The organization of the future.* San Francisco: Jossey-Bass.

This compendium of essays presents a variety of views about how organizations and leaders must evolve to survive and prosper.

Koch, L., Gold, A., & Jacobsma, B. (1990). Setting up a fee for service program for psychiatric liaison nurses. *Clinical Nurse Specialist, 4* (4), 207-210.

This article describes how psychiatric liaison nurses in one facility transformed their services into a revenue-generating service. This same approach could be used by other nurses who want to develop intrapreneurial practices.

Zwanziger, P., Peterson, R., Lethlean, H., Henke, D., et al. (1996). Expanding the CNS role to the community. *Clinical Nurse Specialist, 10* (4), 199-202.

The authors discuss community-based roles for clinical nurse specialists, including that of consultant.

Index

A
"Abilene Paradox," 94
Acceptance
  by group, 92
  consultation role and, 52
Acceptance/openness, 116
Acceptant interventions,
    181–182t
Accountability
  during resistance to
    change, 113–114
  of team members, 98
Action plan
  consultee buying-in of, 185
  developing, 22, 23, 182–185
  facilitating implementation
    of, 22–23, 185–187
  identifying tasks of, 184
  modified Gantt chart for,
    183i
  sample, 183
Action planning phase
  choosing problem solution
    during, 177–182
  conflict during, 188
  described, 21–23
  documentation for, 189–190
  evaluation of, 197
  nurse ethic consultant and,
    304
  nurse legal consultant and,
    292
  overview of, 173–174i
  as participative learning,
    185
  possible difficulties in,
    187–189
  setting goals during,
    175–177
Actions, 162–163
Advocacy role, 46–47
AFFIRM model, 315
Ambivalence
  during action planning, 188

during change process,
    112–113
American Association of
  Counseling and Devel-
  opment, 271
American Association of
  Legal Nurse
  Consultants, 284
American Management Asso-
  ciation, 261
American Nurses Association
  Code for Nurses, 271–272
American Psychological
  Association, 261, 270
American Society for Training
  and Development, 270
Anger, 115–116
Announcement of services,
    232, 233i
Assessment
  agenda for group meeting
    on, 168
  by nurse legal consultant,
    291
  of consultees' perspective
    of change, 118–119
  description, 152
  documentation of, 169
  during problem identifica-
    tion phase, 150t, 151–158
  evaluation and, 198i
  involving consultees in,
    165–166
  of low morale, 161–164
  need, 153
  of organizational culture,
    76–77
  of organization power, 74
  of personal qualities/atti-
    tudes, 132
  purposes of nursing con-
    sultation, 155
  using theoretical
    framework for, 159–165

Assessment activities, 18–20,
    21
Attitude change, 201
Attorney, 285i
Authority
  decision by, 90, 91
  in organizations, 72
  See also Power

B
Bargaining, 114, 116
Behavioral artifacts, 76–77
Behavior patterns
  dysfunction team, 100–101
  malpractice charges related
    to, 254
  obligations of form and,
    266, 268–269
  of open systems, 62–63
  related to nursing consulta-
    tion conduct, 256–257
  related to nursing consulta-
    tion process, 254, 255
Behavior or performance
    change, 201
Blocking, 90
Boundary management func-
    tions, 84, 85
Breach of confidentiality, 256
Breach of contract, 255,
    257–258
Breach of duty, 251
Bringing closure, 25
Brochures, 232, 234i
Building team performance,
    98–99

C
Capability statement, 232,
    236i
Case management, 9–10
Catalytic interventions, 181
Causation, 252
Cause of the problem, 21